Nursing Case Management

From Concept to Evaluation

Nursing Case Management

From Concept to Evaluation

ELAINE L. COHEN, EdD, RN
Private Consultant and Author for
Professional Practice, Outcomes,
and Performance Improvement
Fargo, North Dakota

TONI G. CESTA, PhD, RN
Director of Case Management
St. Vincents Hospital and Medical Center
New York, New York

Illustrated

SECOND EDITION

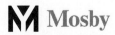 Mosby

St. Louis Baltimore Boston Carlsbad Chicago Naples New York Philadelphia Portland
London Madrid Mexico City Singapore Sydney Tokyo Toronto Wiesbaden

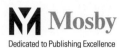
Dedicated to Publishing Excellence

A Times Mirror
Company

Executive Editor: N. Darlene Como
Developmental Editor: Dana L. Knighten
Project Manager: Patricia Tannian
Production Editor: Heidi Fite-Crowley
Book Design Manager: Gail Morey Hudson
Manufacturing Manager: Dave Graybill
Cover Design: Teresa Breckwoldt

SECOND EDITION

Printed in the United States of America
Composition by Graphic World, Inc.
Printing/binding by R.R. Donnelley & Sons Company

Mosby–Year Book, Inc.
11830 Westline Industrial Drive
St. Louis, Missouri 63146

Library of Congress Cataloging in Publication Data

Cohen, Elaine L. (Elaine Liebman)
  Nursing case management : from concept to evaluation / Elaine L.
Cohen, Toni G. Cesta. — 2nd ed.
      p.   cm.
  Includes bibliographical references and index.
  ISBN 0-8151-1906-2
  1. Primary nursing.   I. Cesta, Toni. G.   II. Title.
  [DNLM: 1. Nursing Care—organization & administration. 2. Patient
Care Planning—organization & administration. WY 100 C678n 1997]
RT90.7.C64   1997
362.1′73—dc20
DNLM/DLC
for Library of Congress   96-35125
                              CIP

98 99 00 / 9 8 7 6 5 4 3 2

To
all the pioneers and their efforts in the
development, research, and evaluation of nursing case management.

Contributors

ARTHUR E. BLANK, PhD

Grants Management and Research Support
Beth Israel Medical Center
New York, New York

BILL BRODIE, BSN, RN

Outcome Manager
Brookwood Medical Center
Birmingham, Alabama

TINA GERARDI, MS, RN, CPHQ

Assistant Vice President
HANYS Services, Inc.
Albany, New York

GERRI S. LAMB, PhD, RN, FAAN

Clinical Director for Research and Director,
  Carondelet Community Nursing
  Organization
Carondelet Health Care Corporation
Tucson, Arizona

CATHY MICHAELS, PhD, RN

Professional Nurse Case Manager and
  Nurse Researcher
Associate Director, Community Health
  Services
Carondelet Health Care Corporation
Tucson, Arizona

JEAN NEWSOME, DSN, RN

Outcome Manager
Brookwood Medical Center
Birmingham, Alabama

ROY L. SIMPSON, RN, C, FNAP, FAAN

Executive Director, Nursing Affairs
HBO & Company
Atlanta, Georgia

HUSSEIN A. TAHAN, MS, RN, CNA

Clinical Nurse Manager
Cardiac Care Center
Mount Sinai Medical Center
New York, New York

SISTER CAROL TAYLOR, CSFN, MS, RN

Holy Family College
Philadelphia, Pennsylvania

FOREWORD

In our travels and discussions with health care payors and providers across the country, we have observed the continuing evolution of the professional nurse case manager's role as the managed care environment continues to evolve. Appropriately, Cohen and Cesta have provided the health care market with this timely and proactive second edition of *Nursing Case Management: From Concept to Evaluation.*

Successful health care providers will find that of the many operational initiatives facing them today, their highest priority will be to revisit and refine two crucial imperatives: aggressive concurrent patient care management and accurate concurrent cost management. Both of these imperatives have implications for the organizations in which case managers are employed and, as a result, for the actual role of the case manager.

Aggressive concurrent care management, defined as managing care for the individual patient, per day, per shift, per encounter, will result from organizational changes that affect and are affected by the professional nurse case manager. This timely focused case management requires that provider organizations put into place effective operational infrastructures, create provider financial stability, offer incentives for physical participation and acceptance, establish care protocols and practice guidelines, and control the delivery of services.

The professional nurse case manager must be empowered via enhanced reporting relationships to be the bridge between clinical and financial imperatives while working in a collegial environment with physicians, other health care professionals, facility administrators, and payors. These enhanced reporting relationships will equip the case manager with the authority and resultant accountability for enforcing compliance with care protocols and practice guidelines.

Increased visible participation in the initial design and continual development of the care protocols and practice guidelines, as well as increased flexibility and availability throughout the care continuum, will further provide the nurse case manager with the ability to facilitate aggressive concurrent care management.

Accurate concurrent cost management is a major challenge facing provider organizations and the professional nurse case manager. The evolving financial construct of health care delivery requires an evolution in the current cost accounting systems and the integration of the professional nurse case manager into this unsettled financial arena.

Historically, cost accounting systems used charges as a proxy for identifying the cost of care provided to the patients. Subsequently, cost shifting and cross-subsidization were initiated to maximize revenues. Whereas this was effective in the past for the financial needs of the provider organizations, this revenue maximization strategy left no indicators of true provider costs. These methodologies have already been challenged by various payor groups. Because they do not give the data necessary to concurrently manage the cost of the care, they leave the provider organization unequipped to determine the price to be charged for the service provided.

In a resource-driven, price- and rate-sensitive financial arena the actual cost of each test and each ancillary procedure must be accurately isolated. In addition, increasingly sophisticated cost identification will necessitate "unbundling" of many of the traditional charges. Patient classification systems as the vehicle by which the cost of nursing care is segregated from room and board are but one example of a more accurate cost accounting methodology. The identification of the patient's acuity level further quantifies the cost of providing nursing services and positions provider organizations to more accurately determine the price for services provided. These important organizational cost initiatives are the financial foundations for concurrent cost management and will influence the concurrent care management of both the providers and payors of services.

Consequently, the role and responsibility of the professional nurse case manager will require an increasing level of financial expertise. The nurse case manager must understand the financial materiality of all case management decisions. This begins with an in-depth understanding of the financial implications of practice guidelines and care protocols through and including authorizing the appropriate vendor for home medical equipment.

As the provider organization gains a better understanding of its actual cost of services, the nurse case manager is in the crucial position to assist all care providers in reducing or eliminating cost variance. For the provider organizations with the skill to develop and implement cost identification by test, procedure, and acuity level, the practice guidelines and care protocols will be cost, price, and rate sensitized for the individual patient per day per encounter.

The professional nurse case manager is pivotal in the provider organization's successful implementation of the crucial imperatives of concurrent patient care management and concurrent cost management.

In the first edition of this book, Cohen and Cesta brought to the foreground many of the key issues shaping the emerging role of the nurse case manager. In this second edition the authors have expanded the topic to an even more comprehensive level, offering the reader the opportunity both to revisit and reenvision the care manager's role in this rapidly changing health care marketplace.

Ann Van Slyck, MSN, RN, CNAA, FAAN

President
Van Slyck & Associates, Inc.
Phoenix, Arizona

Thomas W. Van Slyck, MBA

Director, Managed Care Contracting
Mercy Health Care
St. Joseph's Hospital and Medical Center
Phoenix, Arizona

PREFACE

What issues are shaping nursing case management today?

Although nursing case management has grown in sophistication since this book was first published, the second edition of *Nursing Case Management: From Concept to Evaluation* attempts to preserve nurse case management's history by honoring past contributions while at the same time embracing the future by providing updates and changes in model development where appropriate. Most of the developments from which nursing case management grew still remain true and highly relevant when the roots of the model are explored. This information remains in the book for this reason and can be perceived as historical data.

Even though the book's basic structure has remained the same, we have added new voices that lend an even greater dimension and higher level of expertise. These contributors address contemporary issues such as the need for documented information on the measurable outcomes of nursing case management, the importance of future nursing case management research in shaping the structure and process of care, the expanding role and implications of information technology in nursing case management, and the increasing emphasis on ethical competence.

New chapters in the book address each of these trends in turn. New Chapter 11, The Managed Care Market: Nurse Case Management as a Strategy for Success, and new Chapter 17, The Role of the Nurse Case Manager, explore the various roles, responsibilities, and functions of case managers and discuss the skills needed by and the selection criteria for new nurse case managers. New Unit VII, Clinical Outcomes, which comprises Chapters 23, 24, and 25, addresses the need for documented information on nursing case management's outcomes. Chapter 23, Linking the Restructuring of Nursing Care with Outcomes: Conceptualizing the Effects of Nursing Case Management, explains the importance of outcomes, describes the development of valid measures, explores how nursing case management changes the structure and process of care, and suggests directions for future nursing case management research. Chapter 24, Expanding Our Horizons: Managing a Continuum of Care, examines the measurable outcomes of one facility's nursing case management model as used with a population of patients who typically require chronic care (diabetic patients). Chapter 25, Developing Outcome Management Strategies: An Intensive DRG-Focused Study, describes how one facility implemented an intensive DRG-focused outcome study to identify and prioritize opportunities for measurable improvement in delivery of psychiatric patient services. Chapter 28, Case Management and Information Technology, examines the expanding role and implications of information technology in nursing case management. Theoretical and practical approaches to the nurse case manager's role in clinical ethics are the subject of Chapter 29, Ethical Issues in Case Management, which not only presents strategies for developing and evaluating ethical competence but also includes sample case scenarios as a tool to assess the competency of prospective employees.

Although still evolving, case management continues to remain one of the most exciting and pertinent approaches to health care management. We hope that you will share in our vision of forging creative new partnerships for health care and come along with us on this very important journey.

Both of us are deeply grateful to our contributors for sharing their expertise and knowledge. We are also grateful to Darlene Como, executive editor, for staying the course as we have continued to explore case management; to Dana L. Knighten, developmental editor, who besides being a most wonderful D.E., has helped to maintain our perspective with her expert editorial assistance and advice; and to Heidi Fite-Crowley, our production editor, and Mary Espenschied, who kept us on target with all the numerous deadlines and time schedules; and to our families and friends for their continued love and support.

E.L.C. and T.G.C.

CONTENTS

I

EVOLUTION OF CASE MANAGEMENT

1

OVERVIEW OF HEALTH CARE TRENDS

▼ CHAPTER OVERVIEW

Many dramatic changes in the practice and delivery of health services have contributed to the new realities and complexities of the current health care system. This chapter presents nursing as it exists today and shows how the changing health care system and emerging issues have shaped current nursing practices. The chapter also identifies opportunities for innovation and provides an overview of the trends that have led to the development of the nursing case management approach in the delivery of patient care.

This section also discusses the reasons for the success of the nursing case management model in increasing cost-effectiveness, quality of care, and job satisfaction. Included in this discussion are nurse-physician collaborative practice, management of the patient's environment by coordinating and monitoring the appropriate use of patient care resources, monitoring of the patient's length of stay and patient-outcome standards to produce measurements for evaluating cost-effectiveness, and enhanced autonomy and increased decision making by direct health care providers.

Nursing case management offers the nursing profession an opportunity to define its role in the health care industry and challenges the profession to identify the work that nurses do in terms of its autonomous value to the patient. ▲

THE CHANGING CARE CLIMATE

The present health care system is fraught with complications, constraints, and uncertainty. Major shifts in the practice and delivery of health care have moved dramatically toward the proliferation of scientific and technological services, increasing government regulation, greater market competition, and economic constraints. Additional emerging trends affecting care include the following:

- ▼ Rationed and multitiered distribution of health services
- ▼ Increased control mechanisms for quality assurance
- ▼ Greater emphasis on productivity, efficiency, and cost containment
- ▼ Increased demand for concrete, documented information on measurable outcomes
- ▼ Increased ethical and legal concerns
- ▼ Rising prevalence of the human immunodeficiency virus (HIV) and related infections

3

▼ An aging population
▼ Fragmented and dehumanized patient care*

These shifts in the health care industry along with the federal government's prospective payment strategies have raised questions about the quality and effectiveness of health care services. Efforts to control spiraling health care costs have changed the economic position of health care organizations and the delivery of patient services in the acute care setting. Restructured reimbursement and finance mechanisms, which are based on diagnosis-related groups (DRG), have prompted hospitals to establish tighter financial controls over spending and to limit facility services primarily to the acutely ill.

The concomitant effects of these initiatives on nursing practice have resulted in fewer patient admissions, shortened length of stay, increased patient turnover, increased severity of patient condition and case mix complexity, intensified patient case work loads, and renewed emphasis on nursing productivity and efficient utilization of resources (Buerhaus, 1987; Curran, Minnick, & Moss, 1987; Hartley, 1987; Kramer & Schmalenberg, 1987).

Intensity of Service/Severity of Illness

The increases in severity of illness along with greater patient care requirements have resulted in a significant increase in the demand for professional nursing care services in hospitals and other health care settings (Aiken & Mullinix 1987; Iglehart, 1987; McKibbin, 1990; Secretary's Commission on Nursing, 1988). The need for more nurses to practice in a technologically complex and cost-constrained environment is expected to grow and is indicative of an aging and more acutely ill population with more severe and chronic conditions requiring intense nursing care (McKibbin, 1990). Workload statistics reveal that since the late 1970s, the ratio of registered nurses needed to care for the hospitalized patient population has increased. In 1977 there were 61.4 full-time equivalent (FTE) nurses for every 100 hospitalized patients. In 1988 this number grew to 98.0 FTEs per 100 patients (McKibbin, 1990).

The increase in demand for more intense nursing care services provided by registered nurses in hospitals was brought about by the prospective payment system. Institutional responses to the practice constraints inherent in these governmental rate-setting programs have affected nursing services and the environment in which nurses work. The use of the prospective payment system has resulted in discontent among nursing professionals because of the associated decline in autonomy and control over practice, decreased influence over hospital policy and decision-making processes affecting patient care, increased dissatisfaction with the quality of care and inadequate compensation and recognition for services provided (Iglehart, 1987; Styles, 1987).

Organizational variables that influence job satisfaction and the rate of turnover in the nursing profession are well represented in health care literature. This growing body of literature offers nursing suggestions on how to cope with the changing health

---

*Brown & Brown, 1988; Moritz, Hinshaw, & Heinrich, 1989; Mowry & Korpman, 1987; Rosenstein, 1986; Schramm, 1990; Wesbury, 1990.

care environment and how to gain control of nursing practices. Many of the proffered solutions focus on increasing economic rewards, maximizing staff mix and skill, and restructuring the work environment (Aiken & Mullinix, 1987; Barry & Gibbons, 1990; Iglehart, 1987; Strasen, 1988; Styles, 1987; Taft & Stearns, 1991). Emphasis has been placed on fostering nurse involvement in clinical patient care areas and designing better care delivery systems that are more consumer oriented and meet the needs of the patients (Ethridge, 1987; Fagin, 1987; Porter-O'Grady, 1988a; Strasen, 1991). In addition, collaborative practice models between registered nurses and physicians are recommended for enhancing professional satisfaction and improving patient outcomes (Del Togno-Armanasco, Olivas, & Harter, 1989; Ethridge, 1987; Olivas, Del Togno-Armanasco, Erickson, & Harter, 1989a; 1989b; O'Malley, Loverage, & Cummings, 1989; Zander, 1988a).

Both the original Magnet Hospitals Study (McClure, Poulin, Sovie, & Wandelt, 1983) and a follow-up investigation (Kramer, 1990) identify the factors that enhance professional nursing practice within the hospital setting. These factors include maintaining a professional status, having autonomy and control over practice, and upholding quality assurance standards. Nursing care delivery systems based on differentiated practice proved cost effective and provided continuity of care and effective resource utilization. In additon, the interprofessional collaborative relationships associated with differentiated practice had a significant effect on job satisfaction, recruitment, and retention of a professional nursing staff. Nursing care delivery systems based on differentiated practice were later shown to contribute to a hospital's overall productivity and fiscal viability (Cohen, 1991; Ethridge & Lamb, 1989; Fifield, 1988; Sovie, 1984; Tonges, 1989a; 1989b).

Nursing case management, which was introduced in 1985 and is considered an outgrowth of primary nursing, allows for quality care while containing costs. This manangement style has emerged as the professional practice model that increases nurse involvement in decisions regarding standards of practice and integrates the cost and quality components of nursing services (Zander, 1985). Nursing case management provides outcome-oriented patient care within an appropriate length of stay, uses appropriate resources based on specific case types, promotes the integration and coordination of clinical services, monitors the use of patient care resources, supports collaborative practice and continuity of care, and enhances patient and provider satisfaction (Ethridge & Lamb, 1989; Henderson & Wallack, 1987; Stetler, 1987; Zander, 1987; 1988a).

WHAT IS NURSING CASE MANAGEMENT?

The definition of nursing case management varies depending upon the discipline that employs it, the personnel and staff mix used, and the setting in which the model is implemented. Primarily borrowing principles from managed care systems, nursing case management is an approach that focuses on the coordination, integration, and direct delivery of patient services and places internal controls on the resources used for care. Such management emphasizes early assessment and intervention, comprehensive care planning, and inclusive service system referrals.

Several health care settings have adopted unique methods of monitoring patient care activity and resource distribution, such as critical paths (a description of patient care requirements in outline form), case management care plans (similar to the standard nursing care plan but adapted to nursing case management outcome standards), and multidisciplinary action plans (MAPs).

Nursing case management has been described as within the walls (WTW), which emphasizes case management activities in the acute care hospital setting, and as beyond the walls (BTW), which refers to case management in outpatient and community-based environments as well as health maintenance organization (HMO) arrangements (Ethridge, 1991; Ethridge & Lamb, 1989; Rogers, Riordan, & Swindle, 1991).

However one views it, because nursing case management balances the cost and quality components of nursing service and patient care outcomes, it is successfully evolving into a professional model that is both sensitive and responsive to current practice demands. A more detailed and differential analysis of nursing case management models is provided in following chapters of this book.

WHY NURSING CASE MANAGEMENT?

Current models of nursing care delivery are unable to meet many of the challenges and issues posed by the present health care setting and professional practice. When analyzing current models of patient care and studies on recruitment and retention of professional nurses, problem areas emerge. These care systems are based on traditional industrial models that promote conventional practices and regimented reporting structures. The current nursing care delivery approaches do not articulate the association between nursing interventions and patient outcomes; therefore, they are unable to assess the beneficial effects of clinical nursing services in relation to today's costs and reimbursement systems (O'Malley, 1988a; 1988b; Porter-O'Grady, 1988b; Stevens, 1985). In addition, the current unstable economic environment compels providers of health care services to engage in the restructuring and innovative rethinking of priorities related to the delivery and management of patient care. The focus on different approaches to care delivery has prompted health service institutions to look at alternative delivery systems as a means of improving patient outcomes and controlling costs.

Restructured Reimbursement

The current prospective budgeting process rations reimbursement for direct care costs and the patient's anticipated hospital resource use (Joel, 1984). Because payment is predetermined, no allowance is made for expenses incurred above the reimbursable rate. The major indicator of a hospital's financial performance and predictor of resource consumption in this system is the patient's length of stay (Joel, 1984; Shaffer, 1983).

The concept of managed care within the acute care setting has evolved as an alternative approach by which the directives on patient care are determined by predicted patterns of resource use. The managed care system places emphasis on managing the patient's environment by coordinating and monitoring the appropriate use of resources and is an integral component of the nursing case management model (Cohen, 1991). This model seeks to increase accountability for nursing practice and to reduce costs and fragmentation associated with patient care by establishing a mechanism for the regulation and integration of services over the course of an individual's illness (Henderson & Wallack, 1987; Zander, 1988a). Chapter 11, The Managed Care Market: Nurse Case Management as a Strategy for Success, examines case management in the context of the current health care market, expresses the nurse case manager's role within the managed care environment, and discusses new opportunities that managed care has generated for nurses.

Assessment criteria related to hospital-based nursing case management must be able to assess quality while monitoring and evaluating the outcomes of professional practice. The method used demands the following from the provider:

▼ Independent assessment and adjustment to variations in patients' needs as defined in terms of patient diagnosis, severity level, and spiritual, emotional, and family concerns

▼ Identification and utilization of appropriate health care resources

▼ Comprehensive monitoring of patient discharge programs to ensure continuous access to care (Ethridge & Lamb, 1989; Zander, 1988b).

The basic principles used in case management have universal application and are widely used by insurers to control escalating health care costs. These principles are also used by providers in acute care settings to contain inpatient expenditures and provide quality patient care (McIntosh, 1987; Ricklefs, 1987).

The findings of research studies indicate that the changes in inpatient nursing practice patterns associated with nursing case management have helped reduce costs related to the hospitalization of defined groups of patients within certain DRG categories (Cohen, 1991; Ethridge & Lamb, 1989; Zander, 1988b). Nursing case management has also had a positive effect on the demand-induced nursing care shortage by reorganizing delivery systems to maximize professional decision-making opportunities for nurses while allowing for continuity of patient care. These changes have promoted cost-effectiveness, allowed nurses to maintain professional autonomy, improved relationships between nurses and physicians, and improved care provider satisfaction (Cohen, 1991; Ethridge & Lamb, 1989; Olivas et al., 1989a; 1989b; Zander, 1988c).

CURRENT ISSUES IN NURSING CASE MANAGEMENT

Nursing case management continues to evolve in concert with the changing health care marketplace. Among the trends and issues shaping case management today are the need for concrete, documented information on the measurable outcomes of nursing case management and the importance of future nursing case management research in shaping the structure and process of care. Other important influences are the expanding role and implications of information technology and the increasing emphasis on ethical competence in nursing case management. Later chapters address each of these issues in turn.

Traditional nursing care delivery systems are ill equipped to deal with the many constraints, economic limitations, and continual changes in today's health care settings. Cost containment and concerns about quality of care are pushing health care institutions to consider case management as a way to improve patient care and control costs. Assigning a case manager to oversee the provision of patients' care is an increasingly utilized and widely recognized strategy to help ensure that patients receive needed care and services and that those services are delivered in an efficient, cost-effective manner.

REFERENCES

Aiken, L., & Mullinix, C. (1987). The nurse shortage: Myth or reality. *The New England Journal of Medicine, 317*(10), 641-645.

Barry, C., & Gibbons, L. (1990). DHHS nursing roundtable: Redesigning patient care delivery. *Nursing Management, 21*(9), 64-66.

Brown, B., & Brown, J. (1988). The third international conference on AIDS: Risk of AIDS in health care workers. *Nursing Management, 19*(3), 33-35.

Buerhaus, P. (1987). Not just another nursing shortage. *Nursing Economics, 5*(6), 267-279.

Cohen, E. (1991). Nursing case management: Does it pay? *Journal of Nursing Administration, 21*(4), 20-25.

Curran, C., Minnick, A., & Moss, J. (1987). Who needs nurses? *American Journal of Nursing, 87*(4), 444-447.

Del Togno-Armanasco, V., Olivas, G., & Harter, S. (1989). Developing an integrated nursing case management model. *Nursing Management, 20*(5), 26-29.

Ethridge, P. (1987). Building successful nursing care delivery systems for the future. In National Commission on Nursing Implementation Project (Ed.), *Post-conference papers second invitational conference* (pp. 91-99). Milwaukee: W.K. Kellogg Foundation.

Ethridge, P. (1991). A nursing HMO: Carondelet St. Mary's experience. *Nursing Management, 22*(7), 22-27.

Ethridge, P., & Lamb, G. (1989). Professional nursing case management improves quality, access, and costs. *Nursing Management, 20*(3), 30-35.

Fagin, C. (1987). Nurses for the future. *American Journal of Nursing, 87*(12), 1593-1648.

Fifield, F. (1988). What is a productivity-excellent hospital? *Nursing Research, 24*(1), 27-32.

Hartley, S. (1986). Effects of prospective pricing on nursing. *Nursing Economics, 4*(1), 16-18.

Henderson, M.G., & Wallack, S.S. (1987). Evaluating case management for catastrophic illness. *Business and Health, 4*(3), 7-11.

Iglehart, J. (1987). Problems facing the nursing profession. *New England Journal of Medicine, 317*(10), 646-651.

Joel, L. (1984). DRGs and RIMs: Implications for nursing. *Nursing Outlook, 32*(1), 42-49.

Kramer, M. (1990). The magnet hospitals, excellence revisited. *Journal of Nursing Administration, 20*(9), 35-44.

Kramer, M., & Schmalenberg, C. (1987). Magnet hospitals talk about the impact of DRGs on nursing care, Part I. *Nursing Management, 18*(9), 38-42.

McClure, M.L., Poulin, M.A., Sovie, M.D., & Wandelt, M.A. (1983). *Magnet hospitals, attrition and retention of professional nurses.* Kansas City, Mo.: American Nurses Association.

McIntosh, L. (1987). Hospital based case management. *Nursing Economics, 5*(5), 232-236.

McKibbin, R. (1990). *The nursing shortage and the 1990s: Realities and remedies.* Kansas City, Mo.: American Nurses Association.

Moritz, P., Hinshaw, A.S., & Heinrich, J. (1989). Nursing resources and the delivery of patient care: The National Center for Nursing Research perspective. *Journal of Nursing Administration, 19*(5), 12-17.

Mowry, J., & Korpman, R. (1987). Hospitals, nursing and medicine: The years ahead. *Journal of Nursing Administration, 17*(11), 16-22.

Olivas, G., Del Togno-Armanasco, V., Erickson, J.R., & Harter, S. (1989a). Case management: A bottom-line care delivery model: Part I: The concept. *Journal of Nursing Administration, 19*(11), 16-20.

Olivas, G., Del Togno-Armanasco, V., Erickson, J.R., & Harter, S. (1989b). Case management: A bottom-line care delivery model. II: Adaptation of the model. *Journal of Nursing Administration, 19*(12), 12-17.

O'Malley, J. (1988a). Nursing case management. II: Dimensions of the nurse case manager role. *Aspen's Advisor for Nurse Executives, 3*(6), 7.

O'Malley, J. (1988b). Nursing case management. III: Implementing case management. *Aspen's Advisor for Nurse Executives, 3*(7), 8-9.

O'Malley, J., Loveridge, C., & Cummings, S. (1989). The new nursing organization. *Nursing Management, 20*(2), 29-32.

Porter-O'Grady, T. (1988a). From process model to outcome models. *Aspen's Advisor for Nurse Executives, 3*(5), 3-4.

Porter-O'Grady, T. (1988b). Restructuring the nursing organization for a consumer-driven market-place. *Nursing Administration Quarterly, 12*(3), 60-65.

Ricklefs, R. (1987, December 30). Firms turn to case management to bring down health care costs. *Wall Street Journal.*

Rogers, M., Riordan, J., & Swindle, D. (1991). Community-based nursing case management pays off. *Nursing Management, 22*(3), 30-34.

Rosenstein, A. (1986). Hospital closure or survival: Formula for success. *Health Care Management Review, 11*(3), 29-35.

Schaffer, F. (1983). DRGs: History and overview. *Nursing and Health Care, 4*(7), 388-396.

Schramm, C. (1990, January). Healthcare industry problems call for cooperative solutions. *Healthcare Financial Management,* 54-61.

Secretary's Commission on Nursing (1988, December). *Final report (Vol. I).* Washington, D.C.: Department of Health and Human Services.

Sovie, M.D. (1984). The economics of magnetism. *Nursing Economics, 2*(2), 85-92.

Stetler, C.B. (1987). The case manager's role: A preliminary evaluation. *Definition, 2*(3), 1-4.

Stevens, B.J. (1985). *The nurse as executive* (pp. 105-137). Rockville, Md.: Aspen Publication.

Strasen, L. (1988). Designing health delivery systems. *Journal of Nursing Administration, 18*(9), 3-5.

Strasen, L. (1991). Redesigning hospitals around patients and technology. *Nursing Economics, 9*(4), 233-238.

Styles, M. (1987). Nursing today and a vision for the future. *Nursing Economics, 5*(3), 103-106.

Taft, S., & Stearns, J. (1991). Organizational change toward a nursing agenda: A framework from the Strengthening Hospital Nursing Program. *Journal of Nursing Administration, 21*(2), 12-21.

Tonges, M. (1989a). Redesigning hospital nursing practices: The professionally advanced care team (ProAct TM) model, part I. *Journal of Nursing Administration, 19*(7), 31-38.

Tonges, M. (1989b). Redesigning hospital nursing practices: The professionally advanced care team (ProAct TM) model, part II. *Journal of Nursing Administration, 19*(9), 19-22.

Wesbury, S. (1988). The future of health care: Changes and choices. *Nursing Economics, 6*(2), 59-62.

Zander, K. (1985). Second generation primary nursing: A new agenda. *Journal of Nursing Administration, 15*(3), 18-24.

Zander, K. (1987). Nursing case management: A classic. *Definition, 2*(2), 1-3.

Zander, K. (1988a). Managed care within acute care settings: Design and implementation via nursing case management. *Health Care Supervisor, 6*(2), 24-43.

Zander, K. (1988b). Nursing case management: Strategic management of cost and quality outcomes. *Journal of Nursing Administration, 18*(5), 23-30.

Zander, K. (1988c, April 11). Conference held on nursing case management. At Memorial Sloan Kettering Hospital, New York.

2

HISTORICAL PERSPECTIVE OF NURSING CARE DELIVERY MODELS WITHIN THE HOSPITAL SETTING

▼ CHAPTER OVERVIEW

This chapter reviews the history and theory of various models of professional practice and institutional patient care systems used in today's health care environment. The restructuring of health care delivery systems has become a promising and successful solution in dealing with cost containment, patient care, and quality assurance issues. Benefits include managing the appropriate use of health care and personnel resources; providing effective and efficient patient care through comprehensive assessment, planning, and coordination efforts; promoting opportunities for professional development and growth across all health care disciplines through participatory and collaborative practice models; and meeting the needs of both the provider and recipients of care through integrated networks of health services.

▲

EVOLUTION OF NURSING CARE

A historical perspective will help readers see how professional practice and nursing care delivery models evolved and how some of the methodologies used by previous approaches have contributed to the development of nursing case management today.

Various configurations for the delivery of nursing care have evolved within the rapidly changing health care industry. These changes have paralleled major economic, societal, and demographic trends. Most recently, changes in patient requirements have occurred as a result of imposed economic constraints. At present, patients are being discharged with increased severity of illness levels, and alternative access to care is not always available or affordable (Sovie, 1987). The rise of consumerism, with its emphasis on patient involvement, the advances in scientific technology, and the change in societal values and expectations all contribute to the multifaceted nature of nursing care delivery systems. Several approaches have emerged to meet specific market demands. These modes of delivery are defined by patient selection and allocation and assignment systems of personnel (Arndt & Huckabay, 1980; Stevens, 1985).

The case method was one of the earliest staffing assignments developed. It involved the assignment of the nurse to either one patient or a case load of patients to provide complete care. Sometimes referred to as private duty, the case method used a patient-centered approach by giving the professional nurse full responsibility for the care of the patients on an 8-hour basis (Poulin, 1985; Stevens, 1985). This method, considered the precursor of primary nursing (Poulin, 1985), was inefficient because only one nurse provided all direct care for the patient.

The functional method required a division of labor according to specific tasks and was a popular improvement of the case method (Stevens, 1985). The functional model, a task-oriented approach, involved the use of a variety of personnel. It was regarded as a highly efficient, regimented system and was designed to take advantage of different levels of caregiver skill (Stevens, 1985). In functional care the nurse was required to organize and manage a number of given tasks within a certain time.

The issue associated with the functional approach in nursing care delivery was the fragmentation that occurred in the effort to meet the needs of both patient and staff. Components of patient care that were not addressed raised the frustration levels of both the provider and the patient (Poulin, 1985; Stevens, 1985). The sole reliance on regimented tasks was one of the functional model's major drawbacks and resulted in dissatisfaction for both the patient and the nurse. The functional method also did not offer the opportunity to provide comprehensive, continuous care. Nursing's use of the functional method was the adaptation of an industrial mode of practice to a service system (Poulin, 1985; Stevens, 1985).

Team nursing changed the assignment orientation from tasks to patients and addressed the problems of the functional system (Shukla, 1982; Van Servellen & Joiner, 1984). For instance, patient care needs that might have been missed in a functional nursing model could be picked up by the team approach. The team method was developed in the early 1950s by Dr. Eleanor Lambertsen as a way to use all nursing personnel with various skill levels (professional nurses, practical nurses, and nurses' aides). This approach developed in response to the improved technology and shortage of professional nurses (Lambertsen, 1958). The system began to evolve, with greater efforts being made to improve the quality of patient care by focusing on patient outcomes. The professional nurse was responsible for the delivery of patient care services and the supervision, coordination, and evaluation of the outcomes of nursing care provided by the team members.

The advantage of team nursing over functional nursing included increased availability of professional nursing skill for a larger number of patients, greater continuity of care, increased interaction between nurses and patients, and a reduction in the amount of time spent by professional staff on nonprofessional tasks. The anticipated outcome of such a system was cost-effective nursing care (Chavigny & Lewis, 1984; Hinshaw, Chance, & Atwood, 1981; Lambertsen, 1958; Shukla & Turner, 1984).

The team approach was more than a system for the assignment of personnel. The approach relied heavily on the education, experience, clinical skill, and values of all staff involved in the care of patients. The specifics of nursing care were delineated in the nursing care plan, which included therapeutic, preventive, and rehabilitative steps. Because the care plan was initiated upon admission and developed throughout the course of the patient's hospitalization, it was considered cumulative. The plan served as an evaluative measure of patient care and later was adapted as a standard for nursing practice by the Joint Commission on Accreditation of Healthcare Organizations (JCAHO). Although team nursing increased the professional nurse's responsibility for patient outcomes, the limitation in the team approach was related to a greater complexity of role functions and an inability to fit into existing practice systems.

Primary nursing is a configuration of care that promotes greater professional accountability and autonomy and improves continuity of care. This model picks up where team nursing leaves off by having the individual nurse be responsible for the assessment, planning, coordination, and evaluation of the effectiveness of care for a certain number of patients. Primary nursing encourages collaborative practice and promotes patient advocacy (Dieman, Noble, & Russel, 1984; Halloran, 1983; Poulin, 1985; Zander, 1985).

Primary nursing is viewed as a care-planning system rather than a caregiving one. The focus in this model is on the planning process for comprehensive and individualized delivery of care. The process uses the nursing care plan, which outlines preferred patient outcomes (Dieman et al., 1984; Stevens, 1985). Nurses are held responsible and accountable for the outcome of patient care during hospitalization. The nurse is also expected to use the nursing process as a framework for administering professional and direct care responsibilities (Halloran, 1983).

Studies have compared the economic and cost-effective variables of primary nursing (Daeffler, 1975; Felton, 1975; Hancock et al., 1984; Hinshaw et al., 1981). These studies report that primary nursing contributes to greater patient and staff satisfaction and is less expensive than team nursing (Daeffler, 1975; Felton, 1975). However, the validity of these studies has been questioned. It appears that the reported cost savings and improvement in the quality of care are a result of the competency levels of the professional staff rather than the structure of primary nursing (Shukla, 1981).

For primary nursing to be effective, compatible support systems, such as unit secretaries, need to be in place to provide for the routine and nonprofessional activities of the care setting. However, because of current budget constraints, increased severity of patient conditions, and shortened length of stay, hospitals have difficulty maintaining this system of care. Initially, the concept of primary nursing required an all-professional nursing staff. However, a mix of nursing service staff skills and competencies is currently being used successfully in many hospitals (Poulin, 1985; Stevens, 1985). As a result, this patient care delivery system is assuming characteristics of other patient care models and is evolving into a prototype that can be adapted to alternative delivery models of nursing care.

PROFESSIONAL PRACTICE AND ALTERNATIVE PATIENT CARE DELIVERY MODELS

The unstable nature of health care economics has made it necessary to focus attention on developing and implementing alternative systems for delivery of patient care. The need to deliver health care effectively and efficiently has stimulated the promotion of national initiatives directed by the Department of Health and Human Services and supported by the National Commission on Nursing. The purpose of these efforts was to decrease length of stay, reduce costs, and improve the quality of patient care (National Commission on Nursing Implementation Project [NCNIP], 1986; Secretary's Commission on Nursing, 1988).

To achieve these goals while maintaining viability, patient care-delivery systems must be sensitive to limited fiscal and resource appropriation. The systems must also incorporate cost-effective standards and establish quality assurance outcomes of professional practice. To date, several professional practice and alternative care delivery models have been successfully developed and implemented. These models have prompted major adjustments in the practice environments of their settings.

Some of the fundamental characteristics of these professional practice and care delivery approaches are the adaptability and receptiveness of the approaches to differentiated and professional competency levels of practice, the reconfiguration of patient care and maximum use of nursing personnel resources, the use of collaborative practice arrangements among nurses, physicians, and other health care workers, the redesigning of the relationship between the providers and recipients of health care to improve patient care outcomes, and the enhancement of the relationship between the providers of patient care and the organizational culture supporting them. A description of some of the current models used in practice follows.

Integrated Competencies of Nurses Model (ICON)

The ICON models I and II are examples of the earliest alternate care delivery approaches blending the professional and education competency levels of staff with the health care needs and requirements of patients (Rotkovich, 1986). The nursing care responsibilities in these models, which were set up as demonstration projects, are differentiated on the basis of the nurse's educational preparation. Head nurses are required to have a master's degree and are responsible for the management and distribution of personnel and resources and overall quality of care delivered on the unit. Nurses with baccalaureate degrees are accountable for the assessment, planning, and evaluation activities of the nursing process. Nurses with associate degrees complement the professional nurse in patient care and carry out nursing decisions. In the ICON I model, licensed practical nurses (LPN), nurses with diplomas, and nursing assistants are excluded from the staffing complement.

Although ICON I is considered the nursing care delivery system for the future, another model, ICON II, has been implemented and is running concurrently to help LPNs and nurses with diplomas or associate degrees make the transition into their respective practice roles (Rotkovich & Smith, 1987). The goal of this model is to assist through in-service programs, continual education, and clinical preceptors the grandfathering of the associate degree and diploma nurses into the professional nurse's role and the LPNs into the associate nurse's role. This objective is in line with the profession's broader goal of achieving two entry levels of nursing practice.

Cost effectiveness, quality, and job satisfaction variables are measured and evaluated on an ongoing basis. At present no data have been published relating the effects of staff mix and competency levels of nursing staff on the productivity and quality of patient care using the ICON I and II models. Information on nursing personnel satisfaction and retention is also needed.

South Dakota Demonstration Project

Another nursing delivery model expanding on the theme of differentiated practice has been developed and implemented at Sioux Valley Hospital in South Dakota. This hospital is one of several institutions participating in a statewide demonstration project. The project demonstration sites consist of a consortium of institutions including representation from the acute care setting, long-term care (nursing home), and home health agencies (Koerner, Bunkers, Nelson, & Santema, 1989).

This project, directed by Peggy Primm and sponsored by the Midwest Alliance in Nursing (MAIN), differentiates practice at the registered nurse level and uses these levels of competence with a case management delivery system of care. Differentiated job descriptions (developed by MAIN) based on baccalaureate and associate degree nursing competences have been implemented. These descriptions classify the role into the primary and associate nurse positions. "The primary nurse plans care for patients with complex needs from admission through discharge on their unit. The associate nurse provides direct care on a shift-by-shift basis and utilizes Integrated Clinical Pathways to manage patient care. Both groups coordinate resources and discharge planning to facilitate quality patient outcomes and an appropriate length of stay" (Gibson, 1992a; 1992b). Primary nurses at Sioux Valley Hospital are unit based, and one of their duties is to provide phone followup to patients with complex needs. This followup helps evaluate the patient's discharge plan. Most of the primary nurses at Sioux Valley Hospital have bachelor of science in nursing degrees.

The nursing role classification process used by Sioux Valley Hospital is based on a factoring method that takes into account each nurse's experience, desire, motivation, and competence. This process also involves an assessment by the head nurse as well as a self-evaluation. Implementation of the South Dakota project resulted in revised documentation forms that now provide room for interdisciplinary planning and assessments of patient care outcomes (Koerner et al., 1989).

The most recent delineation to the Sioux Valley Hospital model has been the advanced practice nurse (APN) role, including clinical nurse specialists (CNSs) and nurse practitioners (NPs). Building on the differentiated practice model, the APN role is ideal for case management of patients on a longitudinal basis beyond the acute episode of illness (Gibson et al., 1994).

The Center for Innovation at Sioux Valley Hospital provided funding and administrative support for the creation of the Center for Case Management. The following description of the case management model was provided by S. Jo Gibson, Clinical Nurse Specialist and Project Director for the Center for Case Management.

Recognizing that certain patients require more than episodic hospital care, the APN manages the care of these select patients on a continuum. The patients are selected on a case-by-case basis, and each must exhibit at least one of the following:
▼ Chronic illness or catastrophic event (e.g., high-risk pregnancy)
▼ Frequent inpatient admissions or emergency visits
▼ Fixed financial resources (e.g., Medicare, Medicaid, self-pay)
▼ Absent or inadequate caregiver support
▼ Cognitive or developmental deficit
▼ Decreased coping capacity or emotional support

The projected outcomes for case-managed patients include the following:
▼ High quality care
▼ Appropriate use of health care dollars
▼ Decreased length of stay
▼ Decreased readmission rates
▼ Decreased acuity upon readmission
▼ Appropriate use of resources
▼ Enhanced interdisciplinary and interagency collaboration
▼ Client and family, physician, and nurse satisfaction

Sioux Valley Hospital has 17 APNs across three nursing divisions including Critical Care, Adult Specialty Care, and Maternal-Child Health. In addition to case managing patients, the APNs fulfill all the role components defined by the American Nurse Association for a CNS: expert clinician, educator, consultant, and researcher.

Referrals for case management come primarily from the primary nurses. Referrals also come from physicians, social workers, medical records, insurance case managers, employers, trust officers, families, and other nurses and health care workers.

Others who contribute to the success of case management include personnel from finance, medical records, data processing, quality assurance, and utilization review. Case management, therefore, pulls together the resources within the hospital to accurately portray a financial and clinical picture (Gibson, 1992a).

A demonstration project resulted in dramatic results for 35 patients. A significant impact was made in decreasing hospital admissions, mean length of stay, critical care days, and total charges. Satisfaction from a patient and family, physician, other health care provider, and APN case manager perspective was enhanced (Gibson, 1996).

Partners in Practice

The partners-in-practice system, defined by Manthey (1989) as a progression from primary nursing, is a partnership established between an experienced senior registered nurse and an individual who supports the nurse as a technical assistant. The technical assistant is assigned to the nurse, not to a case load of patients. Consequently, by delegating tasks to the technical assistant, the registered nurse is able to concentrate on providing professional patient care.

The registered nurse is responsible for defining the role, standards, and nursing care activities. By providing direction and supervision, the registered nurse is also accountable for the overall care delivered in the partnership. An official contract is used to confirm the relationship, and both members are paired on the same time schedule.

This system of care delivery is highly sensitive to unit-based human resource distribution requirements, skill mix, competence levels, and patient care needs. Because of the emphasis placed on the delivery of productive and efficient health care services, the partners-in-practice system can yield substantial benefits. These benefits include savings in overall budget and personnel salary expenditures as a result of reduced turnover rates, decreased use of staffing agencies, and improved management of supplemental nursing resources. The system enhances nursing staff retention by offering opportunities for advanced clinical training and education.

Contract and Group Practice Models

Contract and group practice models have been implemented at Johns Hopkins Hospital. They focus on building up the relationship among nursing care providers, the organization, and the environments in which they work. The contract model concentrates on promoting job satisfaction and retention by engaging nursing staff in autonomous decision making related to unit-based staffing levels and coverage, scheduling activities, standards of practice, quality assurance, and peer review (York & Fecteau, 1987). Another characteristic of this model is that it uses primary nursing. The staff benefits from the associated practice arrangements, which include salaried (versus hourly wage) compensation programs.

The group practice model is another innovative system developed for nurse practitioners who work in the emergency department and provide services to a group of patients needing primary health care (York & Fecteau, 1987). This model, which is built on the same objectives and goals as the contract model, initiates a productivity incentive that compensates nurse practitioners for the amount of care they provide per patient visit. This model calls for creation of an incentive fund that is allocated as patient target volumes are met.

Both these models prove their economic viability and organizational effectiveness by decreasing costs related to staff turnover and sick time, increasing patient visits and admissions, and decreasing length of stay. Reallocation of staff mix, skill, and competence levels leads to greater productivity and better use of the professional nursing staff. Additional gains include increased job satisfaction because of greater continuity of patient care, increased professional responsibility and autonomy, and reciprocal compensation packages.

The Professionally Advanced Care Team Model (ProACT)

The ProACT model was developed at the Robert Wood Johnson University Hospital to meet the demand-induced nursing shortage, differentiated practice, and prospective payment initiatives (Tonges, 1989a; 1989b). This model expands the role and professional practice of the registered nurse by establishing two roles for the nurse. The first role is that of the clinical care manager (CCM), and the second is that of primary nurse.

The CCM role requires a nurse with a baccalaureate degree who manages the care for a case load of patients throughout their hospitalization. This position involves managerial, personnel, clinical, and fiscal accountability. Primary nurses, who are graduates of accredited registered-nurse programs, are given responsibility for 24-hour management of patients on the unit and all direct and indirect caregiving activities. They are also accountable for the assessment, planning, and evaluation components of patient care as well as the delegation of tasks to LPNs and nursing assistants providing direct patient care.

This system maximizes primary nursing through the redistribution of support staff and a restructuring of ancillary services at the unit level. Patient care services that could be supported by nonnursing departments, such as housekeeping, dietary, supplies, and pharmacy, are assigned to the appropriate unit personnel. For example, support-service hosts are responsible for hotel-type functions such as bed making, and pharmacy technicians are responsible for ordering, obtaining, and preparing medications, among other duties. By placing accountability for nonclinical services on personnel from the respective support departments, nurses are free to provide comprehensive and coordinated patient care.

The traditional reporting structures and organizational processes are altered to adapt to the ProACT model's premise of restructuring care with the patient as the central focus. Luckenbill & Tonges (1990) reported in a preliminary evaluation that job satisfaction increased through collaborative care efforts among nurses, physicians, and other health care workers and through a well-coordinated support-service system for staff and patients. Additional findings included a 10% decrease in length of stay with specific DRG patients and a concomitant increase in patient revenues that are attributable to nursing interventions.

Mercy Health Services Consortium

A major restructuring of nursing services was initiated by 15 institutions within the Mercy Health Service System. This 3-year effort was in response to a grant from the Robert Wood Johnson/Pew Charitable Trusts titled "Strengthening Hospital Nursing: A Program to Improve Patient Care." Demonstration project sites included acute care hospitals and long-term and home-care settings (Beyers, 1991; Porter, 1991).

The goal of this project was to restructure nursing services to meet the challenges presented by cost, quality, and health care provider satisfaction (Beyers, 1991). Various models of patient care delivery were adapted for multidisciplinary involvement in planning and delivery of health care, collaborative relationships between nurses, nursing accountability and autonomy, patient and family participation in health care, continuous quality improvement, support services for physicians and ancillaries, and systems that are responsive to local community needs (Grayson, 1991; Porter, 1991).

Five of the 15 hospitals were designated to start this project. Two of the five hospitals developed case management delivery models of care (St. Joseph Mercy Hospital's Pontiac Project and Mercy Hospital's Port Huron Project), which are discussed in Chapter 5. The remaining three institutions established a combination of collaborative and dyad-system approaches to nursing practice. These health care innovations are highlighted in the following section.

The Catherine McAuley Health System, Ann Arbor Project. This system is a collaborative practice model that was developed to focus on the coordination and planning of services for patients requiring a wide range of medical, social, and psychiatric interventions and care. The patient population consisted of elderly, indigent, chronically ill, and chemically dependent individuals (Hill & Reynolds, 1991).

A designated unit was established within the institution to reduce the fragmentation and meet the health care needs of these patients. A collaborative practice group was also developed and consisted of registered nurses, physicians, social workers, nutritionists, pharmacists, and financial counselors among others. In keeping with the project's goal of maintaining continuous quality care, the responsibilities of this practice group were extended to include services in an outpatient setting. Evaluation data are not yet available.

The Marion Health Center, Sioux City Project. The Sioux City project involved the restructuring of nursing practice and health care delivery on a medical-surgical inpatient unit (Welte, 1991). The project incorporated a collaborative practice arrangement and the reassignment of ancillary staff to assist in the delivery of patient care. The overall design also incorporated a shared governance model.

Changes in nursing practice were realized as programs were developed to reevaluate role functions and support systems for the unit and prehospitalization assessment and evaluation processes, create information and documentation systems to enhance overall delivery and quality patient care, and promote nurse-patient partnerships.

The Saint Joseph Mercy Hospital, Mason City Project. The Mason City project involved development of a dyad model of nursing practice used on an inpatient oncology unit. This approach outlined role functions for the registered nurse, licensed practical nurse, and nursing assistant. Clinical nurse specialists provided overall leadership and management of patient care.

The main goal of this project was to provide continuous, holistic care in a network of hospital-based units and outpatient, hospice, and community resource settings (Schumacher, 1991). Joint planning committees for nurses and physicians promoted collaboration on health care decisions and evaluated outcomes of patient care. Patient and family support groups provided for many housing, educational, and pastoral needs. Again, the data from this project are not yet available.

NURSING CASE MANAGEMENT

A review of the literature indicates that aspects of some of the past and current nursing practice approaches and delivery models of care were incorporated into the development of nursing case management. The strength of nursing case management comes from the philosophy and collaborative practice strategies of both primary and team nursing. In fact, some of the care planning and coordination processes used in these models are reflected in the critical paths and care plans of nursing case management. These plans are used to monitor patient care requirements and activity as well as the resources for meeting those needs.

With former models, nursing care revolved around the nursing care plan, which provided a broad-based outline for the delivery of nursing services for the patient. These plans gave little direction in establishing a structure for achieving expected outcomes of nursing care for each day of hospitalization. The nursing case management model, however, provides a framework for nurses to manage the patient's hospital stay. Directing the delivery of patient care services allows the nurse to anticipate needs, thereby providing the opportunity for overall coordination and integration of outcomes and cost (Cohen & Cesta, 1992; Zander, 1990).

Nursing case management also integrates many of the professional practice demands and initiatives characteristic of alternative patient care delivery models. By emphasizing care that is patient-centered, the nursing case management approach embraces techniques of business in which the patient is seen as a valuable consumer who has the right to demand the best in health care. Placing the patient at the core of nursing's power base authorizes the profession to reconfirm its commitment to society. Nursing case management incorporates a new way of looking at the relationships among cost, quality, and nursing care. It places an emphasis on the autonomy, authority, and accountability of professional nursing practice by promoting an open system of care in which information is shared among all disciplines. The individual method of providing patient care is replaced by a team whose members work collaboratively (Cohen & Cesta, 1992). Because of its universal applicability, an in-depth discussion and treatment of the nursing case management model will be provided in Unit II.

REFERENCES

Arndt, C., & Huckabay, L. (1980). *Nursing administration theory for practice with a system approach* (pp. 65-111). Chicago: American Hospital Association.

Beyers, M. (1991). Restructuring nursing services in the Mercy Health Services Consortium. *Nursing Administration Quarterly, 15*(4), 43-45.

Chavigny, K., & Lewis, A. (1984). Team or primary nursing care? *Nursing Outlook, 32*(6), 322-327.

Cohen, E., & Cesta, T. (1992). *The economics of health care and the realities of nursing in the 1990s.* Manuscript submitted for publication.

Daeffler, R.J. (1975). Patient's perception of care under team or primary nursing. *Journal of Nursing Administration, 6*(3), 20-26.

Dieman, P.A., Noble, E., & Russel, M.E. (1984). Achieving a professional practice model: How primary nursing can help. *Journal of Nursing Administration, 14*(7), 16-21.

Felton, G. (1975). Increasing the quality of nursing care by introducing the concept of primary nursing: A model project. *Nursing Research, 24*(1), 27-32.

Gibson, S. (1992a). *Center for case management Sioux Valley Hospital.* Unpublished manuscript.

Gibson, S. (1992b). Personal communication.

Gibson, S.J., et al. (1994). CNS-directed case management: Cost and quality in harmony. *Journal of Nursing Administration, 24*(6), 45-51.

Gibson, S.J. (1996). Differentiated practice within and beyond the hospital walls. In Cohen, E. (Ed.), *Nurse case management in the 21st century.* St. Louis: Mosby–Year Book, Inc.

Grayson, M. (1991, August 5). System uses financial data and grass roots ideas to restructure care delivery. *Hospitals*, 31-32.

Halloran, E. (1983). Staffing assignment: By task or by patient. *Nursing Management, 14*(8), 16-18.

Hancock, W.N., et al. (1984). A cost and staffing comparison of an all-RN staff and team nursing. *Nursing Administration Quarterly, 8*(2), 45-55.

Hill, B., & Reynolds, M. (1991). The Catherine McAuley Health System, Ann Arbor Project. *Nursing Administration Quarterly, 15*(4), 48-50.

Hinshaw, A.S., Chance, H.C., & Atwood, J. (1981). Staff, patient and cost outcomes of All-RN registered nurse staffing. *Journal of Nursing Administration, 11*(11), 30-36.

Koerner, J.E., Bunkers, L., Nelson, B., & Santema, K. (1989). Implementing differentiated practice: The Sioux Valley Hospital experience. *Journal of Nursing Administration, 19*(2), 13-20.

Lambertsen, E. (1958). *Education for nursing leadership.* Philadelphia: J.B. Lippincott Company.

Luckenbill, J., & Tonges, M. (1990). Restructured patient care delivery: Evaluation of the ProACT TM model. *Nursing Economics, 8*(1), 36-44.

Manthey, M. (1989). Practice partnerships: The newest concept in care delivery. *Journal of Nursing Administration, 19*(2), 33-35.

National Commission on Nursing Implementation Project (1986, November 7). *Invitational Conference.* Milwaukee: W.K. Kellogg Foundation.

Porter, A. (1991). The Consortium Demonstration Project planning. *Nursing Administration Quarterly, 15*(4), 45-48.

Poulin, M. (1985). Configuration of nursing practice. In American Nurse's Association (Ed.), *Issues in professional nursing practice* (pp. 1-14). Kansas City, Mo.: The Association.

Rotkovich, R. (1986). ICON: A model of nursing practice for the future. *Nursing Management, 17*(6), 54-56.

Rotkovich, R., & Smith, C. (1987). ICON I—The future model, ICON II—The transition model. *Nursing Management, 18*(11), 91-96.

Schumacher, L. (1991). The St. Joseph Mercy Hospital, Mason City Project. *Nursing Administration Quarterly, 15*(4), 56-58.

Secretary's Commission on Nursing (1988, December). *Final report (Volume I).* Washington, D.C.: Department of Health and Human Services.

Shukla, R.K. (1981). Structure vs. people in primary nursing: An inquiry. *Nursing Research, 30*(7), 236-241.

Shukla, R.K. (1982). Primary or team nursing? Two conditions determine the choice. *Journal of Nursing Administration, 12*(11), 12-15.

Shukla, R.K., & Turner, W.E. (1984). Patient's perception of care under primary and team nursing. *Research in Nursing and Health, 7*(2), 93-99.

Sovie, M.D. (1987). Exceptional executive leadership shapes nursing's future. *Nursing Economics, 5*(1), 13-20.

Stevens, B.J. (1985). *The nurse as executive* (pp. 105-137). Rockville, Md.: Aspen Publication.

Tonges, M. (1989a). Redesigning hospital nursing practice: The professionally advanced care team (ProACT®) model, part I. *Journal of Nursing Administration, 19*(7), 31-38.

Tonges, M. (1989b). Redesigning hospital nursing practice: The professionally advanced care team (ProACT®) model, part II. *Journal of Nursing Administration, 19*(9), 19-22.

Van Servellen, G.M., & Joiner, C. (1984). Convergence among primary nurses in their perception of their nursing functions. *Nursing and Health Care, 5*(4), 213-217.

Welte, V. (1991). The Marian Health Center, Sioux City Project. *Nursing Administration Quarterly, 15*(4), 54-56.

York, C., & Fecteau, D. (1987). Innovative models of professional nursing practice. *Nursing Economics, 5*(4), 162-166.

Zander, K. (1985). Second generation primary nursing: A new agenda. *Journal of Nursing Administration, 15*(3), 18-24.

Zander, K. (1990). Managed care and nursing case management. In G.G. Mayer, M.J. Madden, & E. Lawrenz (Eds.), *Patient care delivery model* (pp. 37-61). Rockville, MD: Aspen Publishers, Inc.

3

HISTORICAL DEVELOPMENT OF CASE MANAGEMENT

▼ *CHAPTER OVERVIEW*

The case management approach represents an innovative response to the demands of providing care in the least expensive setting and coordinating and planning for needed community resources. For the past 20 years there has been a growth in the variety of case management delivery systems of care.

This chapter reviews the historical development of the case management concept. Descriptions of different nonnursing case management models are given to make the reader aware of the vastness and complexity of this approach. This is not intended to suggest limited use of the case management model. On the contrary, its great potential and applicability should be promoted. Studies show that this model can be an effective and efficient system by focusing on and caring for the health and social needs of the individual.

▲

INTRODUCTION OF CASE MANAGEMENT

Most of the literature on nursing case management practiced in the acute care setting is new. However, case management has been used by mental health and social services for years. For more than two decades the case management approach has been used as an alternate design for the delivery of health care. The first federally funded demonstration project began in 1971 and has been associated with a number of methods to coordinate and provide comprehensive services of care for the individual (Merrill, 1985). Regardless of the different approaches, the main principle underlying case management is ensuring the quality as well as the efficiency and cost-effectiveness of services provided (Weil & Karls, 1985). Emphasis is placed on the recipient of case managed care and the coordination and networking of services (Weil & Karls, 1985; White, 1986).

Research related to the outpatient and community-based population has studied the effects of health care case management in areas other than nursing. The specific target groups included the frail elderly, the chronically ill who are functionally or emotionally challenged, and clients who require long-term care services. These case management projects were designed to use less expensive, community-based services to prevent unnecessary institutionalization (Steinberg & Carter, 1983; Zawadski, 1983). Various services, from companionship to homemaking, were provided to assist individuals in their daily activities.

Findings of these studies show that case-managed, in-home support services, such as mental health, respite care, and homemaker or personal care services, have been effective in improving access (evidenced by shorter service waiting lists), assessment, and care planning needs of elderly clients (EISEP, 1988; Raschko, 1985). Additional studies illustrate the efficacy of case management in coordinating and integrating health and social services for long-term care, assessing quality-of-life outcomes (quality-of-living conditions), and reducing time spent in long-term care facilities (Carcagno & Kemper, 1988; Eggert, Bowlyow, & Nichols, 1980; Sherwood & Morris, 1983).

Because the nursing profession recognizes the need for changes in the system of health care delivery, more and more nurses are being designated as case managers. This change is due to nurses' expertise and knowledge in managing patient care. Case managers are involved in the assessment, coordination, referral, and individualized planning, monitoring, and follow-up activities associated with case management (Grau, 1984; Johnson & Grant, 1985; Mudinger, 1984).

Primarily used with long-term care populations, case management arrangements have been developed by private insurance carriers as cost-containment strategies and have been integrated into the acute care setting (Henderson & Collard, 1988; McIntosh, 1987). Consequently, different models of case management have evolved. Merrill (1985) identified three categories of case management: social, primary care, and medical-social.

SOCIAL CASE MANAGEMENT

Social case management models emphasize comprehensive long-term community care services used to delay hospitalization. Both health and social needs are addressed in this setting. Primarily successful with the elderly population, this model focuses on ensuring the independence of the individual through family and community involvement. It is based on a multidisciplinary approach to coordinate the care of the patient.

A variety of services, from companionship to homemaking, are offered to assist individuals in their daily activities. One example of the social case management approach is the U.S. Department of Housing and Urban Development's Congregate Housing Services Program, in which nonhealth services are provided to the elderly living in a housing project.

PRIMARY CARE CASE MANAGEMENT

Primary care case management takes on the role of gatekeeper based on the medical model of care. This approach focuses on the treatment of a particular health problem and tries to prevent institutionalization. In this model the physician functions as the case manager and has the responsibility of coordinating services and managing the patient (Johnson & Grant, 1985).

Primary care case management emphasizes the need to regulate resource use to assure cost-effectiveness. Examples mentioned include HMOs, which originally served Medicaid beneficiaries and have become increasingly popular among insurance companies as a means of controlling the disproportionate use of medical care.

Since the patient population accommodated by primary care case management is defined by health status, the type of case management services required varies according to the health needs of the patient. The financial imperatives to curtail high-cost medical technology are strong under the primary care case management system. However, a major liability of this approach is the exclusion of necessary medical services and hospitalization. Johnson and Grant (1985) recommend that quality assurance standards be incorporated into this mode of health care delivery.

MEDICAL-SOCIAL CASE MANAGEMENT

The medical-social case management model focuses on the long-term-care patient population at risk for hospitalization. This model combines available resource utilization with additional services, which are not traditionally covered by health insurance, to maintain the individual in the home or community. The case manager(s) in this system may be drawn from nurses, physicians, social workers, and family members who have input into the assessment, coordination, care planning, and care monitoring.

An example of the medical-social case management model is the social-HMO demonstration project, which integrates both medical and social services on a prepaid capitated basis to meet the multiple needs of the chronically ill patient. This model emphasizes providing the least restrictive and least costly long-term care by identifying the appropriate services and coordinating its delivery.

Additional definitions of the case management model are offered by White (1986), who bases the case management approach on a continual process of responsibility and authority for the provision of care and resource appropriation and use. Along this spectrum situations arise that either preclude the use of case management or facilitate case management arrangements with direct health service delivery.

Five case management models were also characterized. These models are differentiated on the basis of authority level of the client, support and financial systems, and payment allocation (White, 1986).

1. Restricted market: In this arrangement the clients become their own case managers and negotiate for services among independent providers.
2. Multiservice agency: This system allows an agency to provide its own health care.
3. Advocacy agency: With this model, some case management is provided along with direct patient care services.
4. Brokerage agency: The agency in this system acts as a broker in coordinating, controlling, and monitoring services and resources.

5. Prepaid long-term-care organization: With this arrangement a company contracts for case management services and coordinates resources on a prepaid, capitated basis.

Weil and Karls (1985) further characterized case management into three practice models: the generalist case manager or broker model, the primary-therapist-as-case-manager model, and the interdisciplinary team model.

The generalist case manager model is structured to provide direct service, access, planning, and monitoring activities to clients. The case manager in this system acts as a broker and is involved in the intake, coordination, and evaluation processes.

A broad range of professional disciplines may be represented; therefore the case managers in this model may include social workers, nurses, and mental health or rehabilitation specialists. Continuous and efficient service is assured because of the close working relationship between the case manager and client. The case manager also benefits from autonomous decision making and other independent management responsibilities.

The primary therapist model emphasizes a therapeutic relationship between the case manager and client. The case manager in this system is required to have a master's degree and training in psychology, social work, psychiatry, or psychiatric clinical nursing specialties.

As in the generalist model the case manager–patient relationship is a close one with the case manager responsible for coordination and evaluation services. Because of this one-on-one relationship, the primary therapist model works well with small, community-based programs and has been successful in coordinating and planning efforts and resources with larger networking systems.

Initiatives to ensure the delivery of case management are strong under the primary therapist model. However, therapeutic services have been known to take precedence at the expense of case management functions. Weil and Karls (1985) recommend the supplementation of case management responsibilities with therapeutic care.

The interdisciplinary team model focuses on providing case management services through a collaborative team approach. The responsibilities and designated case management functions are divided among the team members according to their area of specialization and expertise.

In this system the case managers may include nurses, social workers, or therapists who have accountability and provide services within their own area of concentration. One team member, however, is appointed to maintain overall service coordination and evaluation.

The benefits of the interdisciplinary team approach include improved continuity of care and enhanced coordination of services and staff support systems to promote mutual program planning, problem solving, and client advocacy.

PRIVATE CASE MANAGEMENT

Private case management systems have evolved to meet the needs of clients outside publicly funded programs or those who prefer more personalized services (Parker & Secord 1988). Parker and Secord cite the findings of a major survey conducted by

Inter-Study's Center for Aging and Long-Term Care and funded by the Retirement Research Foundation.

This study investigated the characteristics, services, referral, and funding sources of private geriatric-case-management firms across the United States. According to Parker and Secord (1988), this model evolved as a result of an increase in the elderly population, escalating health care costs, growing need for integrated social and health services for the elderly, and increasing emphasis placed on long-term care issues. Survey findings are discussed in the following five paragraphs.

Private case management firms were in business an average of 3 years, and most (98.9%) were independently owned, run for profit, and self-managed. Some affiliations existed with hospitals, public and private social service agencies, and nursing homes. Clientele consisted of elderly individuals with mean annual incomes ranging from $5,000 to $15,000. Case managers in this system were college graduates who were prepared in social work or nursing and who carried a small case load of clients.

In most instances, private case management functions included coordination of services, social, functional, and financial; mental health assessment and counseling; and referral, monitoring, and evaluation services. Medical assessments were done by physicians in 44% of the private case management businesses. Some of the other services consisted of nursing home and housing placement, retirement planning, companion and homemaker services, and transportation and respite care. These direct services were provided more frequently by for-profit and unaffiliated private case management businesses than by the nonprofit and affiliated companies. Those firms that employed registered nurses as case managers had a tendency to provide more direct care services as well.

Services most often referred by private case managers included home health care, homemaker, and personal care services, family and legal counseling, and physical therapy. Referral sources were composed of physicians, social workers, family members, and self-referrals.

Private case managers were able to provide more individualized services and were also accessible on off hours, weekends, and holidays.

Reimbursement for services provided by private case managers ranged from hourly and set rates per session to service and package rates. Unaffiliated and for-profit businesses used more hourly and set rate methods and also segregated their services to charge for case management functions involving more time and attention. Sliding fee scales were more common in affiliated and nonprofit organizations. Funding sources to private case management businesses included out-of-pocket payments by client or family members, private insurance, Medicare, Medicaid, and other sources that consisted of public funds, trusts, and grants.

Benefits of private case management approaches for staff members include increased flexibility and autonomy in decision making, independent planning and coordinating of services, greater income, and professional satisfaction. Clients and their families also reported improved accessibility to case managers, less duplication and redundancy of services, individualized care, and long-term association with one case manager. However, further evaluation is needed regarding access to other health care services, overall quality of private case management care, cost, and reimbursement issues.

COMPONENTS OF CASE MANAGEMENT

Weil and Karls (1985) extensively outlined the main service components common in all case management models.

Client Identification and Outreach. Individuals who are eligible or need case management services are identified. Admission to a case management program is determined by interview process, referral, and networking systems or by the case manager actively promoting eligibility for individuals who might not inquire about case management services for themselves (for example, individuals who are indigent or have mental illness).

Individual Assessment and Diagnosis. Case managers use their comprehensive knowledge and skill to assess the physical, emotional, and psychological needs as well as the social and support requirements of their clients. This process aids in the coordination, facilitation, monitoring, and access of case management services.

Service Planning and Resource Identification. With the collaboration of the client the case manager assumes the responsibility for coordinating and planning care services. This includes the development of care plans and determining resource and networking systems.

Linking Clients to Needed Services. Case managers act as brokers to expedite and follow through with the coordination and planning needs of the client. Both community and agency resources may be used. In some systems this responsibility involves actually transporting the client to a recommended service.

Service Implementation and Coordination. The case manager ensures that the identified needs are satisfied and follows the formal agreements made with the networking agencies. This is done by extensive documentation and record keeping of the efficiency, effectiveness, and quality of case management care services. A participative relationship of client and case manager and autonomous decision making on the part of the case manager are crucial to both groups' engagement in the system.

Monitoring Service Delivery. The case manager is responsible for directing and overseeing the distribution of services to the client. A multidisciplinary and multiservice relationship is promoted to assure appropriate and effective delivery of case-managed services.

Advocacy. Case managers act on behalf of the client in assuring that needed interventions are obtained and that the client is making progress in the program. As explained by Weil, the advocacy strategy is used not only for the individual client but also for the benefit of all individuals in common predicaments.

Evaluation. The case manager is responsible and accountable for appraising the specific as well as the overall usefulness and effectiveness of case managed services. The evaluation process involves continuous monitoring and analysis of the needs of the individuals and services provided to the clients. Early identification of changes or problems with the client or the provider of services is made, ensuring timely intervention and replanning by the case manager.

REFERENCES

Carcagno, G.J., & Kemper, P. (1988). The evolution of the National Long Term Care Demonstration: An overview of the Channeling Demonstration and its evaluation. *Health Services Research, 23,* 1-22.

Eggert, G.M., Bowlyow, J.E., & Nichols, C.W. (1980). Gaining control of the long term care system: First returns from Access Experiment. *The Gerontologist, 20,* 356-363.

EISEP (1988, November 30). *An evaluation of New York City's home care services supported under the expanded in-home service for the elderly program.* Health Research: New York University. Funded by New York City's Department for the Aging (contract #11000100).

Grau, L. (1984). Case management and the nurse. *Geriatric Nurse, 5,* 372-375.

Henderson, M.G., & Collard, A. (1988). Measuring quality in medical case management programs. *Quality Review Bulletin, 14*(2), 33-39.

Johnson, C., & Grant, L. (1985). *The nursing home in American society* (pp. 140-200). Baltimore: Johns Hopkins University Press.

McIntosh, L. (1987). Hospital based case management. *Nursing Economics, 5*(5), 232-236.

Merrill, J.C. (1985). Defining case management. *Business and Health, 3*(5-9), 5-9.

Mudinger, M.O. (1984). Community based case:

Who will be the case managers? *Nursing Outlook, 32*(6), 294-295.

Parker, M., & Secord, L. (1988). Private geriatric case management: Providers, services and fees. *Nursing Economics, 6*(4), 165-172, 195.

Raschko, R. (1985). Systems integration at the program level: aging and mental health. *The Gerontologist, 25,* 460-463.

Sherwood, S., & Morris, J.N. (1983). The Pennsylvania Domiciliary Care Experiment: Impact on quality life. *American Journal of Public Health, 73,* 646-653.

Steinberg, R.M. & Carter, G.W. (1983). *Case management and the elderly: A handbook for planning and administering programs.* Lexington, Mass.: Lexington Books.

Weil, M., & Karls, J. (1985). Historical origins and recent developments. In M. Weil & J. Karls (Eds.), *Case management in human service practice* (pp. 1-28). San Francisco: Jossey-Bass Publishers.

White, M. (1986). Case management. In G.L. Maddox (Ed.), *The encyclopedia of aging* (pp. 92-96). New York: Springer Publishing.

Zawadski, R.T. (1983). The long-term care demonstration projects: What are they and why they came into being? *Home Health Care Services Quarterly, 4*(3-4), 5-26.

II

CONTEMPORARY MODELS OF CASE MANAGEMENT

4

THE DIFFERENCE BETWEEN MANAGED CARE AND NURSING CASE MANAGEMENT

▼ *CHAPTER OVERVIEW*

As the demand for cost-effective high-quality health care continues to grow, innovative approaches to improving patient care delivery must be explored. These goals can only be achieved within a framework of total organizational commitment to restructuring care to meet the needs of today's health care provider and the present patient population.

Managed care and case management are both effective approaches that can be used in the reorganization process. As discussed, both systems help define the role and scope of the nurse's responsibilities in the delivery setting. These models can enhance the productivity and competence levels of staff by organizing personnel to use their varying skills and expertise in better ways. This could increase professionalism and satisfaction of all providers.

By ensuring that appropriate outcomes are achieved, both managed care and case management provide a framework for continuous and refined planning of nursing and multidisciplinary care and ensure appropriate and cost-effective use of patient resources. Finally, these models can contribute to the foundation of total quality improvement and ensure continued delivery of high-quality patient care. ▲

THE MANAGED CARE/CASE MANAGEMENT ALTERNATIVE

Because the terms *managed care* and *case management* have been used interchangeably in the professional literature, confusion as to the difference between the two concepts arises. Furthermore, managed care and case management share a common ground in their historical development and have similar purposes and goals relating to cost containment and quality care. These similarities add to the confusion.

Cost management issues and quality care, which at one point were on opposite sides of the health care delivery spectrum, are now being integrated into one system. The economic power that had been reserved for physicians and hospitals has been transferred to the purchasers of health services, which include business corporations, insurance companies, and individuals. The buyers' objectives are coordinating and managing the use of health services and allocating resources for future distribution.

Managed care emerged as control shifted from the provider to the purchaser of health services. The managed care system links the provider with the patient to manage cost, access, and quality components of health care delivery. Major health policies like the federal Health Maintenance Organization Act, adopted in the early 1970s, established a trend for the growth of managed care programs. The HMOs and preferred provider organizations (PPO), two popular examples, offered an alternative to costly inpatient care through the provision of cost-effective treatments and multiple preventive and outpatient services.

Case management is used in these managed care plans as a cost-containment initiative. It further grounds the managed care approach by focusing on the individual health care needs of the patient. Case management is effective because it targets the coordination, integration, and outcome evaluation processes of care.

The inherent strengths in both the managed care and case management systems have led to a renewed interest in the utility and effectiveness of such systems. Both systems are currently being used as strategic approaches to the restructuring of the delivery aspects of health care.

DEFINING MANAGED CARE AND NURSING CASE MANAGEMENT

In a traditional context, managed care is viewed as a system that provides the generalized structure and focus for managing the use, cost, quality, and effectiveness of health care services. Managed care then becomes an umbrella for several cost containment initiatives that may involve case management.

On the other hand, nursing case management can be conceptualized as a process model, the underpinnings of which are essential in attending to the many components and services used in the delivery aspects of patient care. The case-managed approach is based on and includes variations on the managed care theme.

Aside from its broader application, managed care has been further diversified as its principles have been adapted to the inpatient, acute care setting. In this setting, managed care has evolved in its own right into a separate professional nursing care delivery model.

Various definitions have been offered in an attempt to distinguish managed care from nursing case management. Managed care is a nursing care delivery system that supports cost-effective, patient outcome–oriented care. It is unit based and structurally designed to promote and support care at the patient's bedside. Patient assignments are not targeted to any particular case type, and critical paths and case management care plans are used to ensure support for standardized patterns of care and length of hospitalization for the individual patient. Managed care can also be used with primary, team, functional, and alternative nursing care delivery systems.

Continuous monitoring and evaluating of the patient's care is maintained through interdisciplinary team meetings, and variances from the plan of care are analyzed by the unit's nurse manager or patient care manager (Cesta, 1991; Etheredge, 1989; Zander, 1991).

One of the strengths of the managed care system is that it can be structured to use staff through differentiated practice arrangements and competence levels of nursing personnel. In short, managed care implies a consistency of plan in that what is done to or for a given patient is consistent even though individual care givers may change (Zander, 1991).

Case management differs from managed care in that the accountability and responsibility for the delivery of care is based on an entire occurrence of hospitalization for a targeted DRG group of patients and is not geographically confined to that patient's unit (Etheredge, 1989; Zander, 1990). This widens the circumscribed area of patient services to include patient care planning and coordination across health care settings. Case management, then, implies consistency of provider: even though different, formal, informal, and even very esoteric resources are used, the coordinator or provider (usually an individual) remains the same (Zander, 1991).

Collaborative practice arrangements in the form of group practice are supported, and interdisciplinary decision making is facilitated to ensure appropriate use of patient resources and achievement of expected clinical outcomes. Collaboration usually includes members of the health care team and the patient or family to help accomplish anticipated care outcomes. Critical paths and case management plans are used by the participants of the health care teams. Variance analysis and evaluation of patient care is expanded beyond the confines of the patient unit and encompasses all patients in the specific case load (Etheredge, 1989; Zander, 1990).

An example of a case management model—the Beth Israel Multidisciplinary Patient Care Model (Appendix 4-1; Cesta, 1991)—was developed for use within an acute care setting. Using the practice concepts of both primary and team nursing, this model supports the coordination and management of the care of patients from admission to discharge. The objectives of the model are as follows:

▼ Improve quality of care
▼ Control resource utilization
▼ Decrease length of stay
▼ Increase patient satisfaction
▼ Increase staff satisfaction

This case management model, which was implemented through a reorganization of the nursing department structure, provides the opportunity for advancement of selected registered nurses working at the bedside. When a case management career ladder is used, nurses who have a baccalaureate degree and who have demonstrated advanced clinical and leadership skills can remain in the direct patient care environment and expand their professional careers by working as case managers.

The case manager is removed from direct care delivery to coordinate overall patient services. This individual is also part of a multidisciplinary team that continually assesses, evaluates, and plans patient care. The assessment is based on expectations regarding outcomes of care of the physician, nurse, and all other individuals involved in the care of the patient.

Case managers assume responsibility for a caseload of patients who meet high-risk criteria developed for each clinical area. Patients are referred to utilization management or social work as needed. Care is managed through prospective protocols called multidisciplinary action plans (MAPs). Outcome data, including variances, are collected and used to improve clinical and system processes.

A MAP projects patient care outcomes for each day of hospitalization. Because the care plan is a group effort, it promotes greater satisfaction for the patient, family, and health team members. These plans involve all patient care areas and specialities and cover a wide range of diagnoses or surgical procedures, such as neurosurgery, orthopedics, AIDS, general medicine, pediatrics, maternal and child health, oncology, detoxification, and rehabilitation. Ultimately the model increases professional development and improves recruitment, motivation, and retention of staff (Ake et al, 1991).

Case managers, who are unit-based, coordinate the care being delivered by the registered nurses and nursing assistants working on the team. The manager also serves as a role model to the novice nurse or orientee. By consulting with less-experienced registered nurses, the manager helps improve the professionalism and clinical skills of the unit's personnel and promotes collegial relationships with all health care providers. Other responsibilities of the case manager include patient and family teaching and support and discharge planning with the social worker.

This model enhances the use of personnel by expanding support or ancillary staff role responsibilities. Because the nursing attendants are included as part of the care team, they better understand the medical and nursing needs of their patients.

The multidisciplinary patient care model is an integral component of the organizational restructuring of patient care delivery. Because it is research based and part of the planned change process, several clinical and quality care indicators are being evaluated to determine the effectiveness of this model. This model requires ongoing assessment of quality improvement data, job and patient satisfaction ratings, and length-of-stay data in order to adapt the practice principles and philosophy of the managed patient care model to the needs of the providers and recipients of acute health care services.

Another example of a comprehensive case management model is the one developed at The Long Island College Hospital, Brooklyn, New York. This model incorporates the same goals as the Beth Israel model, with emphasis on the use of product and personnel resources. Process and structure redesign for this model began with a review of the role functions of nurses, social workers, utilization managers, and discharge planners. The existing care process for each discipline was entered in a flow chart, and process barriers were identified. Each discipline identified ways in which personnel might be redeployed to assure the best use of available personnel as well as to reduce duplication. Interventions were moved to preadmission whenever possible. For example, discharge planning and home care referrals were moved to the preadmission arena. Social workers began to divide their time between the inpatient and outpatient care settings.

Another significant component of this model is the redeployment of the existing clinical nurse specialists as case managers. Long Island College Hospital identified the case manager as an advanced practice role, and the clinical nurse specialists were best prepared to assume the additional responsibilities associated with case management. Generic staff development functions that they were performing were returned to the Department of Nursing Education and Research.

REFERENCES

Ake, J.M., Bower-Ferris, S., Cesta, T., Gould, D., Greenfield, J., Hayes, P., Maislin, G., & Mezey, M. (1991). The nursing initiatives program: Practice based models for care in hospitals. In *Differentiating nursing practice: Into the twenty-first century.* Kansas City, MO: American Academy of Nursing.

Cesta, T. (1991, November). *Managed care,* personal correspondence and paper presented at the Annual Symposium on Health Services Research, New York.

Etheredge, M.L. (1989). *Collaborative care nursing case management.* Chicago: American Hospital Publishing, Inc. (American Hospital Association).

Zander, K. (1990). Managed care and nursing case management. In G.G. Mayer, M.J. Madden, & E. Lawrenz (Eds.), *Patient care delivery models* (pp. 37-61). Rockville, MD: Aspen Publishers.

Zander, K. (1991, April). Presentation at *Nursing care management: Transcending walls opening gates,* Saint Joseph Medical Center, Wichita, Kansas.

APPENDIX 4-1

BETH ISRAEL MEDICAL CENTER

MULTI-DISCIPLINARY ACTION PLAN

DIAGNOSIS: <u>ASTHMA (PEDIATRICS)</u>

MD: <u>PEDIATRIC AMBULATORY GROUP</u>

UNIT: <u>PEDIATRIC - INPATIENT</u>

ADMISSION DATE: _____

DATE MAP INITIATED: _____

DRG #: <u>98/774/775</u>

_____

EXPECTED LENGTH OF STAY: <u>4 DAYS</u>

PATIENT CARE MANAGER: _____

SOCIAL WORKER: _____

PATIENT ALLERGIES: _____

YES/NO | DATE

_____

_____ DNR:

HEALTH CARE PROXY

OR LIVING WILL: _____

```
BETH ISRAEL MEDICAL CENTER
MULTI-DISCIPLINARY ACTION PLAN

        DAY 1 OF 4


MD: _____

DIAGNOSIS: _____

RN/MD REVIEW: _____

                        DATE: _____
```

MAP DOES NOT REPLACE MD ORDERS ·   **VARIANCE**

TESTS/ PROCEDURES/ TREATMENTS	CBC, Theophylline level, SMA6, PPD. Initiate chest PT before NEB TX. Dipstick Urine X1, Check specific gravity X1. Ask for old chart & problem face sheet from clinic chart. When indicated order should include: Peak flow >6yrs. or cooperative qshift., ABG'S, CXR, pulse oximeter, postural drainage
MEDICATIONS	(amt. according to wt. in kg's.) IV Aminophylline and/ or Proventil NEB/PO and/or Steroids (Solucortef, solumedrol, Prednisone and/or Cromolyn and/or Oxygen.)
ACTIVITY	As tolerated
NUTRITION	As tolerated
CONSULTS	None
SOCIAL WORK	
DISCHARGE PLANNING	Determine if Home Care Services were provided prior to admission. Consult with social worker regarding initial screening and projected discharge plan.
PATIENT VARIANCE (On Admission)	

DATE	INITIALS	PRINT NAME	SIGNATURE

BETH ISRAEL MEDICAL CENTER
MULTI-DISCIPLINARY ACTION PLAN

DAY 1 OF 4

MD: _____

DIAGNOSIS: _____

DATE: _____

MAP DOES NOT REPLACE MD ORDERS

PATIENT PROBLEM	EXPECTED PATIENT OUTCOME/ DISCHARGE OUTCOME	NURSING INTERVENTIONS		ASSESSMENT/ INTERVENTION
1. Alteration in breathing pattern	1. Pt. will be free of respiratory distress as evidenced by: A. Resp. rate within normal limits for age. B. Arterial blood gases within normal limits. C. Equal air movement heard on auscultation. D. Clear breath sounds. E. Minimal work effort for breathing.	1A. Auscultate breath sounds: Assess adventitious breath sounds (wheezing stridor, rhonchi, rales). B. Assess color changes of skin, mucous membrane, ex: pallor, cyanosis. C. Assess and observe for retractions and nasal flaring q4 hrs, and more frequently during the acute attack. D. Observe for agitation, anxiety. E. Note changes in VS, BP, or O2 saturation if on oximeter. F. Position in manner most comfortable and to facilitate chest expansion. G. Monitor response to tx. (Report to MD resp. distress, vomiting, headache, agitation, tachycardia) H. Chest P/T once per shft, unless otherwise contraindicated. I. Check specific gravity, dipstick urine X one. J. Enc. fluids if tolerating po. K. Peak flow qshift, if child >6yrs. L. Assess pt's. response to activity.		
2. Knowledge deficit	2. The parent/child will verb. knowledge of teaching done regarding: A. Precipitating factors (Allergens, smoke, sudden changes in temp.). B. Meds, names, dose desired effects, adverse effects, frequency and times. C. Importance of regular follow-up appointments. D. Exercise regimen with breathing exercises.	2A. Orient to room and unit. B. Assess readiness to learn. C. Familiarize with treatment regimen, i.e. IV pump, Medications, respiratory nebulizer treatment, peak flow meter.		
3. Anxiety	3A. De-escalation of anxiety to within coping levels. B. Identify stress factors.	3A. Provide quiet calm environment, minimize anxiety producing situations. B. Explore stressors and coping mechanisms. C. Assess family dynamics.		

```
BETH ISRAEL MEDICAL CENTER

MULTI-DISCIPLINARY ACTION PLAN

        DAY 2 OF 4


MD: _____

DIAGNOSIS: _____

RN/MD REVIEW: _____
```

DATE: _____

MAP DOES NOT REPLACE MD ORDERS   **VARIANCE**

TESTS/ PROCEDURES/ TREATMENTS	Theophylline level, ABG's if indicated. Peak flow every shift if >6yrs "or" cooperative q8 hrs. Chest PT/Postural Drainage	
MEDICATIONS	Steroids could be discontinued within 48 hours or taper over a period of 7-10 days. Assess for change to PO meds.	
ACTIVITY	As tolerated	
NUTRITION	As tolerated	
CONSULTS	None	
SOCIAL WORK	Screen to identify psychosocial and discharge planning needs. Begin social work assessment for hi-risk patients: If patient has been or is being reported to Child Welfare Administration, document all pertinent information, especially registry number.	
DISCHARGE PLANNING	Request Home Health Care evaluation as indicated.	
PATIENT VARIANCE (On Admission)		

DATE	INITIALS	PRINT NAME	SIGNATURE

BETH ISRAEL MEDICAL CENTER
MULTI-DISCIPLINARY ACTION PLAN

DAY 2 OF 4

MD: _____

DIAGNOSIS: _____

DATE: _____

MAP DOES NOT REPLACE MD ORDERS

PATIENT PROBLEM	EXPECTED PATIENT OUTCOME/ DISCHARGE OUTCOME	NURSING INTERVENTIONS		ASSESSMENT/ INTERVENTION
1. Alteration in breathing pattern	1. Pt. will be free of respiratory distress as evidenced by: A. Resp. rate within normal limits for age. B. Arterial blood gases within normal limits. C. Equal air movement heard on auscultation. D. Clear breath sounds. E. Minimal work effort for breathing.	1A. Auscultate breath sounds: Assess adventitious breath sounds (wheezing, stridor, rhonchi, rales). B. Assess color changes of skin, i.e pallor and cyanosis. C. Assess and observe for retractions and nasal flaring q4 hrs. and more frequently during the D. Note changes in VS, BP, or O2 Saturation (if on oximeter) and readiness to D/C pulse Oximetry. E. Chest P/T once per shift, unless otherwise ordered or contraindicated. F. Monitor response to tx. Report to MD increase resp. distress, vomiting, headache, agitation, tachycardia. G. Peak flow every shift if >6 yrs. H. Assess pt's. response to activity. I. Encourage fluids if tolerating po.		
2. Knowledge deficit	2. The parent/child will verb. knowledge of teaching done regarding: A. Precipitating factors (Allergens, smoke, sudden changes in temp.). B. Meds, names, dose desired effects, adverse effects, frequency and times. C. Importance of regular follow-up appointments. D. Exercise regimen with breathing exercises.	2A. Assess family and patients knowledge base of disease process and begin discharge teaching. B. Assess need for VNS (initiate if applicable). C. Community referrals (ex. N.Y. Lung Assoc.)		
3. Anxiety	3A. De-escalation of anxiety to within coping levels. B. Identify stress factors.	3A. Allow for verbalization of feelings, fears, and anxieties. B. Provide emotional support. C. Reevaluate level of anxiety PRN, provide supportive measures. D. Teach regarding guided imagery, diversional activities.		

BETH ISRAEL MEDICAL CENTER

MULTI-DISCIPLINARY ACTION PLAN

DAY 3 OF 4

MD: _____

DIAGNOSIS: _____

RN/MD REVIEW: _____

DATE: _____

MAP DOES NOT REPLACE MD ORDERS   VARIANCE

TESTS/ PROCEDURES/ TREATMENTS	Check PPD, Theophylline level Peak flow every shift if >6yrs "or" cooperative q8 hrs. Chest PT/Postural Drainage	
MEDICATIONS	Assess change to po medications i.e. Slobid, Somophylline, Proventil, Steroids	
ACTIVITY	As tolerated	
NUTRITION	As tolerated	
CONSULTS		
SOCIAL WORK	Continue involvement in discharge planning; ongoing consultation with patient, family, MD, RN, and HHIC. On the day prior to discharge: Finalize D/C plan, verify-parent/caregiver avail., clothing, etc. Confirm trans., home care plans with HHIC & CCMU as needed. Coordinate prep. of req. documents for trans. e.g. inter-institutional transfer form etc.	
DISCHARGE PLANNING	Monitor progress on discharge plan; consult with MD, SW, and HHIC. MD to give 24 hrs. notice to patient and write official discharge order.	
PATIENT VARIANCE (On Admission)		

DATE	INITIALS	PRINT NAME	SIGNATURE

BETH ISRAEL MEDICAL CENTER
MULTI-DISCIPLINARY ACTION PLAN

DAY 3 OF 4

MD: _____

DIAGNOSIS: _____

DATE: _____

MAP DOES NOT REPLACE MD ORDERS

PATIENT PROBLEM	EXPECTED PATIENT OUTCOME/ DISCHARGE OUTCOME	NURSING INTERVENTIONS		ASSESSMENT/ INTERVENTION
1. Alteration in breathing pattern	1. Pt. will be free of respiratory distress as evidenced by: A. Resp. rate within normal limits for age. B. Arterial blood gases within normal limits. C. Equal air movement heard on ausculation. D. Clear breath sounds. E. Minimal work effort for breathing.	1A. Auscultate breath sounds, assess color, observe for retractions, nasal flaring every 8hrs. and PRN B. Vital signs with blood pressure, every 8hrs and PRN. C. Assess with MD readiness for change to po medications. D. Chest physical therapy every shift, unless contraindicated. E. Observe response to Nebulizer treatment and check with MD to decrease frequency. F. Peak flow every shift if >6 yrs. G. Assess pt's. response to activity H. Assess diet tolerance and record		
2. Knowledge deficit	2. The parent/child will verb. knowledge of teaching done regarding: A. Precipitating factors (Allergens, smoke, sudden changes in temp.). B. Meds, names, dose desired effects, adverse effects, frequency and times. C. Importance of regular follow-up appointments. D. Exercise regimen with breathing exercises.	2A. Continue ongoing discharge teaching i.e. medication administration, treatments, importance of follow-up. B. Disc. plan with parents to minimize.allergies in the home. B. Reevaluate for VNS referral.		
3. Anxiety	3A. De-escalation of anxiety to within coping levels. B. Identify stress factors.	3A. Continue allowing verbalization of feelings, fears, and anxieties B. Provide emotional support. C. Reevaluate level of anxiety prn, provide supportive measures i.e. support groups OPD.		

```
BETH ISRAEL MEDICAL CENTER

MULTI-DISCIPLINARY ACTION PLAN


        DAY 4 OF 4


MD: _____

DIAGNOSIS: _____

RN/MD REVIEW: _____

                              DATE: _____
```

MAP DOES NOT REPLACE MD ORDERS   VARIANCE

TESTS/ PROCEDURES/ TREATMENTS	Check theophylline level Peak flow every shift if >6yrs cooperative q8 hrs. Consider discharge if increased peak flow and improved clinical picture	
MEDICATIONS	Consider discharge home within 24 hours of initiation of po medication.	
ACTIVITY	As tolerated	
NUTRITION	As tolerated	
CONSULTS		
SOCIAL WORK	If patient is placed on ALC; all referral materials must be completed to CCMU within 24 hrs.	
DISCHARGE PLANNING	If patient is placed on ALC and is going to LTC faci- lity, transfer summaries must be completed prior to discharge. Prior to discharge confirm Home Care plans with SW and HHIC. Any patient with active CWA case must be cleared by social work.	
PATIENT VARIANCE (On Admission)		

DATE	INITIALS	PRINT NAME	SIGNATURE

```
        BETH ISRAEL MEDICAL CENTER
        MULTI-DISCIPLINARY ACTION PLAN

            DAY 4 OF 4
```

MD: _____

DIAGNOSIS: _____

DATE: _____

MAP DOES NOT REPLACE MD ORDERS

PATIENT PROBLEM	EXPECTED PATIENT OUTCOME/ DISCHARGE OUTCOME	NURSING INTERVENTIONS		ASSESSMENT/ INTERVENTION
1. Alteration in breathing pattern	1. Pt. will be free of respiratory distress as evidenced by: A. Resp. rate within normal limits for age. B. Arterial blood gases within normal limits. C. Equal air movement heard on auscultation. D. Clear breath sounds. E. Minimal work effort for breathing.	1A. Auscultate breath sounds, assess color, observe for retractions, nasal flaring every 8hrs. and prn B. Vital signs with blood pressure, every 8hrs and PRN C. Chest P.T. every shift, unless contraindicated. D. Observe response to Nebulizer treatment and check with MD to decrease frequency. E. Peak flow every shift if >6 yrs. F. Assess pt's. response to activity G. Assess diet tolerance and record. H. Assess clinical picture i.e. increased peak flow, toleration of PO meds., theophyline level between 10 & 20.		
2. Knowledge deficit	2. The parent/child will verb. knowledge of teaching done regarding: A. Precipitating factors (Allergens, smoke, sudden changes in temp.). B. Meds, names, dose desired effects, adverse effects, frequency and times. C. Importance of regular follow-up appointments. D. Exercise regimen with breathing exercises.	2A. Discharge Planning. B. Medications reviewed. C. Signs and symptoms of respiratory distress reviewed. D. Identification of factors that may precipitate asthmatic attacks. E. Exercise regimen, i.e. breathing exercises and rest periods. F. Follow-up care. G. When to call MD/come to E.R.		
3. Anxiety	3A. De-escalation of anxiety to within coping levels. B. Identify stress factors.	3A. Reevaluate level of anxiety and provide support prn. B. Reassure parents/child regarding knowledge of asthma.		

DATE/INITIALS	VARIANCE

5

WITHIN-THE-WALLS CASE MANAGEMENT

A NURSING HOSPITAL-BASED CASE MANAGEMENT MODEL

▼ *CHAPTER OVERVIEW*

This chapter reviews various models of within-the-walls case management. This approach became popular when hospitals began restructuring to improve productivity, manage effective use of resources, lower costs, and maintain quality.

Preliminary findings show that this patient care delivery model can have a great effect on resource use and quality patient care. Daily assessment and evaluation of the patient's clinical care, reduced length of stay and other financial benefits, general applicability of this model, and improved nurse, physician, and patient satisfaction demonstrate the merit and relevancy of this approach to patient care delivery and professional practice.

▲

COST-EFFECTIVE CARE

The changing nature of health care economics has forced hospitals to view case management as an alternative to the delivery of direct care services. Hospital-based case management is founded on traditional approaches. It ensures the most appropriate use of services by patients. A case management system in the hospital setting avoids duplication and misuse of medical services, controls costs by reducing inefficient services, and improves the effectiveness of care delivery (Lavizzo-Mourey, 1987). Lavizzo-Mourey (1987), McIntosh (1987), and Henderson and Collard (1988) reported several advantages of hospital-based case management. First, the hospital setting offers a wide range of specialized skills that can be made available to both the provider and recipient of case management services. Second, because most of the resources needed for patient care are centralized within the acute care setting, early assessment of patient needs, planning and coordination of care delivery, and evaluation of alternative systems are enhanced. Third, because space and overhead costs are factored into hospital-based care, the management of expenditures associated with high-cost patients is minimized. Fourth, systems for monitoring and measuring the cost-effectiveness of case management arrangements are present within the hospital setting.

Many hospital-based case management systems have engaged registered nurses as case managers (Henderson & Collard, 1988; Henderson & Wallack, 1987; McIntosh, 1987). Nurse involvement in case management allows nurses to influence and direct the delivery and quality of patient care. Such involvement allows for more control, visibility, and recognition for nursing services delivered. The involvement also offers more consistent outcome attainment and demonstrates nursing personnel contributions to patient care (Zander, 1988a).

Because it would be virtually impossible to cover all patient models of nursing case management that may currently exist, this chapter will focus on some of the systems that have served as the foundation for the development of within-the-walls case management. The chapter will also highlight those approaches to patient care delivery and professional practice that have been published and have received national attention.

PRIMARY NURSE CASE MANAGEMENT MODEL

Nursing case management has emerged in the acute care setting as a professional model of practice. One model, characterized as a primary nurse case management model, has been used at the New England Medical Center in Boston, Massachusetts. Stetler (1987), Woldum (1987), and Zander (1988a; 1988b; 1990) have identified the following factors that distinguish this case management system of care.

▼ Primary nurse case management is based on the concept of managed care. Managed care is defined as care that is unit based, outcome oriented, dependent on a designated time frame, and focused on the appropriate use of resources for both the inpatient and outpatient population.

▼ Primary nurse case management services and case loads are designated for specific patient case types or case mixes. Some examples of case types coordinated by primary nurse case management are cardiac, leukemia, pediatric gastrointestinal, stroke, craniotomy, and some gynecological.

▼ Nursing case managers are the primary care givers for patients. The managers provide direct care to patients in their case loads while the patients are housed in their units and continue to coordinate the care of these patients throughout hospitalization, regardless of the patient's physical location.

▼ The process of care is monitored by the use of case management plans, which include DRG length of stay; critical path reports, which outline the components of appropriate care; and variance analysis, which ensures the continuous evaluation of patient care activities.

▼ Care is coordinated through collaborative group practice arrangements across geographic units, case consultation, and health care team meetings. Patient discharge planning is outlined before admission and updated throughout hospitalization until the time of discharge.

The New England Medical Center's nursing case management model presents an innovative alternative to the delivery of nursing care within the acute care setting. The model has evolved since its introduction and has been widely adapted.* The development of care multidisciplinary action plans (MAPs) increases the potential for evaluating the cost-effectiveness and quality of care standards proposed by this model. Care MAPS have expanded on case management plans and critical paths by focusing on standards of care and practice for a specific case type, responding to variances in the delivery of care, linking continuous quality improvement (CQI) to practices, and integrating resource allocation, patient care outcomes, and cost reimbursement systems (Zander, 1991; 1992a; 1992b).

The competence and experience of the case manager are critical to the effective delivery of patient care services (Henderson & Wallack, 1987). The case management model at the New England Medical Center, along with most nurse case management programs, primarily uses registered nurses as case managers. A case manager must have at least 1 year of nursing experience and charge responsibilities and must demonstrate leadership ability. Henderson and Wallack (1987) and Henderson and Collard (1988) recommend that to ensure cost-effective care and quality assurance standards, the nurse case manager should have expertise related to the care of designated types of patients and specific diagnostic categories. Because of the model's reliance on a primary nursing care delivery system, staffing mix allocation was not differentiated in the New England Medical Center's model. Some case management programs have successfully employed a variety of personnel other than professional nursing staff. Studies are needed to determine the best staffing mix for nursing case management programs. Contrary to what Zander (1990) reported about the nursing case management model at the New England Medical Center, a study in another institution has shown a preliminary increase in direct nursing care hours and greater use of resources during the initial phase of hospitalization. These changes resulted in an overall decrease in length of stay, an increase in patient turnover, and a potential increase in patient revenues generated for the hospital (Cohen, 1991).

LEVELED PRACTICE MODEL

Another nursing case management model, identified as the leveled practice model, has focused on the management and coordination of patient care needs. This system differs from the primary nurse case management model in that the case manager's functions are focused on the management activities of patient care and not on the responsibility for patient care delivery (Loveridge, Cummings, & O'Malley, 1988; O'Malley & Cummings, 1988). A work group consisting of registered nurses, licensed practical nurses, and nurses' aides provides direct care on a specific patient unit. The professional nurse is designated as the case manager and is responsible for coordinating and monitoring patient care of an assigned case load through collaboration with the work group, patient, family, and interdisciplinary health team members. In addition, the case manager relies on information related to case mix, hospital costs, patient resource use, insurance, and reimbursement data (O'Malley & Cummings, 1988).

Conceptually, case management is now considered a strategy for the coordination of care and is evolving into a sophisticated resource for managing access, quality, and cost (Bower & Falk, 1996).

The leveled case management model has promoted differentiated practice arrangements by delineating functional role responsibility and accountability between those nurses with baccalaureate degrees and those with associate degrees (Loveridge et al., 1988). Differentiated competence levels in nursing practice were classified extensively by Primm (1986). Because of the principles inherent in leveled practice case management, the role of the professional staff nurse changes to an autonomous one. Consequently, this change in practice places different obligations on the nurse manager. The nurse manager's role becomes what MacGregor-Burns (1978) described as transformational leadership, which focuses on teaching, mentoring, and coaching activities. In the leveled practice nursing case management model, management responsibility emphasized overall administrative and fiscal support, as well as patient outcome assessment and quality care improvement (Loveridge et al., 1988; O'Malley & Cummings, 1988).

PRIMARY CASE MANAGEMENT

The primary case management model, which was developed and implemented at Hermann Hospital in Houston, embraced the primary nursing philosophy of care and used a clinical career ladder for registered nurses (Cavouras, Walts, Taylor, Garner, & Bordelon, 1990). The clinical ladder consisted of six levels of clinical expertise, which progressed from a patient-focused orientation at the beginning levels to interdisciplinary and general service practice responsibility and accountability as nurse case managers at the top level.

The primary case management model used unit-based case managers who were responsible for coordinating, developing, and evaluating the delivery and the quality of patient care. Staff nurses and nurse extenders were the ones who provided the care, which was based on standard protocols. The care plans outlined the daily care requirements and activities and served as a mechanism for monitoring and evaluating issues related to quality and as a patient care resource for nursing and hospitalwide support services such as laboratory, pharmacy, and respiratory therapy. Quality improvement was monitored as well through unit-based quality assurance programs.

Cost effectiveness, quality of care, and nurses' job satisfaction were also evaluated through retrospective variance analysis of patient charges and length of hospital stay, quality-assurance monitoring, and nurse satisfaction surveys. To date, no data have been published.

SAINT JOSEPH MERCY HOSPITAL'S PONTIAC PROJECT AND MERCY HOSPITAL'S PORT HURON PROJECT

Both Saint Joseph Mercy Hospital and Mercy Hospital served as case management project demonstration sites and were part of the Mercy Health Services Consortium.

The Pontiac project, a collaborative practice model, implemented case management in the medical-surgical division (Wesley & Easterling, 1991). Critical paths and patient care teaching plans focused care needs and resources on high risk patients. These plans involved patient, family, and care team assessments. Variations in patient care were monitored to ensure continuity. A competence-based clinical advancement design maintained the high level of leadership, commitment, and expertise needed for the case manager role.

Preliminary evaluation of this model revealed increased collaboration and enhanced professional relationships among nurses and physicians. Additional benefits of this collaborative effort included more efficient and improved clinical programs, improved quality care, and greater professional respect and autonomy.

The Mercy Hospital Port Huron Project incorporates a case management approach into a community health care system (McClelland & Foster, 1991). This case management model is used for oncology patients. In this system, health care delivery operates on a continuum and integrates service aspects related to hospitalization, home care, and hospice. Collaborative practice arrangements are interdisciplinary to ensure continuous, quality patient care. Community education programs, home care, and respite services are also provided. Monitoring systems help evaluate job satisfaction, cost, and quality of patient care.

TUCSON MEDICAL CENTER CASE MANAGEMENT MODEL

A case management model developed at Tucson Medical Center addresses the cost and quality aspects of patient care delivery (Del Togno-Armanasco et al., 1989). This approach incorporates elements of the New England Medical Center's case management model and differentiates practice models in addition to basic philosophic practice components of primary nursing and shared governance.

Called collaborative nursing case management, this model primarily focuses on standardizing the use of patient care resources and the delivery of services during the patient's hospitalization for selected DRG case types. Both patient mix and service volume management strategies were used to attain cost-effective, quality patient care (Olivas et al., 1989a).

A collaborative case management plan (CCMP) and a care plan MAP are used to identify the contributions of all health care providers and support a unit-specific standard of patient care. Variations from practice standards are also monitored and evaluated. The care plan MAP (see Appendix 5-1) was revised in 1991 to meet requirements of the Joint Commission on Accreditation of Healthcare Organizations (Gwozdz & Del Togno-Armanasco, 1992). It is also used as a basic documentation form.

Hospitalwide and unit-specific multidisciplinary practice committees were established to assist in clinical decision making and overall evaluation processes of the patient care model. These groups consist of physical therapists, dietitians, social workers, physicians, and home care professionals (Olivas et al., 1989b). Patients are encouraged to participate and are included in the planning of their care regimens, which are carried out on a continuous basis from the time of admission to after discharge.

Various evaluation mechanisms were developed to measure the potential impact of this case management model on outcomes of care. A patient-satisfaction questionnaire and a retrospective chart review have been implemented along with a physician-satisfaction-with-care questionnaire to ascertain variables related to patient care and job satisfaction. Information on cost of care, rate of absenteeism, and staff turnover also are collected. Findings showed increased satisfaction with both nursing and medical care (at the .05 alpha level) for case-managed, total-hip-replacement, coronary bypass, and valvular surgery patients. There was no turnover of nurse case managers, and a marked decrease in turnover rates was demonstrated for nursing staff on the oncology and orthopedic units.

Outcome data also showed a decreased length of stay among patients who underwent total-hip and knee replacements. The decrease was 3.48 and 2.82 days respectively over a 3½-year period. Length of stay for valvular replacement and coronary bypass patients also decreased. In addition, a positive cost variance of $9,273 was realized for the valvular replacement and coronary bypass patient populations (Del Togno-Armanasco, 1992).

SAINT MICHAEL HOSPITAL'S COORDINATED CARE MODEL

Coordinated care, another innovative case management approach, was developed at Saint Michael Hospital in Milwaukee, Wisconsin. Using critical paths and a comprehensive variance analysis system, this model expands on the practice concepts of nursing case management used in the New England Medical Center's model (Sinnen & Schifalacqua, 1991).

The coordinated care approach demonstrated organizational effectiveness through a decrease in costs related to shorter length of stay and a reduction in hospital-associated charges (Sinnen & Schifalacqua, 1991). An additional gain was better communication across all disciplines involved in patient care delivery.

Within the last 3 years the modified primary nursing delivery system has been changed to the dyad model. The dyad care delivery modification involves a partnership between a registered nurse and technical assistant who care for a specific number of patients (see Chapter 2 for description). In addition, Saint Michael's within-the-walls model is in the fourth generation of multidisciplinary critical paths. The patient action plan is a permanent part of the medical record and includes patient outcomes, multidisciplinary interventions, teaching record, and nursing care plan (M. Schifalacqua, 1992).

REFERENCES

Bower, K.A., & Falk, C.D. (1996). Case Management as a response to quality, cost, and access imperatives In E. Cohen (Ed.), *Nurse case management in the 21st century* (pp 161-167). St Louis: Mosby-Year Book, Inc.

Cavouras, C.A., Walts, L., Taylor, S., Garner, A., & Bordelon, P. (1990). Alternative Delivery System: Primary case management. In G. Mayer, M. Madden, & E. Lawrenz (Eds.), *Patient care delivery models* (pp. 275-282), Rockville, Md.: Aspen Publishers, Inc.

Cohen, E. (1991). Nursing case management: Does it pay? *Journal of Nursing Administration, 21*(4), 20-25.

Del Togno-Armanasco, V. (1992). [Collaborative Case Management: Outcome data]. Unpublished raw data.

Del Togno-Armanasco, V., Olivas, G., & Harter, S. (1989). Developing an integrated nursing case management model. *Nursing Management, 20*(5), 26-29.

Gwozdz, D.T., & Del Togno-Armanasco, V. (1992). Developing an integrated nursing case management model. *Nursing Management, 20*(5), 26-29.

Henderson, M.G., & Collard, A. (1988). Measuring quality in medical case management programs. *Quality Review Bulletin, 14*(2), 33-39.

Henderson, M.G., & Wallack, S.S. (1987). Evaluating case management for catastrophic illness. *Business and Health, 4*(3), 741.

Lavizzo-Mourey, R. (1987). Hospital based case management. *DRG Monitor, 5*(1), 1-8.

Loveridge, C., Cummings, S., & O'Malley, J. (1988). Developing case management in a primary nursing system. *Journal of Nursing Administration, 18*(10), 36-39.

MacGregor-Burns, J. (1978). *Leadership.* New York: Harper & Row.

McClelland, M., & Foster, D. (1991). The Mercy Hospital, Port Huron Project. *Nursing Administration Quarterly, 15*(4), 58-60.

McIntosh, L. (1987). Hospital based case management. *Nursing Economics, 5*(5), 232-236.

Olivas, G., Del Togno-Armanasco, V., Erickson, J.R., & Harter, S. (1989a). Case management: A bottom-line care delivery model. 1: The concept. *Journal of Nursing Administration, 19*(11), 16-20.

Olivas, G., Del Togno-Armanasco, V., Erickson, J.R., & Harter, S. (1989b). Case management: A bottom-line care delivery model. 2: Adaptation of the model. *Journal of Nursing Administration, 19*(12), 12-17.

O'Malley, J., & Cummings, S. (1988). Nursing case management. 3: Implementing case management. *Aspen's Advisor for Nurse Executives, 3*(7), 8-9.

Primm, P.L. (1986). Entry into practice: Competency statements for BSNs and ADNs. *Nursing Outlook, 34*(3), 135-137.

Schifalacqua, M. (1992). Personal communication.

Sinnen, M.T., & Schifalacqua, M. (1991). Coordinated care in a community hospital. *Nursing Management, 22*(3), 38-42.

Stetler, C.B. (1987). The case manager's role: A preliminary evaluation. *Definition, 2*(3), 1-4.

Wesley, M.L., & Easterling, A. (1991). The St. Joseph Mercy Hospital, Pontiac Project. *Nursing Administration Quarterly, 15*(4), 50-54.

Woldum, K. (1987). Critical paths: Marking the course. *Definition, 2*(3), 1-4.

Zander, K. (1988a). Managed care within acute care settings: Design and implementation via nursing case management. *Health Care Supervisor, 6*(2), 24-43.

Zander, K. (1988b). Nursing care management: Strategic management of cost and quality outcomes. *Journal of Nursing Administration, 18*(5), 23-30.

Zander, K. (1990). Managed care and nursing case management. In G.G. Mayer, M.J. Madden, & E. Lawrenz (Eds.), *Patient care delivery models* (pp. 37-61). Rockville, Md. Aspen Publishers, Inc.

Zander, K. (1991, Fall). Care Maps TM: The core of cost/quality care. *The New Definition, 6*(3), 1-3.

Zander, K. (1992a, Winter). Physicians, Care Maps and collaboration. *The New Definition, 7*(1), 1-4.

Zander, K. (1992b, Spring). Quantifying, managing, and improving quality. 1: How Care Maps link CQI to the patient. *The New Definition, 1*(2), 1-3.

Appendix 5-1

TUCSON MEDICAL CENTER
DIVISION OF NURSING
COLECTOMY
CarePlan MAP©

NRA 1175 REV 09/92

Developed by: Gail Greene, BSN, RN

NURSING DIAGNOSIS/ PATIENT PROBLEMS	OUTCOME EXPECTATIONS	EXPECTATIONS MET AT DISCHARGE Yes No Nurse's Signature
Pre-Operative		
A. Actual/potential for anxiety related to potential threat to well-being secondary to hospitalization and surgery.	A. Patient will express decreased amount of fear. B. Patient will identify any questions or concerns or needs necessary to decrease anxiety.	A. _____ Date achieved: _____ B. _____ Date achieved: _____
B. Actual/potential knowledge deficit related to surgery.	A. Patient will verbalize an understanding of nursing care. B. Patient will demonstrate compliance with nursing interventions.	A. _____ Date achieved: _____ B. _____ Date achieved: _____
Post-Operative		
1. Actual/potential for volume deficit related to NPO status, nausea and/or emesis.	Patient will obtain and maintain adequate hydration. A. Dressing is dry and intact.	A. _____ Date achieved: _____

Continued.

53

NURSING DIAGNOSIS/ PATIENT PROBLEMS	OUTCOME EXPECTATIONS	EXPECTATIONS MET AT DISCHARGE Yes No Nurse's Signature
Post-Operative—cont'd		
	B. Heart rate within normal limits.	B. _____ Date achieved: _____
	C. B/P within normal limits.	C. _____ Date achieved: _____
	D. Mucosa pink and moist.	D. _____ Date achieved: _____
	E. Skin remains warm and dry without diaphoresis.	E. _____ Date achieved: _____
	F. Electrolyte balance at normal limits.	F. _____ Date achieved: _____
2. Actual/potential ineffective breathing pattern related to anesthesia and surgical pain.	Patient will maintain normal respiration pattern for patient.	_____ Date achieved: _____
3. Actual/potential for alteration in comfort: pain related to surgery.	A. Patient verbalizes absence or decrease in pain level.	A. _____ Date achieved: _____
	B. Participates in exercises and care.	B. _____ Date achieved: _____
	C. Comfortable and oriented to environment.	C. _____ Date achieved: _____
4. Actual/potential injury related to infection.	A. Skin integrity is maintained.	A. _____ Date achieved: _____

5. Actual/potential altered elimination: Constipation related to anesthesia, immobility, narcotics, and surgically changed pathway for stool.

B. Healing occurs without untoward evidence of infection, i.e., increased temperature, increased WBCs, wound redness, edema, or purulent drainage.

B. _____
Date achieved: _____

A. Patient will experience patient's normal bowel elimination pattern and will expel flatus.

A. _____
Date achieved: _____

B. Will be aware of and begin to understand changes regarding bowel function if ileostomy or colostomy are necessary.

B. _____
Date achieved: _____

6. Actual/potential altered elimination: Urinary retention related to anesthesia and surgery.

A. Patient will either:
• Urinate within 6 to 12 hours post surgery or 6 to 12 hours after catheter is discontinued.

A. _____
Date achieved: _____

• Pass 30 ml of urine per hour when patient has a catheter.

Date achieved: _____

B. Will tolerate PO fluids without N/V prior to discontinuing IV fluids.

B. _____
Date achieved: _____

7. Actual/potential for injury.

Free of injuries during hospital stay.

Date achieved: _____

8. Knowledge deficit as related to disease process and convalescent period.

Patient and significant others will verbalize acceptable level of knowledge and sign discharge instructions concerning:
A. Activity
B. Medication regimen

Date achieved: _____

Continued.

NURSING DIAGNOSIS/ PATIENT PROBLEMS	OUTCOME EXPECTATIONS	EXPECTATIONS MET AT DISCHARGE Yes No Nurse's Signature
Post-Operative—cont'd	C. Future doctor appointment D. Diet E. Understanding symptoms requiring attention F. Hygiene changes relative to health status. G. Understand preprinted education materials regarding disease process. H. J.P.Tube care I. Other _____	

Additional Problems

9. _____   _____ Date achieved: _____

10. _____   _____ Date achieved: _____

TUCSON MEDICAL CENTER
DIVISION OF NURSING
COLECTOMY
CarePlan MAP©

NRA 1175 REV 09/92   Developed by: Gail Greene, BSN, RN

PRE-OPERATIVE TEACHING—GUIDELINE AND DOCUMENTATION

Discuss the following with your patient and/or family before sending to surgery.

A. Pre-operative
   1. NPO means "Nothing by Mouth"
   2. Shower/pre-op
   3. Pre-op medication: Causes relaxation, dry mouth, drowsiness. Patient is to remain in bed after getting this medication.
   4. Transportation to holding areas.
   5. Disposition of valuables.
   6. Use of call bell systems.
   7. Turn, coughing, deep breathing.
   8. JP tube care

B. Intro-operative
   1. Recovery Room (PACU)—after surgery until awake and reacting (usually 1 to 2 hours)
   2. Frequent vital signs.
   3. Lots of people, no need for concern.

C. Post-operative
   1. Diet
   2. Activity
   3. Special checks or treatments
   4. Restriction, if any
   5. Exercises, breathing, extremities

Continued.

PRE-OPERATIVE TEACHING—GUIDELINE AND DOCUMENTATION—cont'd

6. Pain medicine—need to request
7. I.V.
8. Location after surgery
9. Voiding/catheterization
10. Possible tubes (i.e., foley, CT, NG, ET, invasive lines)
11. Possibility of colostomy or ileostomy

D. Fears, concern or other information requested: _____

_____

_____

E. Response to teaching: _____

_____

F. Additional reinforcement needed on: _____

_____

_____

Nurse's Signature _____ Date _____

NRA 1175 REV 09/92

TUCSON MEDICAL CENTER
DIVISION OF NURSING
COLECTOMY
CarePlan MAP©

Developed by: Gail Greene, BSN, RN

INDEPENDENT ACTIONS BASED UPON THE HUMAN RESPONSE TO ACTUAL OR POTENTIAL PROBLEMS

Hospital Day	Consults	Tests	Activity/Rest	Medical Interventions	Medications	Nutrition	Nurses' Signatures
PTA or Day of Admit Date ___	-Anesthesia	-CBC -Urinalysis	-Up ad lib		-Own, if any	-NPO	_____
Surgery Date: ___		-Lytes if NG -H&H or CBC	-Up in PM to bathroom with help -If A-line; bedrest, turn, cough, & deep breath q 2 hours -Bed side commode with help	-IV -JP tube(s) -NG suction -Foley -Possible A-line	-Analgesics IM, IV, epidural -Antibiotics	-NPO, I&O	_____ _____ _____
Day 1 Date: ___		-Lytes if NG -H&H or CBC	-Walk in hall 4 times with assistance -If A-line: turn, cough, & deep breathe q 2 hours when in bed -Up in chair	-IV -JP tube(s) -NG to suction -Foley -A-line	-Analgesics IM, IV epidural -Antibiotics	-NPO, I&O	_____ _____

All items not provided as planned. Enter explanation in the individualization/variance section on the last page.
DRG Number: 148/149. Expected LOS: 6-8 days.

TUCSON MEDICAL CENTER
DIVISION OF NURSING
COLECTOMY
CarePlan MAP©

NRA 1175 REV 09/92   Developed by: Gail Greene, BSN, RN

INDEPENDENT ACTIONS BASED UPON THE HUMAN RESPONSE TO ACTUAL OR POTENTIAL PROBLEMS

Hospital Day	Assessment	Discharge Planning	Teaching	Psycho Social	Self Care	Nurses' Signatures
PTA or Day of Admit Date: ___	-Lung status -Location and nature of pain		Reinforce pre-op teaching -Reassure and encourage patient that numerous people have ostomies and still enjoy active, happy and productive lives	-Assess anxiety level	-ADLs	
Surgery Date: ___	-Lung status -Bowel sounds		-Reinforce post-teaching	-Continue to assess anxiety level -Inform of colostomy/ileostomy immediately post-op if one way constructed	-Assisted ADLs	
Day 1 Date: ___	-Lung status -Bowel sounds	-Assess at home needs	-Continue to reinforce post-op teaching	-Continue to assess anxiety level -Patient to look at ostomy area during AM care and ostomy care. If no ostomy, look at incision area/dressing	-Assisted ADLs	

All items not provided as planned. Enter explanation in the individualization/variance section on the last page.
DRG Number: 148/149. Expected LOS: 6-8 days.

TUCSON MEDICAL CENTER
DIVISION OF NURSING
COLECTOMY
CarePlan MAP©

NRA 1175 REV 09/92   Developed by: Gail Greene, BSN, RN

INDEPENDENT ACTIONS BASED UPON THE HUMAN RESPONSE TO ACTUAL OR POTENTIAL PROBLEMS

Hospital Day	Consults	Tests	Activity/Rest	Medical Interventions	Medications	Nutrition	Nurses' Signatures
Day 2 Date: ___	-If ordered, internist for resumption of usual meds	-Lytes if NG -H&H or CBC	-Walk in hall at least 4 times with help	-JP tube(s) -NG to suction -possible to go to clamping schedule, if ordered	-Analgesics PO -IM, IV, epidural, antibiotics	-NPO, I&O -Possible clear liquid (if ordered) -If total clamping scheduled (if ordered)	_____ _____
Day 3 Date: ___			-Walk in hall at least 4 times with help	-Possible discontinue NG if ordered. Clamping schedule for NG if ordered -JP -IV	-IV, PO, IM, epidural. Antibiotics	-I&O -Clear liquid → full liquid late in day if tolerated clear liquids.	_____ _____
Day 4 Date: ___			-Walk in hall at least 4 times (self ambulation)	-Possible Heparin well -JP tubes -Colostomy or ileostomy	-Analgesics PO or IM -Antibiotics	-Full liquid to diet as tolerated	_____ _____

All items not provided as planned. Enter explanation in the individualization/variance section on the last page.
DRG Number: 148/149. Expected LOS: 6-8 days.

NRA-1175 REV 09/92

TUCSON MEDICAL CENTER
DIVISION OF NURSING
COLECTOMY
CarePlan MAP©

Developed by: Gail Greene, BSN, RN

INDEPENDENT ACTIONS BASED UPON THE HUMAN RESPONSE TO ACTUAL OR POTENTIAL PROBLEMS

Hospital Day	Assessment	Discharge Planning	Teaching	Psycho Social	Self Care	Nurses' Signatures
Day 2 Date:___	-Lung status -Bowel sounds	-Assess at home needs -Ostomy to see patient if has ostomy.	-Continue to reinforce post-op teaching -Begin ostomy self-care teaching if has ostomy	-Continue to assess anxiety level -Begin handling ostomy equipment, possibly refer patient to ostomy client if available to decrease sense of isolation	-Assisted ADLs	
Day 3 Date:___	-Lung status -Bowel sounds	-Assess at home needs	-Continue to reinforce post-op & ostomy teaching -If path report indicates malignancy, give 1-800-4-CANCER number of patient access to more information	-Continue to assess anxiety level -Patient may choose to look at incision when dressing is changed -Empty own ostomy pouch	-Self ADLs	
Day 4 Date:___	-Lung status -Bowel sounds	-Assess at home needs	-Continue to reinforce post-op teaching -Continue ostomy teaching and assess patient response	Continue to assess anxiety level -Patient may choose to look at incision when dressing is changed -Empty own ostomy pouch	-Self ADLs	

All items not provided as planned. Enter explanation in the individualization/variation section on the last page.
DRG Number: 148/149. Expected LOS: 6-8 days.

TUCSON MEDICAL CENTER
DIVISION OF NURSING
COLECTOMY
CarePlan MAP©

NRA-1175 REV 09/92   Developed by: Gail Greene, BSN, RN

INDEPENDENT ACTIONS BASED UPON THE HUMAN RESPONSE TO ACTUAL OR POTENTIAL PROBLEMS

Hospital Day	Consults	Tests	Activity/Rest	Medical Interventions	Medications	Nutrition	Nurses' Signatures
Day 5 Date: ___			-Walk in hall at least 4 times (self ambula-tion)	-Possible heparin line -JP tube(s) -Colostomy or ileostomy	-Analgesics PO -Antibiotics	Diet as tolerated	
Day 6 Date: ___				-Heparin line -Colostomy/ ileostomy			
Day 7 Date: ___							
Day 8 Date ___							

All items not provided as planned. Enter explanation in the individualization/variation section on the last page.
DRG Number: 148/149. Expected LOS: 6-8 days.

TUCSON MEDICAL CENTER
DIVISION OF NURSING
COLECTOMY
CarePlan MAP©

NRA 1175 REV 09/92   Developed by: Gail Greene, BSN, RN

INDEPENDENT ACTIONS BASED UPON THE HUMAN RESPONSE TO ACTUAL OR POTENTIAL PROBLEMS

Hospital Day	Assessment	Discharge Planning	Teaching	Psycho Social	Self Care	Nurses' Signatures
Day 5 Date: _____	-Lung status -Bowel sounds	-Assess at home needs -Continue Ostomy teaching and assess patient response	-Continue to reinforce post-op teaching	-Continue to assess anxiety level -Begin/continue self stoma care including changing bag, skin care as per ostomy if applicable	-Self ADLs	_____ _____ _____
Day 6 Date: _____	-Lung status -Bowel sounds	-Assess at home needs -Continue Ostomy teaching and assess patient response	Ascertain that patient & family are competent to handle ostomy care (if applicable)	-Continue to assess anxiety level -Continue assisted/self stoma care if applicable	-Self ADLs	_____ _____ _____
Day 7 Date: _____	-Lung status -Bowel sounds	-Assess at home needs -Continue Ostomy teaching and assess patient response	-Continue to assess for ostomy teaching	-Continue to assess anxiety level -Continue assisted/self stoma care if applicable	-Self ADLs	_____ _____ _____
Day 8 Date: _____	-Lung status -Bowel sounds	-Assess at home needs -Continue Ostomy teaching and assess patient response	-Continue to assess for ostomy teaching -Review availability of Cancer Society as a resource if patient's surgery was due to a malignancy	-Continue to assess anxiety level -Continue assisted/self stoma care if applicable	-Self ADLs	_____ _____ _____

All items not provided as planned. Enter explanation in the individualization/variance section on the last page.
DRG Number: 148/149. Expected LOS: 6-8 days.

NRA 1175 REV 09/92

TUCSON MEDICAL CENTER
DIVISION OF NURSING
COLECTOMY
CarePlan MAP©

Developed by: Gail Greene, BSN, RN

Date	Individualization/Variation	Cause	Action Taken	Signature

MAP Reviewed by:

Date: _____
Nurse Case Manager

Date: _____
Associate Case Manager

Date: _____
Associate Case Manager

Date: _____

All items not provided as planned. Enter explanation in the individualization/variance section on the last page.
DRG Number: 148/149. Expected LOS: 6-8 days.

6

BEYOND-THE-WALLS CASE MANAGEMENT

▼ *CHAPTER OVERVIEW*

Nursing case management approaches have grown in sophistication and diversity as evidenced by their emergence in community-based programs and capitated system arrangements. A beyond-the-walls program offers magnificent opportunities for professional nursing to control and manage health care resources and quality of patient care. Such a program also provides multiple advantages for the coordination and integration of outcomes and costs. The nursing profession's emphasis on the patient strengthens its power base and reconfirms its professional commitment to society.

Beyond-the-walls case management represents yet another example of the versatility and applicability of the case management model. This community-based approach has shown great promise in reshaping nursing practice and health care management. Examples of some of the more prominent models are presented in the next section. ▲

NURSING CASE MANAGEMENT ACROSS CARONDELET'S CONTINUUM OF CARE

CATHERINE MICHAELS AND GERRI LAMB

Carondelet Health Care—A Network of Nurse Partnerships and Care Coordination Strategies

Over the past 10 years, nursing case management and other nursing partnerships have evolved, preparing Carondelet for today's managed care environment. In 1985, at the onset of nursing case management beyond the walls of Carondelet St. Mary's Hospital & Health Center, Tucson, Arizona, Carondelet began developing nurse partnerships to assist people at varying levels of risk for managing their health care. Initially, nurse case managers partnered across time and across health care settings with people at high risk. Then, nurse practitioners together with other nurses and disciples partnered with people at moderate risk in nurse-managed and neighborhood-accessible community health centers. More recently, based on Carondelet's experience of creating and maintaining integrated services of nursing case management and home health, respite, and home infusion therapy (Burns, Lamb, & Wholey, 1996; Michaels, 1991), Carondelet was selected as one of the four national

66

demonstration sites for the Health Care Financing Administration (HCFA)–funded Community Nursing Organization, a risk-adjusted, capitated, nurse-managed ambulatory system of care. In this research program, Carondelet provided nurse partnerships and nurse-authorized services to Medicare enrollees at high, moderate, and low risk. Today, Carondelet offers a system of care coordination and case management.

In the Past

Carondelet's model of professional nursing case management evolved from a decentralized home care program and nursing network that provided a multitude of services in a variety of settings (Ethridge, 1987; 1991; Ethridge & Lamb, 1989). The services available in the original system included acute or inpatient care, long-term extended care, home health care, and hospice, rehabilitation, primary prevention, and ambulatory care (Ethridge, 1991; Ethridge & Lamb, 1989). Nursing case management reduced the fragmentation associated with preadmission assessment, discharge planning, postdischarge follow-up, and hospital readmission (Health Care Advisory Board, 1990). The foundation for this work was partnership based on mutual respect. By helping people to understand the relationship between the choices they made and the consequences of their actions, nurse case managers not only translated the illness experience into learning about self and others but also acknowledged the patient as responsible for outcomes and the nurse for facilitating the process. In this regard, Carondelet nursing case management was one of the first models to relate practice to nursing theory, specifically Newman's Health as Expanding Consciousness (Newman, Lamb, & Michaels, 1991).

　　　　Two areas of evaluation predominated: the benefit of partnership and the impact of that partnership on use of hospital services. Qualitative findings supported a strong base in the nurse case manager–client relationship (Lamb & Stempel, 1994; Newman et al., 1991). Quantitative evaluation demonstrated reduced hospital use. The nursing case management process of assessing, coordinating, planning, and monitoring through partnership reflected appropriate use of medical intervention technology, reduced severity of illness when hospitalization was required, subsequent decreases in bed days, and increased accessibility to hospital alternatives (Ethridge, 1991; Ethridge & Lamb, 1989; Health Care Advisory Board, 1990).

　　　　Building on the success of this service, Carondelet established a nursing HMO to provide health care and support services to elderly, chronically ill, and disabled individuals within a Medicare Senior Plan Contract (Ethridge, 1991; Michaels, 1991; 1992). If considered high risk, enrollees in this senior plan received integrated, community-focused nursing services: nursing case management and home health, respite, and home infusion therapy. Enrollees who did not match the high-risk profile were often referred to the Carondelet Community Health Centers for health monitoring, teaching, and care coordination. Overall, hospital bed days for the high-risk senior enrollees were significantly reduced (Burns et al., 1996), and enrollees served expressed high levels of satisfaction.

　　　　In 1992, Carondelet was selected as one of the four national sites to establish a Community Nursing Organization. A 3-year program funded by HCFA, the Community Nursing Organization, is a research program based on experimental design. Indeed, the first outcome for this program was meeting the enrollment targets of 2000 in the experimental program called the Healthy Seniors Program and 1000 in the control group.

Carondelet's initial nursing HMO experience focused on people at high risk for managing their health care; the Healthy Seniors Program offers enrollment to Medicare beneficiaries whatever their risk for managing their health. Hence, nurse partnerships were established for enrollees at low, moderate, and high risk. Building even further on Carondelet's nursing HMO experience, the Healthy Seniors Program is based on a broader array of integrated ambulatory services: community health center, respite, home health, outpatient behavioral health and rehabilitation services, prosthetics, durable medical equipment, respiratory therapy, medical supplies, and ambulance services. This risk-adjusted, capitated, nurse-managed ambulatory system of care for Medicare beneficiaries is slated to end in December 1996 (Lamb, 1995). Although official evaluation is contracted by HCFA, Carondelet is currently exploring program outcomes.

Today

In 1997, Tucson is one of the most heavily penetrated managed care markets in the nation. To provide case management services and other nurse partnerships across Carondelet's full continuum of care, a system of case management has evolved to coordinate care for those at high risk. Community-focused or continuum nurse case managers continue to partner with people at high risk for managing their health concerns across the continuum of care and over time. In general, the people served face life-threatening chronic illness, such as congestive heart failure and end-stage chronic obstructive pulmonary disease. The community-focused nurse case managers link with clinical nurse case managers within the hospital (Mahn, 1993). Clinical nurse case managers serve patients at high risk during hospitalization, and like clinical nurse specialists, they have a specialty focus.

Social workers are also available as consultants or as the primary case manager for clients whose situations are confounded by complex shelter, financial, legal, or behavioral issues. Lastly, case managers for behavioral health and rehabilitation also offer services to clients needing their specialized continuum of care.

Today, except for behavioral health, payment for case management services comes from the global capitation rate that covers hospitalization and that is negotiated in the contract. Behavioral health services are also capitated but are contracted for separately.

The Future

In the future, Carondelet will fully implement a risk identification process recently piloted to evaluate a person's risk for managing his or her health care as people shift into Carondelet's integrated delivery network. Through risk screening and identification of modifiable risk factors, people at high, moderate, and low risk will be identified earlier. Then there will be targeted interventions, framed in terms of primary, secondary, and tertiary prevention and health promotion and based on Carondelet's nurse partnerships, care coordination strategies, practice guidelines, and system of case management. As in the past, Carondelet's goal is to offer service that people believe improves their health and well-being or that brings a peaceful death.

The future will also call for increased integration with primary care providers. For people at moderate risk, especially at the high end, the primary care site is accessible during teachable moments. Targeted intervention may enable people through partnerships with physicians and nurses and other disciplines to stop progression to a higher risk status. As the future builds on experience from the past and the practices of today, Carondelet's goal is constant: through partnership, to offer health services that people believe improve their health and well-being or that facilitate a peaceful death.

SAINT JOSEPH MEDICAL CENTER'S COMMUNITY-BASED NURSING CASE MANAGEMENT

A community-based nursing case management system modeled after the system at Carondelet Saint Mary's has been implemented at Saint Joseph Medical Center in Wichita, Kansas. This system maintains a multidisciplinary, multiservice responsibility for the coordination of services and management of the patient (see Appendix 6-1 for an example of Saint Joseph's nursing critical pathway for cerebral vascular accident [CVA]). The system originally included only those at high risk, the frail elderly, and the chronically ill (Rogers, Riordan, & Swindle, 1991). "[The system] is now addressing several other patient populations including psychiatric, high-risk pregnancy and neonates, and chronically ill younger adults and children. Staff have also done considerable work on collaboration with local schools of nursing on educational issues and on the incorporation of other disciplines into the model. These include social work, respiratory care, dietitians, and a protocol for hospital chaplaincy students who also do rotations with them" (Rogers, 1992).

Outcome variables related to the number of hospital readmissions, length of stay, reimbursement or payment arrangements, and referral relationships are analyzed through a fully automated data base. *Preliminary results* demonstrated cost savings related to reduction in hospital admissions and length of stay. Other projects that integrate nursing diagnosis and standards of care have been designed to create a national nursing data base retrieval system that will enhance the documentation and analysis of this model (Rogers et al., 1991).

REFERENCES

Burns, R., Lamb, G., & Wholey D. (1996). Impact of integrated community nursing services on hospital utilization and costs in a medicare risk plan. *Inquiry, 16*(1), 1,30-41.

Ethridge, P. (1987). Building successful nursing care delivery systems for the future. In National Commission on Nursing Implementation Project (Ed.), *Post-conference papers second invitational conference* (pp. 91-99). Milwaukee: W.K. Kellogg Foundation.

Ethridge, P. (1991). A nursing home: Carondelet St. Mary's experience. *Nursing Management, 22*(7), 22-27.

Ethridge, P., & Lamb, G. S. (1989). Professional

nurse case management improves quality, access and costs. *Nursing Management, 20*(3), 30-35.

Health Care Advisory Board (1990). Tactic #6 "home-based" case management. Superlative clinical quality: Special review of pathbreaking ideas. *Clinical quality* (Vol. 1, pp. 71-74). Washington, D.C.: The Advisory Board Company.

Lamb, G. S. (1995). Case management. *Annual Review of Nursing Research, 13,*117-136.

Lamb, G. S., & Stempel, J. (1994, Jan./Feb.). Nurse case management from the client's view: Growing as insider-expert. *Nursing Outlook,* 7-13.

Lamb, G. S. (1992). Conceptual and methodological issues in nurse case management research. *Advances in Nursing Science, 15*(2), 16-24.

Mahn, V. (1993). Clinical nurse case management: A service line approach. *Nursing Management, 24*(9), 48-50.

Michaels, C. (1991). A nursing HMO—10 months with Carondelet St. Mary's hospital-based nurse case management. *Aspen's Advisor for Nurse Executives, 6*(11), 1.3-4.

Michaels, C. (1991). Carondelet St. Mary's nursing enterprise. *Nursing Clinics of North America, 27*(1), 77-86.

Newman, M., Lamb, G., & Michaels, C. (1991). Nurse case management: The coming together of theory and practice. *Nursing & Health Care, 12,* 404-408.

Rogers, M. (1992). Personal communication.

Rogers, M., Riordan, J., & Swindle, D. (1991). Community-based nursing case management pays off. *Nursing Management, 22*(3), 30-34.

Appendix 6-1

MEDICAL REHABILITATION SERVICES
NURSING CRITICAL PATHWAY/CVA

St. Joseph Medical Center
3600 East Harry/Wichita, Kansas 67218/(316) 685-1111

Patient Name	Date of Admission
L or R CVA	Date of Discharge

ACTIVITY	DATE	VARIANCE
PREADMISSION		
• Introduction of patient/family to rehabilitation program		
• Give Stroke Packet		
Discuss Rehabilitation Concepts		
Clothing/laundry needs		
Conferences		
Family involvement		
Patient rights		
• Tour of department for family (patient if possible)		
• Introduction to Primary/Associate Nurse		
• Other _____		
ADMISSION DAY		
• Orientation to room		
Bedrails		
Call light system		
Emergency call system		
Bath/shower		
Toilet		
• Orientation to Rehab. 1A		
Dining room		
Therapies		
Library		
Conference room		
Other _____		
• Assess for prevention of falls		
• Rehab Nursing Admission Assessment completed in 8 hours		
• Identify problems and patient/family goals		
• Initiate Care Plan and complete Kardex		
• Identify patient/family educational needs		
• Other _____		
• List educational needs for Day 2		
Treatment Day 2		
• Educational needs		
_____		
_____		
_____		
• Review nursing assessment		

Continued.

ACTIVITY	DATE	VARIANCE
• Evaluate and update Care Plan and Kardex		
• Review and implement educational plan:		
Medications		
Elimination		
Skin		
Safety		
Other _____		
• Review Rehab. Nursing Care Plan/Goal with patient		
Set short term goals		
• Review Rehab. Nursing Care Plan/Goals with family		
Set short term goals		
• Alter nursing treatment plan, utilizing patient/family input		
• Nursing Care Plan completed		
• Patient/family signature on Care Plan		
• Other _____		
• List educational needs for Day 3		
Treatment Day 3		
• Educational needs		
• Review therapy goals		
• Incorporate support for therapy goals into Plan/Kardex		
• Review Nursing Care Plan		
• Initial Progress Note completed		
• Other _____		
• List educational needs for Day 4		
Treatment Day 4		
• Educational needs		
• Evaluate physical status:		
Medications/effects		
Weight		
Hydration		
Skin integrity		
Pressure areas		
Weight shifting		
Vital signs		
Other _____		
• Set long term goals with patient/family		
• Evaluate and update Care Plan and Kardex		
• Other _____		
• List educational needs for Day 5		

Continued.

ACTIVITY	DATE	VARIANCE
Treatment Day 5		
• Educational needs		
• Establish estimated length of stay		
• Verbal/written communication with case manager		
• Evaluate and update Care Plan and Kardex		
• Other _____		
• List educational needs for Days 6-7		
Treatment Days 6-7		
• Educational needs		
• Evaluate and update Care Plan and Kardex		
• Patient/family updated regarding plan		
• Introduce patient/family to library		
• Provide one educational opportunity in library		
• Other _____		
• List educational needs for Week Two		
WEEK TWO		
• Educational needs		
• Review/adjust B & B retraining program Patient is greater than 25% continent: Bladder Yes/No Bowel Yes/No		
• Review and adjust safety needs		
• Review and set up support systems for therapy goals (Care Plan, Kardex, signage, etc.)		
• Weekly Progress Note completed		
• Evaluate and update Care Plan and Kardex		
• Patient/family updated regarding plan		
• Evaluate therapeutic day pass		
• Evaluate physical status:		
Medications/effects		
Weight		
Hydration		
Skin integrity		
Pressure areas		
Weight shifting		
Vital signs		
Other _____		
• Other _____		

Continued.

ACTIVITY	DATE	VARIANCE
• List educational needs for Week 3		
WEEK THREE		
• Educational needs 		

• Review/adjust B & B retraining program
     Patient is greater than 50% continent:
          Bladder   Yes/No
          Bowel Yes/No		

• Review safety needs		
• Review and provide support systems for therapy goals		
• Weekly Progress Note completed		
• Evaluate and update Care Plan and Kardex		
• Patient/family updated regarding plan		
• Finalize continuing nursing recommendations		
• Community outing		
• Evaluate physical status:		
Medications/effects		
Weight		
Hydration		
Skin integrity		
Pressure areas		
Weight shifting		
Vital signs		
Other _____		
• Other _____		
• List educational needs to be completed and time frame		
LAST 4 DAYS		
• Completed educational needs: 		
• Educational materials to be sent with patient: 		

• Review B & B retraining program progress:
     Patient is continent of:
          Bladder   _____%
          Bowel   _____%
      Followup plan includes:		

• Weekly Progress Note completed		
• Patient/family updated regarding plan		
• Discharge plan completed		
• Final instructions discussed with patient/family		

Continued.

ACTIVITY	DATE	VARIANCE
• Instructions documented		
• Following physicians notified of dismissal: _____ _____ _____		
• Prescriptions to patient/family		
• Other_____ _____ _____ _____		

MEDICAL REHABILITATION SERVICES
PHYSICAL THERAPY CRITICAL PATHWAY/CVA

St. Joseph Medical Center
3600 East Harry/Wichita, Kansas 67218/(316) 685-1111

Patient Name   Date of Admission
L or R CVA   Date of Discharge

ACTIVITY	DATE	VARIANCE
WEEK ONE **Admission Day**		
• Introduction to patient/family and brief orientation to P.T.—if orders written by 1:00 pm. (N/A for Sunday/holiday admissions). Issue wheelchair and cushion, if appropriate.		
Treatment Day 2 Evaluation		
• Begin initial evaluation		
• Issue appropriate wheelchair and cushion, if not seen on Admission Day		
Treatment Day 3 Evaluation		
• Continue with evaluation		
• Instruct nursing and/or family in PROM to LE, if applicable		
• Document in Kardex the amount of assistance patient requires to do functional activities and issue appropriate equipment, if needed		
Treatment Day 4 Evaluation and Treatment		
• Complete evaluation		
• Set treatment goals/plan and discuss with patient/family		
• Initiate electrical stimulation program to shoulder, if subluxed		
Treatment Day 5 Treatment		
• Initiate treatment		
• Establish estimated length of stay		
• Written/verbal communication with case manager		
Weekend Days No OT, PT, Speech on Saturday or Sunday.		
Family Education Program available on Saturday mornings.		
WEEK TWO		
• Continue treatment and modify as needed		
• Determine need for Home Evaluation and complete. Copy to patient/family and case manager		
• Determine appropriateness for Community Outings		
• Initiate patient/family education—(i.e., bed mobility, transfers, wheelchair mobility, and car transfers, as appropriate)		
• Determine/order bracing, if needed		
• Evaluate therapeutic day pass, as appropriate		
WEEK THREE		
• Continue patient/family education (i.e., ambulation, floor transfers)		
• Finalize equipment recommendations by first of week		
• Finalize continued therapy recommendations		
• Community outing, if appropriate		
• Fit and train with orthosis, if applicable		
LAST 4 DAYS		
• Re-evaluation as indicated		
• Patient/family education completed		
• Home program completed, if indicated		

MEDICAL REHABILITATION SERVICES
OCCUPATIONAL THERAPY CRITICAL PATHWAY/CVA

St. Joseph Medical Center
3600 East Harry/Wichita, Kansas 67218/(316) 685-1111

Patient Name	Date of Admission
L or R CVA	Date of Discharge

ACTIVITY	DATE	VARIANCE
WEEK ONE **Admission Day**		
• Introduction to patient/family and brief orientation to O.T.— if orders written by 1:00 pm. (N/A for Sunday/holiday admissions).		
Treatment Day 2 Evaluation and Treatment • Evaluate ADLs		
• Evaluate and treat need for sling, lap tray, splints and other devices		
• Start evaluation of sensorimotor status		
Treatment Day 3 Evaluation and Treatment • Continue sensorimotor evaluation		
• Evaluate visual perceptual skills/cognition		
• Continue basic ADL evaluations		
Treatment Day 4 Evaluation and Treatment • Continue basic ADL evaluation		
• Continue visual perceptual skills/cognition evaluation		
• Set treatment goals/plan and discuss with patient/family		
Treatment Day 5 Treatment • Complete evaluations, if needed		
• Initiate treatment		
• Establish estimated length of stay		
• Written/verbal communication with case manager		
Weekend Days No OT, PT, Speech on Saturday or Sunday. Family Education Program available on Saturday mornings.		
WEEK TWO • Continue treatment and modify as needed		
• Determine need for Home Evaluation and complete. Copy to patient/family and case manager		
• Determine appropriateness for Community Outings		
• Initiate patient/family education—(i.e., SROM, toilet transfers, as appropriate)		
• Evaluate therapeutic day pass, as appropriate		
WEEK THREE • Continue patient/family education		
• Finalize equipment recommendations by first of week		
• Finalize continued therapy recommendations		
• Community outing, if appropriate		
• Evaluate homemaking skills, as needed		
• Evaluate complex ADLs, as needed		
LAST 4 DAYS • Re-evaluation as indicated		
• Patient/family education completed		
• Home program completed, if indicated		

MEDICAL REHABILITATION SERVICES
SPEECH THERAPY CRITICAL PATHWAY/CVA

St. Joseph Medical Center
3600 East Harry/Wichita, Kansas 67218/(316) 685-1111

| Patient Name | Date of Admission |
| L or R CVA | Date of Discharge |

ACTIVITY	DATE	VARIANCE
WEEK ONE **Admission Day**		
• Introduction to patient/family and brief orientation to Speech Therapy—if orders written by 1:00 pm. (N/A for Sunday/holiday admissions).		
Treatment Day 2		
• Assess swallowing, if ordered		
• Contact Physician or Physician's Assistant to make diet recommendations, if indicated		
• Post sign with diet/swallowing instructions in patient's room, if indicated		
• Discuss swallowing/diet recommendations with patient/family, if available		
• Discuss diet recommendations/special needs with nurse		
• Issue one-to-one communication device for amplification, if indicated		
• Determine need for modified barium swallow study		
• Initiate Speech/language evaluation		
Treatment Day 3		
• Continue Speech/Language evaluation		
Treatment Day 4		
• Continue evaluation		
• Set treatment goals/plan and discuss with patient/family		
Treatment Day 5		
• Initiate treatment		
• Continue in-depth evaluations, as indicated		
• Establish estimated length of stay		
• Written/verbal communication with case manager		
Weekend Days No OT, PT, Speech on Saturday or Sunday. Family Education Program available on Saturday mornings.		
WEEK TWO		
• Continue treatment and modify as needed		
• Re-assess swallowing/diet recommendations		
• Discuss updated recommendations regarding diet with nursing/patient/family		
• Determine appropriateness for Community Outings		
• Continue patient/family education regarding speech/voice/language/swallowing, as indicated		
• Evaluate therapeutic day pass, as appropriate		

Continued.

ACTIVITY	DATE	VARIANCE
WEEK THREE		
• Continue treatment and modify as needed		
• Re-assess swallowing/diet recommendations		
• Discuss updated recommendations regarding diet with nursing/ patient/family		
• Community outing, if appropriate		
• Finalize continued therapy recommendations		
• Continue patient/family education		
LAST 4 DAYS		
• Re-evaluation as indicated		
• Patient/family education completed		
• Home program completed, if indicated		

MEDICAL REHABILITATION SERVICES
CASE MANAGEMENT/SOCIAL WORK CRITICAL PATHWAY/CVA

 St. Joseph Medical Center
3600 East Harry/Wichita, Kansas 67218/(316) 685-1111

Patient Name	Date of Admission
L or R CVA	Date of Discharge

ACTIVITY	DATE	VARIANCE
WEEK ONE **First 48 Hours** • Initial contact made by SW/CM. Explanation of SW/CM roles, family conferences and discharge planning		
Within 72 Hours After Admission • Social history dictated		
Within First 7 Days • Initial family conference scheduled and communicated to patient and family		
• Evaluate discharge plan, financial resources and/or psychosocial concerns. Based on evaluation, action plan developed and implementation began (ongoing process)		
• Evaluate need for referral to Vocational Rehabilitation Services		
• Evaluate need for referral to Rehab Engineering		
WEEK TWO • Evaluate need for community resource referrals (ongoing)		
• Initiate and assist patient/family with application for financial assistance, if needed		
• Recertify with insurance company, if required		
WEEK THREE • Receive DME recommendations from team and evaluate insurance coverage for DME, if necessary		
• Obtain post-discharge therapy recommendations from team		
• Meet with patient/family regarding discharge plan, DME, and post-discharge therapy		
• Arrange acquisition of DME needs		
• Recertify with insurance company, if required		
• If extended care placement is recommended, evaluate availability and financial resources and communicate with family		
• Evaluate discharge transportation needs		
LAST 4 DAYS • Meet with patient/family to finalize discharge planning		
• Place Interagency and other communication forms on chart 48 hours prior to discharge		

MEDICAL REHABILITATION SERVICES
RECREATIONAL/ACTIVITY THERAPY CRITICAL PATHWAY/CVA

St. Joseph Medical Center
3600 East Harry/Wichita, Kansas 67218/(316) 685-1111

Patient Name	Date of Admission
L or R CVA	Date of Discharge

ACTIVITY	DATE	VARIANCE
WEEK ONE **Admission Day** • Introduction to patient/family and brief orientation to R.T./Activities		
Treatment Day 2 • Begin initial evaluation		
• Complete Leisure Interest Survey		
Treatment Day 3 • Complete evaluation		
• Set treatment goals/plan and discuss with patient/family		
Treatment Day 4 • Orientation to the available leisure programs, facilities and resources in the Medical Center		
• Encourage patient participation in scheduled weekly activities		
Treatment Day 5 • Encourage patient participation in scheduled daily activities		
• Determine adaptations of activities to compensate for physical and/or cognitive limitations		
Weekend Days Encourage patient participation in scheduled activities/outings. Family Education Program available on Saturday mornings.		
WEEK TWO • Encourage patient participation in scheduled weekly activities		
• Determine appropriateness for community outings		
• Home evaluation, if appropriate		
• Continue patient/family education		
WEEK THREE • Encourage patient participation in scheduled weekly activities		
• Community outing, if appropriate		
• Provide information regarding community based support systems		
• Provide information regarding appropriate community recreation resources		
LAST 4 DAYS • Re-evaluation as indicated		
• Patient/family education completed		
• Recommendations for post discharge/transition planning		

III

COST-EFFECTIVENESS OF CASE MANAGEMENT AND MAINTAINING CONTROL

SOCIOECONOMIC AND POLITICAL IMPLICATIONS

7

PATIENT DEMOGRAPHICS AFFECTING HEALTH CARE

▼ *CHAPTER OVERVIEW*

Recent shifts in the nation's demographics are causing substantial changes in the delivery of health care. Both the growing elderly population and the AIDS epidemic have prompted health care workers to look for alternatives to the traditional approaches of acute patient care and have fostered the growth of integrative models such as case management. The prevalence of chronic illness and disability associated with demographic changes is also influencing public health policy as we shift our resources from acute to chronic care.

Recently enacted legislation has provided for the civil rights and liberties of individuals with chronic illness and has supported much needed community-based, long-term health care delivery systems. Many businesses and corporations have begun to develop programs and services that will help them adapt to the long-range social, economic, and health care implications of the growing number of elderly and those with acquired immunodeficiency syndrome (AIDS). ▲

AGING PATIENT POPULATION

The Department of Health and Human Services (1990) predicts that by the year 2020, 7 million Americans will be older than 85 years of age. In the 1990s the percentage of men and women who are 80 years old is expected to increase 30% to 45% for men and 24% to 36% for women (Dimond, 1989; Exter, 1990). This increase in the number and percentage of older individuals primarily is due to advances in research, technology, and preventive treatments that have markedly reduced mortality rates associated with cancer, cardiovascular disease, diabetes, stroke, and hypertension (National Center for Health Statistics, 1985; Olshansky, 1985).

Rogers, Rogers, and Belanger (1989) found a correlation between dependency and age. Their study indicates that with an increase in age there is a corresponding rise in functional dependency related to basic activities of daily living. Furthermore, once dependency sets in, the likelihood of returning to an independent status decreases. An example of this is that although women have a longer life expectancy than men, much of that time is spent in dependent situations, which increases the morbidity of this population group (Manton, 1988; Schneider & Brody, 1983).

The 1992 DHHS estimates of years of healthy life showed a decline in health-related quality of life despite increases in life expectancy (U.S. Department of Health and Human Services, 1995a). Statistical projections show that by the year 2044, 7.3 million people will have dependent lifestyles (Rogers et al., 1989). Another projection indicates that by the year 2040, the elderly population will account for 45% of health care expenditures (Callahan, 1987).

With advanced age there is also a proportionate growth in the incidence of chronic and degenerative illnesses. These factors, along with increased dependency and disability, intensify the need and demand for health care services (Goldsmith, 1989; Guralnik, Yanagishita, & Schneider, 1988).

As highlighted by the National Center for Health Statistics (1987), 1.3 million of those older than 65 live in nursing homes. Of those, 46% are older than 85 years of age. It is estimated that by the year 2040, 2.8 million people, age 85 and older, will require institutional care (Guralnik et al., 1988). These data indicate that the aging population will have a significant effect on long-term and skilled nursing care.

Increased longevity and its concomitant effects have encouraged new approaches to the delivery of health care services. Nursing case management, managed care programs, and community-based home care are some examples of alternative approaches to meeting the health care needs of the elderly. These approaches lend themselves to scrutiny and analysis related to cost-effectiveness and the value and quality of services delivered.

In an extensive review of home- and community-based long-term care programs, Weissert, Cready, and Pawelak (1988) found that there were greater total expenditures and no statistically significant cost savings related to home- and community-based care. In fact, an analysis of the effectiveness of various programs showed that even though there were reductions in admissions to institutional care settings, these findings were significant for only a small group of patients who had an obvious need for home-based care. This group consisted of the disabled, chronically ill, and frail elderly.

The study showed, however, that within this patient population, preadmission assessment and screening of those individuals at risk for institutionalization effectively reduced nursing home use. This finding was supported in studies that evaluated the effectiveness of community-based programs in preventing hospitalization. Again, it was shown that more specific identification and evaluation of patient requirements of care decreased the need for and length of inpatient treatment and hospitalization.

One major benefit of community- and home-based care was found in its beneficial and significant effect on the psychosocial well-being and satisfaction of patients and care providers. The community- or home-based care proved better at meeting the patients' needs for physical and social activities as well as medical, mental health, and educational requirements (Weissert, 1985).

Another study, conducted by Roos, Shapiro, and Tate (1989), indicated that only 5% of the elderly are extensive users of health care in the inpatient acute care and nursing home settings. The expenditures associated with this care are higher during the individual's last year of life. However, 45% of the elderly population make large demands on the health care system, and these demands entail greater expenditures.

One recommendation for decreasing the chance of hospitalization is to provide the elderly with a geriatric specialist. Early assessment and evaluation by such a specialist might help reduce the incidence of hospitalization, which in turn decreases costs. In addition, continuous monitoring of discharged patients through home care, community-based care, long-term care, and primary preventive services can be cost effective and aid in the transition to a more independent lifestyle.

It is clear that to plan effectively for future health care needs of the elderly and disabled population, changes in the delivery of health care services and benefits are needed. Resources are now being shifted from acute care and long-term institutional care to home care, community-based services, respite centers, nurse-run HMOs and care centers, case management, and rehabilitation programs (Dimond, 1989; Hollinger & Brugler, 1991; Maraldo & Solomon, 1987).

To maintain control of some of the long-range, economic and social implications, major business groups and corporations are beginning to develop and offer resource and referral services to employees who have caretaking responsibilities for elderly and dependent family members (Buchsbaum, 1991; Peterson, 1992). Called eldercare, these programs provide a range of services including counseling, family leave plans, position reinstatement, flexible work schedules, automated office arrangements that make it possible for employees to work at home, subsidized health care benefits, and reimbursement for adult day care.

Benefits of such an approach include decreased work-related conflicts; lowered costs associated with recruitment, training, and absenteeism of personnel; and increased productivity, loyalty, and commitment to the organization. Referral services have also helped decrease the costs of health services associated with deferred spending, out-of-pocket expenses, lost time, and stress (Buchsbaum, 1991; Peterson, 1992).

HIV INFECTION

Surveillance data from the Centers for Disease Control and Prevention show that over one-half million Americans have contracted AIDS and that of these persons, 62% have died. HIV infection is currently considered the leading cause of death in men ages 25 to 44 years and the third leading cause of death in women of the same age group (U.S. Department of Health and Human Services, 1995b).

There is substantial evidence that the rapid spread of HIV will increase hospitalizations and use of more complex health care resources.

Several studies indicate that the United States will spend about $10 billion in direct cost (i.e., hospitalization, home and hospice care) for the treatment of AIDS in 1991 (American Hospital Association, 1986; Lyon, 1988; Scitovsky & Rice, 1987). This estimate includes the cost of hospitalization, home health care, hospice, and outpatient care as well as costs related to disability and chronicity.

The initial length of hospitalization averages 30 to 60 days, with cumulative acute-care treatment lasting up to 170 days (Hardy, Rauch, Echenberg, Morgan, & Curran, 1986; Sedaka & O'Reilly, 1986). On average, a person with AIDS is hospitalized three to four times. These hospitalizations occur in the early and late stages of illness (Scitovsky, Cline, & Lee, 1986).

Because AIDS is chronic, debilitating, and terminal, it places a substantial burden on the health care system (Benjamin, 1988). Home care, community-based services, hospice, and case management provide alternatives to hospitalization. The availability and applicability of these resources are being considered in the formulation of public policy regarding the delivery of health care services for individuals with AIDS (Fox, 1989).

Various strategies are under consideration to improve accessibility of AIDS care settings. Hospitals have created designated AIDS units where registered nurses coordinate, plan, and evaluate the delivery of care (Chow, 1989; Fox, Aiken, & Messikomer, 1990). Some institutions, such as the San Francisco General Hospital, have implemented comprehensive care programs through multidisciplinary, collaborative efforts with outpatient and community-based services, and home care agencies (Volberding, 1985). These initiatives, along with the improvement in the treatment and management protocols, have worked toward decreasing the length of stay for AIDS patients, thereby affecting the overall care and cost-effectiveness of this group (Fox, 1986).

The effectiveness of ambulatory and community-based programs for AIDS care is being evaluated in many federal, state, and private foundation–sponsored projects (Benjamin, 1988; Fox, 1986). The programs could reduce cost by reducing the need for inpatient hospital care resources and services.

Hospice care is another promising alternative for AIDS treatment. Using a multidisciplinary team approach, the hospice setting provides for the psychosocial needs of both the patient and caregiver (Benjamin, 1988). The emphasis of hospice care is on reducing time spent in institutional care and eliminating the need for acute medical intervention.

Studies done by Mor and Kidder (1985) on the cost-effectiveness of hospice care show savings related to decreases in inpatient length of stay and use of hospital resources. Such decreases possibly are due to the shift in caregiving responsibility to the patient's community, family, and significant others.

Case management presents an additional option for planning nonacute care services and interventions for individuals with AIDS. Capitman, Haskins, and Bernstein (1986) and Spitz (1987) demonstrated the effectiveness and efficiency of a well-integrated case management system. Their studies show that through comprehensive targeting and planning and integration of inpatient, ambulatory, and community-based services, the medical and social needs of AIDS patients can be met. Case management also provides flexibility in service options and reduces the inappropriateness, overuse, and inefficiency associated with hospital and medical care of the chronically ill (Schramm, 1990). Other hospital-based nursing case management models dedicated to AIDS care have also been effective in delivering less-expensive quality care (American Nurses Association, 1988).

Since AIDS presents enormous acute and long-term care needs, business firms have begun to develop and provide employee education and assistance programs, counseling services, nondiscriminatory employment policies, and flexible work schedules. Corporations have also begun to comply with federal, state, and local infection control guidelines (McDonald, 1990; Mello, 1991).

The passage of the Americans with Disabilities Act (ADA) in 1992 has also helped to ensure the rights of HIV- and AIDS-infected people in the workplace. The benefits and entitlements under this act include opportunities for employment, access to public services, accessible transportation, and a mechanism of communication with employers to support nondiscriminatory policies, confidentiality, and ongoing education (Feldblum, 1991; LaPlante, 1991).

REFERENCES

American Hospital Association (1986). *Infection Control and Environmental Safety Committee. AIDS.* Chicago: American Hospital Association.

American Nurses Association (1988). *Nursing case management.* Kansas City, MO.: American Nurses Association.

Benjamin, A.E. (1988). Long-term care and AIDS: Perspectives from experience with the elderly. *The Milbank Quarterly, 66*(3), 415-443.

Buchsbaum, S. (1991). Sending "care" packages to the workplace. *Business and Health, 9*(5), 56-69.

Callahan, D. (1987). *Setting limits: Medical goals in an aging society.* New York: Simon and Schuster.

Capitman, J.A., Haskins, B., & Bernstein, J. (1986). Case management approaches in community oriented long-term care demonstrations. *Gerontologist, 26,* 398-404.

Chow, M. (1989). Nursing's response to the challenge of AIDS. *Nursing Outlook, 37*(2), 82-83.

Dimond, M. (1989). Health care and the aging population. *Nursing Outlook, 37*(2), 76-77.

Exter, T. (1990, June). How big will the older market be? *American Demographics,* 30-36.

Feldblum, C. (1991). Employment protections. *The Milbank Quarterly, 69*(Suppl. 1/2), 81-110.

Fox, D. (1986). AIDS and the American health policy: History and prospects of a crises of authority *The Milbank Quarterly, 64,* 7-33.

Fox, D. (1989). Policy and epidemiology: Financing health services for the chronically ill and disabled, 1930-1990. *The Milbank Quarterly, 67*(Suppl. 2, Part 2), 257-287.

Fox, R., Aiken, L., & Messikomer, C. (1990). The culture of caring: AIDS and the nursing profession. *The Milbank Quarterly, 68*(Suppl. 2), 226-256.

Goldsmith, J. (1989). Radical prescription for hospitals. *Harvard Business Review, 89*(3), 104-111.

Guralnik, J., Yanagishita, M., & Schneider, E. (1988). Projecting the older population of the United States: Lessons from the past and prospects for the future. *The Milbank Quarterly, 66*(2), 283-308.

Hardy, A., Rauch, K., Echenberg, D., Morgan, W., & Curran, J.W. (1986). The economic impact of the first 10,000 cases of acquired immunodeficiency syndrome in the United States. *Journal of the American Medical Association, 225,* 209-211.

Hollinger, W., & Brugler, K. (1991). Managing resource use. *Healthcare Forum, 34*(6), 45-47.

LaPlante, M. (1991). The demographics of disability. *The Milbank Quarterly, 69*(Suppl. 1/2), 55-77.

Lyon, J. (1988). AIDS: What are the costs? Who will pay? *Nursing Economics, 6*(5), 241-244, 274.

Manton, K.G. (1988). A longitudinal study of functional change and mortality in the United States. *Journal of Gerontology, 43*(5), 153-161.

Maraldo, P., & Solomon, S. (1987). Nursing's window of opportunity. *Image,19*(2), 83-86.

McDonald, M. (1990). How to deal with AIDS in the workplace. *Business and Health, 8*(7), 12-22.

Mello, J. (1991, September). Getting to know about AIDS. *Business and Health, 9*(9), 88-89.

Mor, V., & Kidder, D. (1985). Cost savings in hospice: Final results of the National Hospice Study. *Health Services Research, 20,* 407-421.

National Center for Health Statistics. (1985). *Vital Statistics of the United States, 1980.* 2(pt. A., mortality). DHHS pub. no. (PHS) 85-1101. Washington, D.C.

National Center for Health Statistics. (1987). Use of nursing homes by the elderly, preliminary data from the 1985 National Nursing Home Survey, by E. Hing. *Vital and Health Statistics,* no. 135. DHHS pub. no. (PHS) 87-1250. Washington, D.C.

Olshansky, S.J. (1985). Pursuing longevity: Delay vs. elimination of degenerative diseases. *American Journal of Public Health, 75,* 754-757.

Peterson, H. (1992, February). Eldercare: More than company kindness. *Business & Health, 10*(2), 54-57.

Rogers, R., Rogers, A., & Belanger, A. (1989). Active life among the elderly in the United States: Multistate Life-table estimates and population projections. *The Milbank Quarterly, 67*(3-4), 370-411.

Roos, N., Shapiro, E., & Tate, R. (1989). Does a small minority of elderly account for a majority of healthcare expenditures? A sixteen-year perspective. *The Milbank Quarterly, 67*(3-4), 347-369.

Schneider, E., & Brody, J. (1983). Aging, natural death, and the compression of morbidity: Another view. *New England Journal of Medicine, 309*(14), 854-855.

Schramm, C. (1990). Health care industry problems call for cooperative solutions. *Healthcare Financial Management,* 54-61.

Scitovsky, A.A., Cline, M., & Lee, P.R. (1986). Medical care costs of patients with AIDS in San Francisco. *Journal of the American Medical Association, 256,* 3103-3106.

Scitovsky, A.A., & Rice, D. (1987). Estimates of the direct and indirect costs of acquired immunodeficiency syndrome in the United States, 1985, 1986, and 1991. *Public Health Reports, 102*(1), 5-17.

Sedaka, S., & O'Reilly, M. (1986). The financial implications of AIDS. *Caring, 5*(6), 38-44.

Spitz, B. (1987). National survey of medicaid case management. *Health Affairs, 6,* 61-70.

U.S. Department of Health and Human Services. (1990). *Healthy People 2000.* Washington, D.C.: DHHS.

U.S. Department of Health and Human Services. (1995a). *Healthy people 2000: Midcourse review and 1995 revisions* (p. 6). Washington, D.C.: DHHS.

U.S. Department of Health and Human Services. Centers for Disease Control and Prevention. (1995b). *HIV/AIDS surveillance report: U.S. HIV and AIDS cases reported through December 1995, 7*(2), 1-39.

Volberding, P.A. (1985). The clinical spectrum of the acquired immunodeficiency syndrome: Implications for comprehensive patient care. *Annals of Internal Medicine, 103,* 729-732.

Weissert, W.G. (1985). Seven reasons why it is so difficult to make community-based long term care cost effective. *Health Services Research, 20*(4), 423-433.

Weissert, W.G., Cready, C., & Pawelak, J. (1988). The past and future of home- and community-based long term care. *The Milbank Quarterly, 66*(2), 309-388.

8

THE BUSINESS OF HEALTH CARE AND THE PROSPECTIVE PAYMENT SYSTEM

▼ CHAPTER OVERVIEW

Changes in consumer behavior, along with various government and private industry strategies, have started to change the health care delivery environment. Programs are being developed to increase access to care and to evaluate and monitor cost-effective outcomes. National health reform initiatives address universal access to care by working for changes in insurance coverage and benefits, reimbursement regulation, and alternative care arrangements. Quality and cost are also addressed through managed care and capitated payment approaches. Long-term care services are being sponsored both publicly and privately.

Collaboration among health care providers for policy formation and implementation, public and private support for health care planning and outcome research, and further development of alternative care delivery and clinical resource models are among the crucial factors needed to develop an accessible, effective, and socially responsive health care system. ▲

COST CONTAINMENT

The incentives promoted by the prospective payment system not only affect the efficiency, safety, and quality of health care in the inpatient setting but also have a direct relationship to the cost containment efforts present in managed care arrangements (Jones, 1989; Sloan, Morrisey, & Valvona, 1988). Increased enrollment in HMOs and other prepaid, coordinated health care plans, restructuring of the physician fee and payment schedule to provide incentives for the delivery of primary care services, the national drive for health care reform, and competition among alternative delivery systems to improve cost-effectiveness and quality all influence prospective payment initiatives (Enthoven & Kronick, 1989a; 1989b; Ginsburg & Hackbarth, 1986; Swoap, 1984; Waldo, Levit, & Lazenby, 1986; Wilensky, 1991).

Prospective payment has also promoted a more efficient use of health care resources and encouraged the study of outcomes to evaluate accessibility, management, and economic effectiveness of care (Jones, 1989; Sloan et al., 1988).

91

The economic effect of rising health care costs has taken its toll on the private sector through increases in group health insurance premium rates and changes in the structure of employee health care benefits. Mullen (1988) and Traska (1989) reported that employers experienced rate increases of 15% to 29% in their efforts to cover health care costs. According to the Hewitt Associates' survey, the double-digit inflation was due to an estimated 21.5% increase by insurance carriers in medical benefit costs (Hewitt Associates, 1989). Increases in premiums were driven primarily by rises in the cost, volume, and variations in health services and were fostered by medical technologic change, an inadequate reimbursement system, demographic changes of an aging population, AIDS, and chronic illness (Kramon, 1989; Welling, 1990).

The issue of escalating health care costs has entered both the political and economic arenas and has prompted furious debates in the public and private sectors over the provision of basic health care services (Hospitals, 1992). Advocates for a national health care policy have locked horns with those who support the rationing of health services. Attempts have been made by Congress to institute a national health insurance plan to ensure equal access to care (Altman & Rodmin, 1988; Reinhardt, 1987a; 1987b). Legislative mandates and congressional bills that would provide health care coverage have been introduced as a means of rationing care through regulation and achieving control over government expenditures. State-mandated benefit laws offer a broad range of service coverage and access to mental health and substance abuse care, prenatal care, mammography, cancer screening, and major organ transplants (Brown, 1988; Davis, 1985; Dwyer, 1991; Eckholm, 1991; Frieden, 1991; Tallon, 1991; Thorpe, 1991; Traska, 1989).

Major health care reform for America began in 1993 with the introduction of the *Health Security Act* (HR3600, 1993), a President Clinton initiative. For almost a year the administration sought information about the existing health care system through task forces, committees, and town meetings directed by the First Lady, Hillary Rodham Clinton. This data collection process stimulated discussions nationwide about the present and future health care systems. The momentum created by a national discussion on health care reform gave the change process a life of its own, separate from the administrative and legislative agendas. Health care providers, health care agencies, and state governmental agencies began to design new systems based on a shifting paradigm—even before federal laws were enacted. The basic premise of the new paradigm, which continues to unfold, is a focus on health and care replacing or augmenting the old paradigm of illness and cure (DeBack & Cohen, 1996).

Many special interest groups have joined forces to propose reform in the current health care system. One such group, the American Medical Association, supports an employer-based health care plan, and another group from organized nursing, has endorsed a proposal titled *Nursing's Agenda for Health Care Reform*. The latter plan supports a consumer partnership with the health care provider regarding decisions about care; access to primary health care services via community-based settings; allocation of more resources to chronic and long-term care; increased access to nonphysician providers, such as nurse practitioners; wellness and prevention classes, public and private sector review and financing of health care; and managed care and case management arrangements (National League for Nursing, 1991).

Changes in payment structure have taken place in almost every sector of the health care industry. Many different strategies aimed at cost containment have been adopted by private corporations and insurance providers. Various efforts have focused on the redesigning of health insurance plans and policies, shifting the direct financial burden of health care expenditures to the federal government and individual payer. This approach includes the following: a single-payer plan, which is a government-financed plan that insures all individuals; introduction of copayments and deductibles applied to health care services; cost sharing, in which employees share the costs of health care by paying for the care of convalescing patients and hospice care for the terminally ill; catastrophic health plans, which provide coverage for high cost illnesses; second opinions for surgical interventions; and primary prevention and stress management programs aimed at controlling smoking, alcohol use, and hypertension (Brown, 1988; Frieden, 1991; Gilman & Bucco, 1987; Herzlinger & Calkins, 1986; Herzlinger & Schwartz, 1985; Peres, 1992).

As an effective strategy for controlling health care costs, major corporations have also encouraged participation in comprehensive, capitated rate plans, such as HMOs and PPOs. In these managed care plans, providers set an amount to cover all of their enrollees' health care needs. A percentage of that payment is put into a risk pool as insurance against unexpected expenditures. Providers assume a certain element of risk in exchange for the opportunity to benefit from lower costs, an integrated care system, and management savings (Brown, 1988; Christensen, 1991; Hicks, Stallmeyer, & Coleman, 1992; O'Connor, 1991).

Another initiative, called *managed competition*, finances health insurance coverage through large businesses. The employer is required to purchase insurance or pay a payroll tax for a public (government) sponsor. This system promotes competition among private insurers and ensures quality improvement standards (Enthoven & Kronick, 1989a; 1989b; Garland, 1991). All these health care delivery arrangements focus on both primary and secondary prevention, thereby increasing positive health outcomes and reducing costs (Hospitals, 1988; Luft, 1978; 1982; Rosenberg, Perlis, Lynne, & Leto, 1991; Sloss et al., 1987).

Another response to the problems of financing health care benefits is assuring the employer's involvement in managing the delivery of health care services. Providers are developing and participating in corporate health care programs that monitor cost and use of health care services. Those services that are monitored include preadmission testing, which has been shown to reduce inpatient stays, utilization review, monitoring of catastrophic illness and injury through medical case management programs, and mandatory employer-sponsored health insurance that would extend both private and public employer-sponsored health insurance that would extend both private and public insurance coverage through various financial arrangements (Aaron, 1991; Brown, 1988; Dalton, 1987; Dentzer, 1991; Herzlinger, 1985; Herzlinger & Calkins, 1986; Herzlinger & Schwartz, 1985; Peres, 1992). Such monitoring programs have helped reduce and eliminate medical inefficiency and have improved the effectiveness of care delivery.

Businesses have also begun to form health care coalitions that purchase health care services and offer them at a discount to their members. These coalitions guarantee accessible health care services, cost-effective delivery, and quality care. Some of the services provided by the coalitions include workers' compensation, inpatient and outpatient programs, primary prevention and treatment, and case management services (Bell, 1991).

NONNURSING CASE MANAGEMENT MODELS

The primary focus of the case management model is to improve patient outcomes and control costs through the organization and coordination of health care services. The underlying economic premises of case management are dependent on the linkage to managed care strategies developed by the private sector and insurance provider groups. Managed care programs became popular when private corporations and industry affiliations took an active part in maintaining control over soaring health care expenditures (Federation of American Health Systems Review, 1988).

Medical case management has become an effective way for private industry groups to maintain control over the use and costs of health care and to develop effective management and intervention methods (Califano, 1987; Dentzer, 1991; Katz, 1991). Case management identifies procedures used excessively that involve extended hospital stays and evaluates uncoordinated health care delivery systems, which promote duplication and fragmentation of services. Medical case management controls both the demand for and the supply of health care by identifying potential high-cost cases (appropriate targeting); by coordinating and channeling the delivery of care among providers, patients, insurers, and agencies that may be involved; and by evaluating and managing the patient's existing benefits plan to cover needed services (Dentzer, 1991; Henderson, Bergman, Collard, Souder, & Wallack, 1987; Henderson & Collard, 1988).

Until recently, the cost-effectiveness of the case management method has not been implicitly justified. Past research investigations were concerned with process and structured measures of efficiency. Such investigations sought to discover whether the use of a physician as a case manager or an HMO as an insurer and provider of care actually reduced health care expenditures and increased quality assurance (Austin, 1983; Manning, Liebowitz, Goldberg, Rogers, & Newhouse, 1984).

In 1986, researchers at the Bigel Institute for Health Policy Studies at Brandeis University undertook a major study to evaluate medical case management for catastrophic illnesses. This 2-year project was supported by funding from The Robert Wood Johnson Foundation (Henderson et al., 1987; Henderson & Collard, 1988; Henderson & Wallack, 1987). Specifically the project involved the evaluation of a case management program offered by a predominantly private insurance group and was representative of other case management arrangements offered by other major insurers (Henderson et al., 1987).

Patient case load was identified by five diagnostic categories, which included the high-risk infant, head trauma, spinal cord injury, cancer, and AIDS (Henderson et al., 1987; Henderson & Wallack, 1987). Cost criteria were developed that incorporated the economic rationale of limiting inappropriate use of high-cost procedures and unnecessary ancillary resources. The factors contributing to high costs that were evaluated were patient length of stay that exceeded predefined limits, evidence of complications indicated by the primary and secondary diagnoses, a repeat admission within a set time frame, and total patient charges exceeding a certain limit (Henderson & Wallack, 1987).

Cost-effectiveness was determined when the case management program initiated and implemented an alternative plan that decreased the patient's length of stay in the hospital, facilitated patient transfer to a less costly facility, and decreased expenditures associated with home care services (Henderson et al., 1987).

Case management responsibilities in this study were assigned to registered nurses who were accountable for the assessment, care planning, monitoring, and evaluation activities. A case management plan was developed that incorporated the input of the physician provider and used appropriate resources to meet the individual needs of the patient and family (Henderson & Collard, 1988). Henderson and Collard found that the successful implementation of the case management plan required the cooperation of the attending physician. For the most part, case management was seen as a comprehensive plan for ensuring patients would receive health care services that would not ordinarily be reimbursable.

The Brandeis study found that use of the medical case management model significantly reduced costs. Several factors contributed to the effectiveness of this program:

▼ Early patient identification and intervention assure access to the most appropriate and least restrictive care.
▼ Appropriate resource use helps maintain cost-effective care.
▼ Alternative treatment programming and benefit management allow for flexibility in the payment structure.
▼ Directing of the case management approach to specific patient groups helps achieve significant gains from services.
▼ A cooperative and supportive relationship develops between the care provider and case recipients.
▼ Interpretable, standardized reporting mechanisms help relate program objectives to patient care delivery.
▼ Case management integrates the case planning process with resource allocation based on a patient classification system or DRG methodology.
▼ A computerized information system allows for continuous data monitoring and analysis (Henderson et al., 1987; Henderson & Collard, 1988; Weisman, 1987; White, 1986).

CASE MANAGEMENT AND CATASTROPHIC ILLNESS

The case management model used depends on the patient population it serves. Such adaptability makes it possible to match a particular patient's needs with the appropriate case management approach. For example, the primary care case management model, when used for treating chronically ill patients, may require the addition of medical or social case management services (Merrill, 1985).

Although no one model of case management is applicable in all circumstances, medical case management programs recently have been adapted for use in the management of care associated with catastrophic illness or injury (Brown, 1988;

Henderson & Wallack, 1987). Traditionally, care of those with catastrophic illnesses has been expensive because of a lack of coordination and fragmentation of services. Duplication of patient services and failure to work out alternative care arrangements have also added to the cost of treating catastrophic illness (Henderson & Collard, 1987). The medical case management model focuses cost containment efforts on a small percentage of the patient population that contains frequent users of hospital and medical technology services (Rosenbloom & Gertman, 1984; Zook & Moore, 1980). Zook and Moore identified two types of catastrophic cases that used a considerable amount of health care resources. The first group consisted of unanticipated illnesses such as spinal cord injury, head trauma, neonatal complications, cancer, cardiac disease, and stroke. The second type of catastrophic illness includes chronic medical or psychiatric conditions.

The rationale behind using the medical case management model with catastrophic illness is based on a study by the Health Data Institute of the medical care patterns of major businesses in the United States. This investigation showed that in more than 1 million episodes of hospital care between 1980 and 1983, there were consistent patterns of high-cost illness. This study revealed that a large proportion of health care costs were attributable to only 5% to 10% of health-insured individuals (Rosenbloom & Gertman, 1984). Because catastrophic illness occurs less frequently than ordinary ailments, cost containment efforts should be directed to some of these high-cost illnesses. The Health Data Institute study indicates that medical, social, and financial consequences of catastrophic illness and injury can be controlled through a systematic effort characteristic of the case management approach.

REFERENCES

Aaron, H. (1991). Choosing from the health care reform menu. *The Journal of American Health Policy, 1*(3), 23-27.

Altman, S.H., & Rodmin, M.A. (1988). Halfway competitive markets and ineffective regulation: The American health care system. *Journal of Health Politics, Policy and Law, 13*(2), 323-339.

Austin, C.D. (1983). Case management in long-term care: Options and opportunities. *Health and Social Work, 8*(1), 16-30.

Bell, N. (1991). From the trenches: Strategies that work. *Business and Health, 9*(5), 19-25.

Brown, R. (1988). Principles for a national health program: A framework for analysis and development. *The Milbank Quarterly, 66*(4), 573-617.

Califano, J. (1987). Guiding the forces of the health care revolution. *Nursing and Health Care 8*(7), 400-404.

Christensen, L. (1991). The highs and lows of PPOs. *Business and Health, 9*(9), 72-77.

Dalton, J. (1987). Alternative delivery systems and employers. *Topics in Health Care Financing, 13*(3), 68-76.

Davis, R.G. (1985). Congress and the emergence of public health policy. *Health Care Management Review, 10*(1), 61-73.

DeBack, V., & Cohen, E. (1996). The new practice environment. In E. Cohen (Ed.), *Nurse case management in the 21st century* (pp. 3-9). St. Louis, MO: Mosby–Year Book, Inc.

Dentzer, S. (1991, September 23). Agenda for business: How to fight killer health costs. *U.S. News and World Report*, 50-58.

Dwyer, P., & Garland, S. (1991, November 25). A roar of discontent: Voters want health care reform now. *Business Week*, 28-30.

Eckholm, E. (1991, May 2). Rescuing health care. *The New York Times*, A 1, B 12.

Enthoven, A., & Kronick, R. (1989a). A consumer-choice health plan for the 1990s, part I. *New England Journal of Medicine, 320*(1), 29-37.

Enthoven, A., & Kronick, R. (1989b). A consumer-choice health plan for the 1990s, part II. *New England Journal of Medicine, 320*(2), 94-101.

Federation of American Health Systems Review (1988, July/August). Special report: The facts of life about managed care. Author, 20-49.

Frieden, J. (1991). Many roads lead to health system reform. *Business and Health, 9*(11), 38-66.

Garland, S. (1991, October 7). The health care crises: A prescription for reform. *Business Week,* 59-66.

Gilman, T., & Bucco, C. (1987). Alternate delivery systems: An overview. *Topics in Health Care Financing, 13*(3), 1-7.

Ginsburg, R. B., & Hackbarth, G.M. (1986). Alternative delivery systems and medicare. *Health Affairs, 5*(1), 6-22.

Henderson, M., Bergman, A., Collard, A., Souder, B., Wallack, S. (Draft, May 1, 1987). *Private sector medical case management for high cost illness.* Brandeis University Heller Graduate School Health Policy Center, Waltham, Massachusetts.

Henderson, M.G., & Collard, A. (1988). Measuring quality in medical case management programs. *Quality Review Bulletin, 14*(2) 33-39.

Henderson, M.G., & Wallack, S.S. (1987). Evaluating case management for catastrophic illness. *Business and Health, 4*(3), 7-11.

Herzlinger, R. E. (1985). How companies tackle health care costs: Part II. *Harvard Business Review, 63*(5), 108-120.

Herzlinger, R.E., & Calkins, D. (1986). How companies tackle health care costs: Part III. *Harvard Business Review, 64*(1), 70-80.

Herzlinger, R.E., & Schwartz, J. (1985). How companies tackle health care costs: Part I. *Harvard Business Review, 63*(4), 68-81.

Hewitt Associates. (1989). *Salaried employee benefits provided by major U.S. employers.* Lincolnshire, Ill.: Hewitt Associates.

Hicks, L., Stallmeyer, J., & Coleman, J. (1992). Nursing challenges in managed care. *Nursing Economics, 10*(4), 265-275.

Hospitals (1988, April 5). Managed care: Whoever has the data wins the game. *Hospitals,* 50-55.

Hospitals (1992, January 20). Health care reform a priority in the legislative years. *Hospitals,* 32-50.

Jones, K. (1989). Evolution of the prospective payment system: Implications for nursing. *Nursing Economics, 7*(6), 299-305.

Katz, F. (1991). Making a case for case management. *Business and Health, 9*(4), 75-77.

Kramon, G. (1989, January 8). Taking a scalpel to health costs. *The New York Times,* pp. 1,9.

Luft, H.S. (1978). How do health maintenance organizations achieve their savings? Rhetoric and evidence. *New England Journal of Medicine, 298*(11), 1336-1343.

Luft, H.S. (1982). Health maintenance organizations and the rationing of medical care. *The Milbank Quarterly, 60*(2), 268-306.

Manning, W.G., Leibowitz, A., Goldberg, G., Rogers, W., & Newhouse, J. (1984). A controlled trial of the effect of a prepaid group practice on the use of services. *New England Journal of Medicine, 310*(23), 1505-1510.

Merrill, J.C. (1985). Defining case management. *Business and Health, 3*(5-9), 5-9.

Mullen, P. (1988, December 27). Big increase in health premiums. *Health Week, 2*(26), 1, 26.

National League for Nursing (1991). *Nursing's agenda for health care reform.* New York, N.Y.: NLN.

O'Connor, K. (1991). Risky business: HMOs and managed care. *Business and Health, 9*(6), 30-34.

Peres, A. (1992). Business must act now to shape reform. *Business and Health, 10*(1), 72.

Reinhardt, U.E. (1987a, January 11). Toward a fail-safe health-insurance system. *The Wall Street Journal.*

Reinhardt, U.E. (1987b). Health insurance for the nation's poor. *Health Affairs, 6*(1), 101-102.

Rosenberg, S., Perlis, H., Lynne, D., & Leto, L. (1991). A second look at second surgical opinions. *Business and Health, 9*(2), 14-28.

Rosenbloom, D., & Gertman, P. (1984). An intervention strategy for controlling costly care. *Business and Health, 1*(8), 17-21.

Sloan, F., Morrisey, M., & Valvona, J. (1988). Effects of the medicare prospective payment system on hospital cost containment: An early appraisal. *The Milbank Quarterly, 66*(2), 191-220.

Sloss, E.M., Keeler, E.B., Brook, R.H., Operskalski, B.H., Goldberg, G.A., & Newhouse, J.P. (1987). Effect of a health maintenance organization on physiologic health. *Annals of Internal Medicine, 106*(1), 130-138.

Swoap, D. (1984). Beyond DRGs: Shifting the risk to providers. *Health Affairs, 3*(4), 117-121.

Tallon, J.R. (1991). A report from the front line: Policy and politics in health reform. *The Journal of American Health Policy, 1*(1), 47-50.

Thorpe, K. (1991). The national health insurance conundrum: Shifting paradigms and potential solutions. *The Journal of American Health Policy, 1*(1), 17-22.

Traska, M.R. (1989). What 1989 holds for health benefits. *Business and Health, 1*(1), 22-30.

Waldo, D.R., Levit, J.R., & Lazenby, H. (1986). National health expenditures, 1985. *Health Care Financing Review, 8*(1), 1-21.

Weisman, E. (1987). Practical approaches for developing a case management program. *Quality Review Bulletin, 13*(11), 380-382.

Wellinga, K. (1990, June 11). The sickening spiral: Health-care costs continue to grow at an alarming rate. *Barron's,* 8.

White, M. (1986). Case management. In G.L. Maddox (Ed.), *The encyclopedia of aging* (pp. 92-96). New York: Springer Publishing.

Wilensky, G. (1991). Treat the causes, not the symptoms of the health care cost problem. *The Journal of American Health Policy, 1*(2), 15-17.

Zook, C.V., & Moore, F.D. (1980). High-cost users of medical care. *New England Journal of Medicine, 302*(18), 996-1002.

9

PATIENT MIX AND COST RELATED TO LENGTH OF HOSPITAL STAY

▼ CHAPTER OVERVIEW

Prospective payment systems have influenced the development of innovative care delivery models by placing limits on the use of hospital resources. Because the length of time an individual spends in the hospital affects the appropriation of services and costs involved in that care, the number of hospitalized days becomes an important variable in assessing and measuring the institution's financial outcome.

The effects of care delivery models on health care services provided an important strategy for evaluating system effectiveness, efficiency, and quality. The coordination and integration required for case management are two reasons why such a health care delivery model maximizes the use and allocation of available resources and services.

Nursing case management methods provide indicators that help assess the effectiveness of patient care delivery. By focusing on the coordination and integration of inpatient services, nursing case management can reduce the patient length of stay while keeping it within medically appropriate boundaries.

With the implementation of DRG strategies, patient length of stay has become an overall indicator of a hospital's financial performance and cost-effectiveness. Numerous variables that have an effect on the cost and length of stay have been identified. This chapter reviews and analyzes studies related to patient length-of-stay variables.

The chapter is divided into three general categories: (1) patient demographics, such as age and gender variables; (2) related variables, such as diagnosis and comorbidity, discharge planning, patient care delivery systems, and nursing intensity and workload (a critique of the nursing intensity and workload studies is provided); and (3) nonclinical variables that affect patient length of stay, such as day-of-the-week admission (weekday versus weekend) and organizational factors. ▲

PATIENT DEMOGRAPHICS

Certain patient characteristics, such as age, were reported to be important in judging the postoperative recovery time of patients undergoing surgical procedures, such as a hernia repair or a cholecystectomy (Kolouch, 1965). Although the reasons for a correlation between age and length of surgical convalescent time were not provided, the finding was anticipated because of the close association between age, chronicity, hospital-induced infections, age-related risk factors, patient dependency needs, and increased time required for postoperative healing.

In this study, however, age did not account for all the variations in average length of stay reported by surgical case mix. Other variables existed that were not subject to control such as postoperative surgical complications, patient rehabilitation time, method of payment (i.e., third-party, Blue Cross, or charity), and type of hospital (i.e., teaching or nonteaching).

In another study by Marchette and Holloman (1986), age was the significant variable in prolonging the length of stay of cerebral vascular accident (CVA) patients. On average the CVA patients were older and had the longest hospital stays. Again, as in the Kolouch (1965) study, age did not account for all of the diversity attributed to length of stay. Other intervening variables, such as severity of illness, discharge planning, and social consults, also affected the average length of stay of the hospitalized patients.

Posner and Lin (1975) studied the age variable in association with predicted length of stay for medical patients. In this study, age was evaluated in terms of its effects on comparable diagnoses. The study also evaluated the effect of various hospital settings (voluntary or municipal) on the length of patient stay. It was found that the hospital length of stay was not exclusively affected by the age of the patient. Wide variations were found in length of stay within age groups even when diagnostic categories and hospital variables were controlled.

The unreliability of age as a predictor of hospital length of stay was confirmed in another study by Lave and Leinhardt (1976). This study placed emphasis on case-mix factors and variables that related to the patient's medical condition and that contributed to changes in the patient's length of stay.

Both Lave and Leinhardt (1976) and Marchette and Holloman (1986) looked at the effect of gender on patient length of stay. Findings showed that male patients have shorter lengths of hospital stay than female patients and that single women have the longest stays. Several explanations of these findings were offered. First, because women live longer than men, women will experience more hospitalizations. Second, single women have longer stays because they less often have adult family members available to care for them. Although all these findings are associated with longer than average hospital stays, the effect of patient gender could not be validated. Lave and Leinhardt (1976) advised that although patient demographic variables may be statistically significant in some situations, such variables may have minimal effect on the overall variability of the patient's length of stay.

CLINICALLY RELATED VARIABLES

The patient's primary diagnosis, number of surgical procedures, and number of secondary diagnoses were factors that had a significant effect on patient length of stay (Lave & Leinhardt, 1976; Lew, 1966; McCorkle, 1970; Ro, 1969). These variables were found to account for 38% of the variation in length of stay, with primary diagnosis alone accounting for 27% of the variability in patient length of stay (Lave

& Leinhardt, 1976). Patients diagnosed with acute myocardial infarction had the longest hospital stays, whereas patients with hyperplasia of the prostate had shorter lengths of stay. The findings indicate that patients with urgent or emergent status had longer hospital stays. In addition, the poor health of such patients on admission and the unscheduled nature of these admissions resulted in delays and inefficient mobilization of hospital services.

In two earlier studies, Riedel and Fitzpatrick (1964) and Mughrabi (1976) concluded that the primary diagnosis and the concomitant levels of severity are the most important factors contributing to the length of a patient's hospitalization. Additional studies indicated that comorbidity and related complications resulted in significantly longer lengths of stay (Berki, Ashcraft, & Newbrander, 1984; Grau & Kovner, 1986).

In an investigation conducted by Marchette and Holloman (1986), discharge planning (nurses' and social workers') was found to affect patient length of stay. This study demonstrated a decrease of 0.8 day of hospitalization for those patients who received discharge planning early in their hospital stays. Conversely, the length of stay increased by 0.8 day for those patients who received discharge planning later in their hospitalization. In addition, a decrease of 2 days of hospitalization was shown because of nurses' discharge planning activities with patients diagnosed with CVA. This finding demonstrates that the effect of discharge planning is indicative of individual patient diagnoses (Cable & Mayers, 1983).

Timely social service planning and early referral programs were shown to shorten a patient's length of stay. Factors associated with changes in patients' Medicaid status, a lack of alternate care resources, failure of medical staff to complete transfer and referral forms, and other confounding variables delayed patient discharge (Altman, 1965; Boone, Coulton, & Keller, 1981; Schrager, Halman, Myers, Nichols, & Rosenblum, 1978; Schuman, Ostfeld, & Willard, 1976; Zimmer, 1974).

The nursing case management model for patient care delivery has been recognized for its significant effect on decreasing patient length of stay (Zander, 1988). Through the coordination and monitoring of resources needed for patient care, ischemic stroke patients' length of stay was reduced by 29%, and adult leukemia patients' length of stay decreased from an average of 6 to 8 weeks to 32 days.

Rogers (1992) makes a distinction between the way that beyond-the-walls (BTW) and within-the-walls (WTW) models affect length of stay (LOS):

> Both models involve nurses in relatively autonomous positions that use a holistic nursing approach, "system savvy," collaboration to coordinate professional care team functions, and individualized care planning to achieve reductions in resource utilization while enhancing actual, as well as perceived, quality of care. The reduction in patient anxiety and increased patient compliance when they are more involved in the process and assured that someone they know is watching over things is attested to almost daily. These translate to reduced demands on nursing time during a given stay and in reductions in the actual length of stay.
>
> Beyond this, our experience has been that enhanced transit through the course of a stay and improved discharge planning, particularly with acute cases, takes days off of the end of the stay. This phenomenon is a hallmark of the WTW model.

On the other hand, the forte of the BTW models is care of the chronically ill. The impact of these models on LOS tends to be on the beginning of the stay. This occurs because the BTW nurse case managers know their patients' patterns and disease processes very well. They tend to get these patients into the hospital earlier in an exacerbation than they previously were. Being admitted "less sick" tends to keep these patients out of high-cost emergency and critical care departments and keep the overall LOS down. This phenomenon was noted by Ethridge and Lamb (1989) and alluded to by Rogers, Riordan, and Swindle (1991). St. Joseph Medical Center in Wichita, in an unpublished internal management analysis, has since documented an overall reduction in the admission acuity for their BTW patients.

A major problem with studies relating to patient care delivery systems is the lack of uniformity and sophistication in defining costs. Variations exist as to what factors should be included in direct and indirect cost categories. Some studies included supplies and equipment, while other investigations allocated costs based on overhead expenses from ancillary and support services and general hospital operations. In some studies, nursing costs included the professional services of registered nurses. In other studies, nursing costs included all of the costs of providing nursing care to hospitalized patients (Edwardson & Giovannetti, 1987). Further research is needed to determine the applicability of cost accounting approaches to nursing models of care with the expected clinical and financial outcomes.

Nursing intensity, which is the amount of nursing care provided per patient day, along with various nursing interventions and staffing levels, was cited as reducing length of stay and costs associated with hospitalization. In an investigation done by Halloran (1983a, 1983b), nursing diagnoses were used to classify patients according to their nursing care requirements and to describe the time spent by professional nurses in caring for patients. Nursing diagnoses describe patient conditions and problems that require nursing intervention. It was found that a predominantly registered nurse staff, versus a staffing mix of registered nurses, licensed practical nurses, and nursing attendants, decreased costs associated with patient care. The investigation showed that an all-registered-nurse staff would be more likely to deal with total patient needs than a staff composed of various skill mixes. Halloran also proposed that nursing care costs should be identified and defined according to nursing diagnoses (unit of service) instead of the medical diagnosis-related group (DRG) currently in use.

In another study, Halloran and Kiley (1984) proposed a nursing information system model that allocated staffing and resources using nursing diagnoses. This process was based on a nursing workload unit of analysis that calculated costs using a patient classification system for staffing. The reason for using a patient classification system was that such a system made it possible to measure the nursing workload and allocate costs in order to distinguish the costs of nursing care services from the cost of the hospital's room and board rate.

As outlined by Edwardson and Giovannetti (1987), the patient classification system makes it possible to calculate the hours of care used during a patient's hospitalization. Once the number of patient care hours is identified, this number is translated into a dollar amount. Patients are then classified into DRG categories, and nursing care costs for patients are aggregated and analyzed.

Although patient classification systems offer a more reliable representation than traditional methods of identifying the nursing care needs of patients (i.e., global averages, such as the average amount of care required per day by the typical patient), there are still some inherent problems. As identified by Giovannetti (1972) and Edwardson and Giovannetti (1987) the problems associated with this system include the inadvisability of comparing a patient classification system developed in one hospital with that in another because of the differences in treatment modalities, architectural structure and design of the inpatient units, and standards and policies of the institution. Some of the factors used to weigh the categories are subjective, which results in problems of reliability. Furthermore, methods of validating the system and workload indexes are not transferable. In spite of these difficulties, the method of staffing by workload index has been a generally accepted mode by health care institutions across the country.

An investigation done by Halloran and Halloran (1985) found that nursing diagnoses were accurate for predicting nursing workload and quantity of nursing care. In addition, nursing diagnoses contributed to some of the variation in patient length of stay. It was suggested that nursing instead of medical needs kept patients in the hospital. Nursing diagnoses that dealt with the patient's psychosocial needs and self-care requirements were found to be significant in increasing nursing workload. In another study, nursing workload activities correlated with 77% of the patient's length of hospitalization. These findings imply that variations in length of stay within specific DRG categories can be explained by the clinical management of patient care by nurses (Halloran & Kiley, 1986).

Ventura, Young, Feldman, Pastore, Pikula, and Yates (1985) found that nursing interventions associated with health protection activities for patients with peripheral vascular disease significantly decreased the patient's length of stay and lowered hospitalization costs, which were based on a fixed per diem rate. Mumford, Schlesinger, and Glass (1982) and Devine and Cook (1983) demonstrated that psychological and educational interventions (i.e., patient teaching related to pain prevention and complications) with postsurgical patients reduced the length of stay and improved patient recovery time.

Flood and Diers (1988) identified the effect of professional nurse staffing levels on length of stay. According to the study, decreased nurse staffing levels could lead to a reduction in productivity and inadequate patient care resulting in longer hospitalization. Patients whose case mixes included gastrointestinal hemorrhages and CVAs and who had been located on a unit with significant staffing shortages were found to have longer lengths of stay, 3.8 and 4.14 days respectively, when compared with patients on a unit that had adequate staffing levels. The increase in length of stay was attributed to patient-related complications and nosocomial infections and resulted in the use of high levels of nursing care resources.

However, the findings of the Flood and Diers study are speculative, because many of the variables associated with patient length of stay, for example, primary diagnosis, comorbidity, medical complications, and discharge planning factors, had not been controlled. Because these variables were not controlled, the study is not adequate for showing a significant correlation between nurse staffing levels and length of stay.

The results of the nursing intensity and workload investigations support the premise that patient care requirements, nursing interventions, and level of staff affect the delivery of care. However, other variables, that have a profound effect on the delivery of nursing care services were not accounted for. Some of these variables were identified by Edwardson and Giovannetti (1987) and include service standards of the institution, physician practice patterns, nature and extent of support services, adequacy of the physical plant, and quality-of-care indexes. The last variable would have to be studied with various mixes of staffing personnel to determine the efficacy of patient care delivery.

The general findings of the nursing intensity and workload studies take on a different perspective when viewed in light of the investigations done by the Prospective Payment Assessment Commission (ProPAC). ProPAC was established as an independent advisory board to the Department of Health and Human Services (HHS) and Congress to report on issues surrounding the impact of the prospective payment system on health care delivery and finance. ProPAC's responsibilities include annual recommendations to HHS regarding appropriate changes in Medicare payments for inpatient hospital care and changes in the relative weights of DRGs. ProPAC is also required to report to Congress its evaluation of any adjustments made to DRG classifications and weights (Price & Lake, 1988).

ProPAC focused its research efforts on the DRG allocation method as it related to the intensity of nursing care. The nursing intensity and workload studies done over the last few years established that inaccuracies existed in the allocation of DRG weights to nursing costs. In the past, nursing service in health care institutions was calculated as part of the room and board rate and did not directly affect patient charges. Variations in the patient's nursing care and attributable costs were strictly related to the patient's length of stay and routine and intensive care levels (Cromwell & Price, 1988; Young, 1986).

Accounting for the amount of time spent and for the type of care delivered by nursing is one problem generated by the nature of the services offered. Defining nursing care through a patient classification system became one way of alleviating this difficulty. Matching the type of care a patient will need with a specific category on the patient classification instrument and then determining the amount of nursing resources needed for that patient category provided the foundation for establishing the costs of nursing services and developing a basis for charges to patients. The patient classification system was used as an instrument to measure the severity level of patients (in terms of nursing workload) as well as variations in nursing care. However, studies have shown that because of systematic errors (i.e., quantity of care and level of care are both objective and subjective estimates), a lack of cross-institutional comparability and generalizability, and lack of on-going validity and reliability, patient classification systems were not accurate resources for determining the cost of nursing services (Dijkers & Paradise, 1986). In addition, the wide variations in the methodologies used in the numerous nursing intensity studies question the appropriateness and applicability of using nursing patient classification systems to account for DRG-specific nursing intensity values (Price & Lake, 1988).

In view of these limitations, a major research effort directed by ProPAC to provide national adjustments of DRG weights based on nursing intensity variations was abandoned (Cromwell & Price, 1988; Price & Lake, 1988). Recommendations from ProPAC for further research included:

▼ Developing nursing intensity adjustments for selected DRGs on a case-by-case basis
▼ Documenting nursing intensity variation with DRGs over a patient's length of stay by identifying factors related to patient complexity, changes in staff volume, and skill mix
▼ Establishing uniformity among patient classification systems
▼ Establishing the cost base used to allocate DRG weights

ProPAC also said that the effects of nursing intensity on DRG weights would be greater if applied to all routine and department costs rather than just direct nursing care (Cromwell & Price, 1988; Price & Lake, 1988).

NONCLINICAL VARIABLES

Lew (1966) studied how the day of the week that a patient was admitted affected the average length of stay. Patients who came in for medical admissions on Sunday had the lowest average length of stay, 10.83 days, and those admitted on Friday had the highest average length of stay, 13.81 days. For surgical patients, those admitted on Wednesday had the lowest average length of stay, 9.88 days, and those admitted on Friday had the highest average length of stay, 11.85 days. When medical and surgical admissions were combined, those patients admitted on Friday had the highest average length of stay and those admitted on Sunday had the lowest average length of stay. Reasons for the variations in the lengths of weekday stay were attributed to the availability of resources—such as personnel, operating rooms, equipment, and procedures—and services needed for the care of the patient.

Day-of-the-week variables were found significant in studies conducted by Lave and Leinhardt (1976) and Mughrabi (1976). However, these variables did not account for a large portion of the variation in average length of stay.

Institutional practices related to management, patient care delivery, and use of facility resources (e.g., laboratory, radiology) were among the many variables that affected length of stay. Becker, Shortell, and Neuhouser (1980) identified managerial and organizational factors that had significant effects on overall patient length of stay. In this study, reductions in patient length of stay and increases in the quality and efficiency of services were attributable to the following variables:

▼ Administrative and clinical managers' awareness of traditional outcome measurements of patient care (i.e., length of stay, infection and mortality indexes, and preventable complications) compared with other hospitals
▼ The degree of professional autonomy related to hospital operations and clinical decision making
▼ Interdisciplinary as well as interdepartmental collaboration and accountability for the efficient use, coordination, and monitoring of hospital resources including nursing services, radiology, and laboratory

Decreased length of hospital stay facilitated by interdepartmental coordination and integration of patient services was achieved by regularly scheduled meetings among radiology, nursing service, and laboratory personnel.

Another study, conducted by Berki, Ashcraft, and Newbrander (1984), showed that with certain DRG classifications, patient length-of-stay variations were related to use and consumption of hospital services. Increases in laboratory and radiology services were found to be associated with longer lengths of stay in those DRG categories, such as diabetes and arthritis, that required intensive use of ancillary services. Other DRG categories, for example, eye disease, which requires reattachment of the retina and repair of the cornea, increased nursing service intensity and resulted in decreased patient length of stay.

REFERENCES

Altman, I. (1965). Some factors affecting hospital length of stay. *Hospitals, 39(7),* 68-176.

Becker, S., Shortell, S., & Neuhouser, D. (1980). Management practices and hospital length of stay. *Inquiry, 17,*318-330.

Berki, S., Ashcraft, M., & Newbrander, W. (1984). Length of stay variations within ICDA-8 diagnosis related groups. *Medical Care, 22(2),* 126-142.

Boone, C., Coulton, C., & Keller, S. (1981). The impact of early and comprehensive social work services on length of stay. *Social Work in Health Care, 7(1),* 1-9.

Cable E., & Mayers, S. (1983). Discharge planning effect on length of hospital stay. *Archives of Physical Medicine and Rehabilitation, 64(2),* 57-60.

Cromwell, J., & Price, K. (1988). The sensitivity of DRG weights to variation in nursing intensity. *Nursing Economics, 6(1),* 18-26.

Devine, E., & Cook, T. (1983). A meta-analytic analysis of effects of psychoeducational interventions on length of postsurgical hospital stay. *Nursing Research, 32(5),* 267-274.

Dijkers, M., & Paradise, T. (1986). PCS: One system for both staffing and costing. Do services rendered match need estimates? *Nursing Management, 17(1),* 25-34.

Edwardson, S., & Giovannetti, P. (1987). A review of cost accounting methods for nursing services. *Nursing Economics, 5(3),* 107-117.

Ethridge, P., & Lamb, G. (1989). Professional nursing case management improves quality, access and costs. *Nursing Management, 20(3),* 30-35.

Farren, E., (1991). Effects of early discharge planning on length of hospital stay. *Nursing Economics, 9(1),* 25-30.

Flood, S., & Diers, D. (1988). Nurse staffing, patient outcome and cost. *Nursing Management, 19(5),* 34-43.

Giovannetti, P. (May 1972). *Measurement of patient's requirements for nursing services.* Paper presented to the National Institute of Health Conference, Virginia.

Grau, L., & Kovnor, C. (1986). Comorbidity one length of stay: A case study. In F.A. Shaffer (Ed.), *Patients and purse strings: Patient classification and case management* (pp. 233-242). New York: National League for Nursing.

Halloran, E. (1983a). Staffing assignment: By task or by patient. *Nursing Management, 14(8),* 16-18.

Halloran, E. (1983b). RN staffing: More care less cost. *Nursing Management, 14(9),* 18-22.

Halloran, E. & Halloran, D. (1985). Exploring the DRG/nursing equation. *American Journal of Nursing, 85(10),* 1093-1095.

Halloran, E., & Kiley, M. (1984). Case mix management. *Nursing Management, 15(2),* 39-45.

Halloran, E., & Kiley, M.L. (1986). The nurse's role and length of stay. *Medical Care, 23(9),* 1122-1124.

Kolouch, F. (1965). Computer shows how patient stays vary. *The Modern Hospital, 105(5),* 130-134.

Lave, J., & Leinhardt, S. (1976). The cost and length of a hospital stay. *Inquiry, 13,* 327-343.

Lew, I. (1966). Day of the week and other variables affecting hospital admissions, discharges and length of stay for patients in the Pittsburgh area. *Inquiry, 3,* 3-39.

Marchette, L., & Holloman, F. (1986). Length of stay variables. *Journal of Nursing Administration, 165(3),* 12-19.

McCorkle, L. (1970). Duration of hospitalization prior to surgery. *Health Services Research, 5,* 114-131.

Mughrabi, M.A. (1976). The effects of selected demographic and clinical variables on the length of hospital stay. *Hospital Administration in Canada, 18,* 82-88.

Mumford, E., Schlesinger, H., & Glass, G. (1982). The effects of psychological intervention on recovery from surgery and heart attacks: An analysis of the literature. *American Journal of Public Health, 72*(2), 141-151.

Posner, J., & Lin, H. (1975). Effects of age on length of hospital stay in a low income population. *Medical Care, 13*(10), 855-875.

Price, K., & Lake, E. (1988). ProPAC's assessment of DRGs and nursing intensity. *Nursing Economics, 6*(1), 10-16.

Riedel, D., & Fitzpatrick, T. (1964). *Patterns of patient care: A study of hospital use in six diagnosis.* Ann Arbor: The University of Michigan Graduate School of Business Administration.

Ro, K.K. (1969). Patient characteristics, hospital characteristics and hospital use. *Medical Care,* 7(4), 295-312.

Rogers, M., Personal communication. (August 1992).

Rogers, M., Riordan, J., & Swindle, D. (1991). Community-based nursing case management pays off. *Nursing Management, 22*(3), 30-34.

Schrager, J., Halman, M., Myers, D., Nichols, R., & Rosenblum, L. (1978). Impediments to the course and effectiveness of discharge planning. *Social Work in Health Care, 4*(1), 65-79.

Schuman, J., Ostfeld, A., & Willard, H. (1976). Discharge planning in an acute hospital. *Archives of Physical Medicine and Rehabilitation,* 57(7), 343-347.

Ventura, M., Young, D., Feldman, M.J., Pastore, P., Pikula, S., & Yates, M.A. (1985). Cost savings as an indicator of successful nursing intervention. *Nursing Research, 34*(1), 50-53.

Young, D. (1986). ProPAC: Future Directions. *Nursing Economics, 4*(1), 12-15.

Zander, K. (1988). Nursing care management: Strategic management of cost and quality outcomes. *Journal of Nursing Administration, 18*(5), 23-30.

Zimmer, J. (1974). Length of stay and hospital bed misutilization. *Medical Care, 12*(5), 453-462.

10

POLICY AND LEGISLATION

▼ CHAPTER OVERVIEW

Because the prospective payment system gave hospitals the incentive to shorten length of stay, strategies using case management are being developed to focus on postdischarge planning and community-based long-term care. Case management has also demonstrated its applicability as a resource in the development of health legislation and policy in regard to the delivery of patient care. The usefulness of case management is an integral part of the administration and management of health care and is also a vital cost containment measure.

▲

HISTORICAL LEGISLATION

In 1992, 37 states had Medicaid provisions for case management. Legislation for governing the practices of case managers and for developing national certification and specific state requirements was also considered (National Case Management Task Force Steering Committee, 1992; Sager, 1992).

Case management has been integrated into many of the federal and state policies associated with the delivery of health care and social support services. The overall goal is to reduce the use and costs of expensive treatments. Case management is used in these situations to reduce institutionalization, increase and monitor access of needed services, and expand alternative community resources such as home and long-term care (Boling, 1992; Capitman, 1986; Kane, 1985; Strickland, 1992).

Case management has also been a major component in several federally funded demonstration projects.

The Triage demonstration project provided case management and health care services outside the traditional Medicare benefits. These services include adult day care, companion homemaking services, counseling, transportation, pharmaceuticals, and access to residential care. To be eligible for these services, persons had to be 65 years of age or older, had to have medical, social, and financial problems and a failing support system, and had to be at risk for institutionalization. Case management services were provided by a professional team consisting of registered nurses, physicians, and social workers (O'Rourke, Raisz, & Segal, 1982).

People eligible for the Wisconsin Community Care Organization included those individuals who were at risk for institutionalization as determined by the Geriatric Functional Rating Scale. This scale rated individuals' ability to perform functional and cognitive activities.

Services included companion and home-health-aide services, medical supplies and equipment, transportation, respite care, and skilled nursing care (Applebaum, Seidl, & Austin, 1980; Seidl, Applebaum, Austin, & Mahoney, 1983).

The On Lok demonstration project provided case management to dependent and elderly individuals eligible for skilled nursing or intermediate nursing home care. Acute care services, including hospitalization, were also provided in addition to other services. These other services included adult and social day care, dental care, home health care, optometry, and occupational and pharmaceutical services. Case management is provided by registered nurses, physicians, social workers, physical and occupational therapists, and dietitians (Zawadski, Shen, Yordi, & Hansen, 1984).

The New York City Home Care program offered services to chronically ill and elderly individuals residing in the New York City area. The program provided homemaker and personal care, transportation assistance, and various medical therapies (Sainer et al., 1984).

The Long-Term Care Channeling Demonstration Project provided case management services to dependent and chronically ill individuals. Services included mental health counseling, homemaking, personal care, supportive services, such as adult foster care and day care, skilled nursing, transportation, medical therapies, and equipment (Applebaum, Harrigan, & Kemper, 1986; Kemper et al., 1986; Wooldridge & Schore, 1986).

Those who were eligible for Access, Medicare's long-term care demonstration project, included all individuals 18 or older and Medicare beneficiaries older than 65 who needed long-term, skilled nursing care. Services ranged from case management, skilled nursing and home care, and Medicaid-waived services. Waived services included community health nursing, home health aide, medical and nursing consultations and therapies, personal care, equipment and supplies, respite care, and transportation (Berkeley Planning Associates, 1987; Eggert, Bowlyow, & Nichols, 1980).

LEGISLATION AFFECTING HEALTH CARE

Despite the defeat of health care reform measures proposed at the start of the Clinton administration, several legislation and health care reform proposals have pointed to principles of managed or coordinated care for providing a framework for cost-effective health care delivery. By focusing on case management and long-term care, an alternative to costly hospital and institutional care can be found. These legislative proposals have sought to reduce unneeded care and the use of expensive inpatient services through preventive and primary care interventions. They have also supported comprehensive community-based services and initiatives to improve overall health status and prevent inappropriate hospitalizations (Blankenau, 1992; Pollack, 1992; Strickland, 1992; Wagner, 1991).

Targeted populations included, among others, the chronically ill elderly, young and middle-age individuals with chronic illness and disabilities, the uninsured, and the impoverished. It was also suggested that resources be directed to reducing infant mortality and improving maternal health status (Darman, 1991; Hospitals, 1992a; Wagner, 1991).

Managed care has played a major role in proposals to expand Medicare and Medicaid. The social HMO (SHMO) is a national managed-care demonstration program initiated in 1985 to provide and finance long-term care services for the elderly. The program includes four nonprofit sites and has recently been approved by Congress for six additional locations. Sponsored by the Health Care Financing Administration (HCFA) in cooperation with the Health Policy Center of Brandeis University, this initiative uses case management and integrated service delivery as key features at each of the demonstration sites. The SHMO is recognized as one of the only national demonstration projects to successfully integrate acute and chronic care using existing funding resources (Abrahams, 1990; Abrahams, Macko, & Grais, 1992; Yordi, 1988).

Managed Medicaid legislation, passed in 1987, makes recommendations for a flat payment for Medicaid beneficiaries in need of medical and long-term care. This plan reduces hospital stays and excessive use of services, increases affordable access, and strengthens community-based services and resources (Hospitals, 1992b; McNeil, 1991; "Medicaid-Mandated Managed Care," 1992).

Another example of how the concept of case managed care is used is with the legislation of the CHAMPUS (Civilian Health and Medical Program of the Uniformed Services) Reform Initiative (CRI). This plan extends coverage under a case managed structure for military dependents and retirees younger than 65 (Burke, 1992). It also helps reduce health care expenditures and increase access by encouraging the use of military medical services and facilities (Burke, 1992).

Tricare, introduced as an alternative to CHAMPUS, is structured to be a more efficient, cost-effective system of delivering care. It offers three options for medical care: (1) services can be obtained from a government-approved network; (2) users can choose their own medical providers; and (3) inpatient care can be obtained at an out-of-network facility (CHAMPUS, 1995).

Of the major reform plans introduced in the 102nd Congress, six addressed long-term care policies and legislation. It is important to note that these health reform proposals were ground breaking legislation for case management.

The 1990 Pepper Commission Proposal, developed by the Bipartisan Commission on Health Care, suggested extending Medicare's long-term care initiatives to all disabled individuals. Under the proposal, which was introduced in the Senate by Senator Jay Rockefeller (D-W.Va.), eligibility would be determined by state, local, or federally funded agencies and based on standardized assessments of the beneficiary's resources and support systems.

It was proposed that case managers be used to evaluate and monitor the services provided. Benefits were to include comprehensive home- and community-based services that involve skilled nursing; physical, occupational, and speech therapies; personal care; homemaker services; adult and social day care; respite care for caregivers; hospital care; primary and preventive care; and support counseling (Darman, 1991; Harrington, 1990; Pepper Commission, 1990).

Coverage structure would have incorporated a play or pay plan requiring employers to provide health insurance to employees and their dependents or pay into a public tax plan. A provision was made in this plan for the phasing in of small businesses. Federal and state financing was to have been made available to cover home- and community-based care programs and nursing home care.

Quality-of-care issues were addressed through standardized practice guide-lines, outcome research, and peer review. Overall costs for this proposal included $24 billion for home care and $18.8 billion for nursing home care (Darman, 1991; Frieden, 1991).

The Long-Term Home Care Act (HR 2263), introduced by Senator Claude Pepper (D-Fla.), proposed to provide coverage for the chronically ill or disabled elderly and children younger than 19 with cognitive and functional impairments. It also included individuals with severe functional disabilities.

Benefits included skilled nursing care, homemaker and personal care services, physical, occupational, speech, and respiratory therapies, medical supplies and equipment, caregiver education, support and counseling, and adult day care. Eligi-bility determination was to be made by a long-term care management agency or private nonprofit agency along with the individual's physician.

Patient care management was to be provided through case management agencies that did not have affiliations or control interest in the referral facilities. Estimated costs for this plan were $8.9 billion (Darman, 1991).

The Elder Care Program (HR 3140), proposed by Representative Harry Waxman (D-Calif.), was to provide for Medicare beneficiaries and disabled individu-als. Eligibility determination was to be made by community assessment and review agencies that were restricted in affiliation and ownership to community or nursing care facilities.

Home and community-based services were to include adult day care, skilled nursing, homemaker, and personal care services, medical and social services, diag-nostic tests, medical supplies and equipment, caregiver education and training, and physical and occupational therapy. Estimated costs ranged from $50 billion to $60 billion in 1992 (Darman, 1991; Hospitals, 1992a).

Life Care (S2163/HR4093), sponsored by Senator Edward Kennedy (D-Mass.) and Representative Edward Roybal (D Calif.), proposed extending eligibility to the chronically ill older than 65 or younger than 19, all disabled and dependent individuals, and people with a life expectancy of 1 year or less.

Federally funded case management agencies were to determine eligibility and provide patient management. Benefit coverage was to include up to the first 6 months of nursing home care with extended nursing home coverage provided through a federal long-term care insurance program.

Proposed financial structure included Medicaid and income-related subsidies. Services provided included skilled nursing, adult day care, primary and preventive care, transportation to health and social care facilities, respite care, institutional or noninstitutional care, nutrition and dietary counseling, and physical, occupational, and speech therapies. The estimated cost of such a program was $20 billion (Darman, 1991; Harrington, 1990; Hospitals, 1992a).

Similar to Life Care, the Comprehensive Health Care Plan (HR 4253), proposed providing for the chronically ill older than 65 or younger than 19. The plan also was to provide for Medicare-eligible disabled individuals of all ages and insure those with a life expectancy of 1 year or less.

Eligibility and patient care were to be determined by federally funded case management agencies. Benefits were to include nursing home coverage and income assistance programs.

Home- and community-based services were to include skilled nursing; physical, occupational, and speech therapies; homemaker services; medical and social work care; transportation; adult day care and respite care; and counseling services. The estimated cost of this plan was $258 billion, which included universal health care and preventive and long-term care provisions (Darman, 1991).

MediPlan (HR 5300), sponsored by representative Pete Stark (D-Calif.), suggested that Medicare benefits be extended to chronically ill and disabled individuals of all ages. This plan also included primary and preventive care for children in addition to well-baby care.

It was proposed that eligibility determination and patient management be conducted by case management agencies, which were to have provider and ownership restrictions. A full range of home- and community-based services were to be provided, including skilled nursing; counseling services; medical supplies; adult day care; physical, occupational, and respiratory therapies; medical and social services; caregiver education and training; homemaker and personal care services; and prescription-drug coverage.

The plan's financing structure incorporated payroll tax increases and state contributions. The estimated cost of such a program was $120 billion, which included universal health care provisions and long-term care arrangements (Darman, 1991; Frieden, 1991; Hospitals, 1992a).

Additional legislative initiatives have indicated case management as an integral component of health care delivery and policy formation. This plan was one of several state assembly and senate bills developed in California that would have affected case management (Kowlsen, 1991). An overview of three such bills follows.

California Assembly Bill 1341 was to provide for a 3-year demonstration project to provide case management to children at risk for abuse and neglect. Case management services were to be provided by public health nurses. The goal of this project was to reduce shelter or foster care placement and decrease emergency room visits and hospitalizations among children.

California Senate Bill 1108 established the Primary Care Case Management Advisory Board as part of the California Department of Health Services. It also provided for the delivery of case management services for Medicaid-eligible individuals to promote and increase accessibility to affordable health care resources.

California Assembly Bill 14 would have ratified primary health care coverage to all individuals. Cost containment strategies were to include managed care principles such as case management.

REFERENCES

Abrahams, R. (1990, August). The social/HMO: Case management in an integrated acute and long-term care system. *Caring Magazine,* 30-40.

Abrahams, R., Macko, P., & Grais, M.I. (1992). Across the great divide: Integrating acute post-acute, and long-term care. *Journal of Case Management, 1*(4), 124-134.

Applebaum, R., Seidl, F.W., & Austin, C.D. (1980). The Wisconsin community care organization: Preliminary findings from the Milwaukee experiment. *Gerontologist, 20,* 350-355.

Applebaum, R.A., Harrigan, M.N. & Kemper, P. (1986). *The evaluation of the national long-term care demonstration: Tables comparing channeling to other community care demonstrations.* Princeton, N.J.: Mathematica Policy Research, Inc.

Berkeley Planning Associates (1987). *Evaluation of the Access: Medicare long-term care demonstration project. Final Report.* Berkeley, California.

Blankenau, R. (1992, January 6). Health-reform bills top 1992 agendas of Hill health leaders. *AHA News.*

Boling, J. (1992). An American integrated health care system? Where are we now? *The Case Manager, 3*(3), 53-59.

Burke, M. (1992, January 20). Armed services are marching toward managed care alternatives. *AHA News, 28*(3), pg. 6.

Capitman, J.A. (1986). Community-based long-term care models, target groups, and impacts on service use. *Gerontologist, 26*(4), 389-397.

CHAMPUS (1995, March 13). *CHAMPUS user's guide* (pp. 1-28). Author (special section to Army Times, Navy Times, and Air Force Times).

Darman, R. (1991, October 10). *Comprehensive health reform: Observations about the problem and alternative approaches to solution. Presented to the House Committee on Ways and Means.* Washington, D.C.: Executive Office of the President, Office of Management and Budget.

Eggert, G., Bowlyow, J., & Nichols, C. (1980). Gaining control of the long-term care systems: First returns from the access experiment. *Gerontologist, 20,* 356-363.

Frieden, J. (1991). Many roads lead to health system reform. *Business and Health, 9*(11), 38-66.

Harrington, C. (1990). Policy options for a national health care plan. *Nursing Outlook, 38*(5), 223-228.

Hospitals (1992a, January 20). Health care reform a priority in the new legislative year. 32-50.

Hospitals (1992b, March 20). Managed care in the 1990s: Providers' new role for innovative health delivery. 26-34.

Kane, R. (1985). Case management in health care settings. In M. Weil & J. Karls (Eds.), *Case management in human service practice* (pp. 170-203). San Francisco: Josey Bass Pub.

Kemper, P., Brown, R., Carcagno, G., Applebaum, R., Christianson, J., Carson, W., Dunstan, S., Grannemann, T., Harrigan, M., Holden, N., Phillips, B., Schore, J., Thornton, C., Wooldridge, J., & Skidmore, F. (1986). *The evolution of the national long-term care demonstration: Final report.* Princeton, N.J.: Mathematica Policy Research, Inc.

Kowlsen, T. (1991, October). California dreaming. *Washington Health Beat,* 28-29.

McNeil, D. (1991, November 17). Washington tries to sort out health insurance proposals. *New York Times,* 2.

Medicaid-mandated managed care. (1992, June). *Nursing & Health Care, 13*(6), p. 288.

National Case Management Task Force Steering Committee (1991-1992, February 9). *Work summary and survey of case management toward medical case manager certification.* Little Rock, Ark.: Systemedic Corporation.

O'Rourke, B., Raisz, H., & Segal, J. (1982). *Triage II: Coordinated delivery of services to the elderly: Final report.* Volume 1-2. Plainville, Conn.: Triage, Inc.

Pepper Commission (1990, March 2). *Access to healthcare and long-term care for all Americans.* Washington, D.C.: U.S. Bipartisan Commission on Comprehensive Health.

Pollack, R. (1992, January 13). Hospitals ready for reform of national health care system. *AHA News.*

Sager, O. (1992). Certification: From need to reality. *The Case Manager, 3*(3), 81-84.

Sainer, J.S., Brill, R.S., Horowitz, A., Weinstein, M., Dono, J.E., & Korniloff, N. (1984). *Delivery of medical and social services to the homebound elderly: A demonstration of intersystem coordination: Final report.* New York: New York City Department for the Aging.

Seidl, F.W., Applebaum, R., Austin, C., & Mahoney, K. (1983). *Delivering in-home services to the aged and disabled: The Wisconsin experiment.* Lexington, Mass.: Lexington Books.

Strickland, T. (1992, April, May, June). Profile [Interview with Gail R. Wilensky, Deputy Assistant to the President for Policy Development]. *The Case Manager, 3*(2), 72-81.

Wagner, L. (1991, December 9). Cost containment: Carrot or the stick? *Modern Healthcare,* 36-40.

Wooldridge, J., & Schore, J. (1986). *Evaluation of the national long-term care demonstration: Channeling effects on hospital, nursing home, and other medical services.* Princeton, N.J.: Mathematica Policy Research, Inc.

Yordi, C. (1988). Case management in the social health maintenance organization demonstration. *Health Care Financing Review* (Annual Supplement), 83-88.

Zawadski, R.T., Shen, J., Yordi, C., & Hansen, J.C. (1984). *On Lok's community care organization for dependent adults: A research and development project (1978-1983): Final report.* San Francisco: On Lok Senior Health Services.

11

THE MANAGED CARE MARKET

NURSE CASE MANAGEMENT AS A STRATEGY FOR SUCCESS

TINA GERARDI

▼ *CHAPTER OVERVIEW*

Managed care has become the latest *buzz word* in health care policy making in the United States. Coupled with capitation—fixed per member–per month payments—managed care is supposed to solve all of the U.S. health care problems, from rocketing health care costs to perceived shortcomings in health care quality. A whole new industry of specialized managed care periodicals, resource manuals, and conferences has arisen. Remarkably there is little consensus, especially among the public, as to just what managed care actually is. Nurse case managers must understand managed care if they are to navigate the health care delivery system to meet the complex needs of their patients. This chapter describes the basics of managed care and interprets concepts as they relate to the current marketplace. The role of case management as a strategy for success in the managed care market is also discussed.   ▲

WHY MANAGED CARE?

Before World War I, hospitals were only for the most seriously ill patients. Babies were born at home, and family doctors made house calls. The center of care was the home, and financing was pay-as-you-go. Costs were relatively low, since medicine was not that sophisticated. Also, most people could not afford high fees. Only the very wealthy could afford a specialist.

After World War II, antibiotics made advanced surgery and long-term survival possible. New technologies made hospitals the centers of care, where patients came to see specialists. The federal government, through the Hill-Burton Act in 1946, subsidized hospital construction, which led to a hospital construction boom. With the passage of the Medicare and Medicaid bills in 1965, health care became an industry. The incentives were to fill beds and perform more procedures, and hospitals competed to have the best and most advanced facilities, creating a "technological race." Meanwhile, because most of the public were covered by some sort of indemnity insurance coverage, they were insulated from the true cost of care.

The traditional fee-for-service reimbursement system encouraged overutilization. With this type of reimbursement, hospitals and health care providers were reimbursed for each service provided; therefore the more you ordered or provided, the more you were paid. In the 1960s, health industry leaders began to recognize the potential of prepaid group practice plans as mechanisms to contain the dramatic rise in health care costs. The federal government provided the impetus for expanding the number of prepaid health plans through legislation enacted in 1973. The term *health maintenance organization (HMO)* was coined during the Nixon administration.

Soaring insurance premiums in the 1980s caused businesses to reexamine the system for delivering and financing health care. Commercial insurance plans sought to protect their revenue base by writing narrower policies and raising group premiums based on the experience of one individual in the group. Use of services was discouraged by high deductibles and copayments. Staff were hired to review and approve individual cases to reduce inappropriate services. The diagnosis-related group (DRG)–based payment, a fixed rate for specific diagnoses or procedures, was also introduced as a means of controlling escalating health care costs. The utilization review programs and DRG system have been unsuccessful in reducing health care costs.

The predecessors of the HMO include organizations that mutualized costs and provided direct health care services for Venetian seaman in the thirteenth century, for British seamen in the sixteenth century, and for American merchant seamen in 1798. Kaiser-Permanente, the major prototype of the HMO, traces its origins to the 1930s. It developed from a system serving workers building the Los Angeles Aqueduct in 1933, construction workers and their families at the Grand Coulee Dam project in eastern Washington in 1938, and, on a larger scale, Kaiser shipyard employees in and around Portland, Oregon, and San Francisco, and employees of the Kaiser steel plant at Fontana, California, during World War II. The system was open to the public in 1945. Organized consumers formed the Group Health Cooperative of Puget Sound in 1946, and the Health Insurance Plan of Greater New York was organized in 1947.

Several advantages were identified as these organizations emerged:

▼ Assured availability of and access to services through integrated group practices
▼ Evolution and creation of prepaid insurance plans
▼ Budgeting for provision of services
▼ Incentives for health maintenance and preventive health services
▼ Assurance of quality care through the group practice of physicians offering multiple specialties

To control escalating health care costs, payment systems and cost control measures have been discussed, and managed care programs have been reexamined by both the business community and health economists. Managed care is not a new idea, but it will definitely have new implications, particularly for nursing.

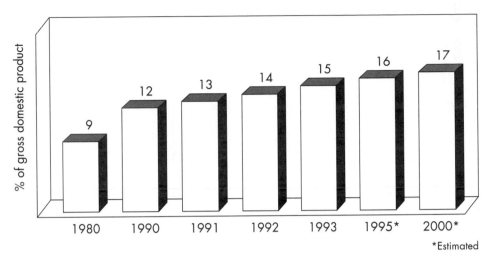

Fig. 11-1   The increase of health care expenses as a percentage of the gross domestic product. (From U.S. Department of Health and Human Services, 1995.)

HOW DOES MANAGED CARE WORK?

Patient care has somehow always been "managed." In many cases, human illness has been managed by the patient and family alone. At other times it has been managed for the patient and family by the health care professional (a gatekeeper) accountable for coordinating all patient health care services and also supplying certain aspects of the patient's health services.

Managed care in its broadest form currently refers to any health care delivery system in which a party other than the health care giver or the patient influences the type of health care delivered. A managed care provider takes the risk for the patient's health care. In this way, rather than simply approving or denying the health benefit, the managed care provider will intervene to provide what it considers to be appropriate health care for the patient.

A montage of managed care organizations has evolved in response to the steady rise in health care costs as a percentage of our gross national product (GNP) (see Fig. 11-1). If health care costs continue to rise at the current level, they will account for 17% of our GNP by the year 2000. Society has decided that the current growth of health care as a proportion of the GNP is more than it is willing to pay. Our average health benefits have increased in a similar vein. The average cost per employee for annual health benefits today is approximately $4,000, as compared to $600 in 1976. Managed care is viewed as an answer to the problems of increasing price, decreasing access, and uncertain quality. In response to these escalating costs, purchasers of health plans, mainly local businesses, have embraced the tenets of managed care and are rapidly making arrangements with HMOs or independent managed care companies.

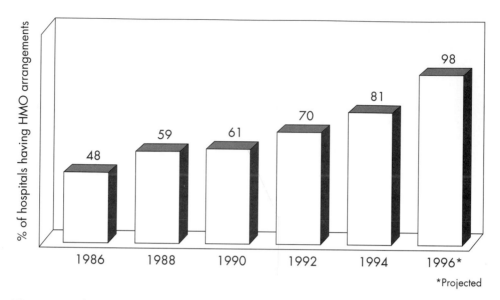

Fig. 11-2   The increase in the percentage of hospitals with HMO arrangements between 1986 and 1996. (Based on data cited in Deloitte & Touche, LLP & HCIA, Inc. *The Comparative performance of U.S. hospitals: The sourcebook* (p. 15). Baltimore: Author.)

According to the Comparative Performance of U.S. Hospitals, the percentage of hospitals with arrangements with HMOs has increased from 48% in 1986 to 98% in 1996 (Fig. 11-2). In traditional fee-for-service plans an individual encounter between a covered individual and the health care system is compensated for by the insuror, if the encounter represents a covered benefit of the patient's plan, subject to deductibles or other contractual reductions in benefits. If the patient does not have insurance coverage or the encounter is not a covered benefit, the patient is liable for the bill. The patient chooses the health care professional or hospital to provide the service based on his or her own criteria. On the other hand, the managed care organization generally presents the patient with a list of health care professionals from which to choose the one to supply a covered benefit. Many managed care plans have specified times during which patients can change health care professionals; therefore once a provider is chosen, it may be difficult to change. Depending on the plan, the patient may be required to see a primary care provider who will be responsible for making all assessments and determinations as to health care needs. Referrals must be initiated by the primary care provider. The patient is likely to have a fixed copayment or fee for every visit, regardless of its complexity, and will probably not need to file insurance papers or be responsible for any other payment. Hospitalizations are likely to be covered entirely with the exception of certain medically unnecessary amenities. Prevention visits such as immunizations, well-baby visits, Pap smears, and mammograms are likely to be covered benefits, with a copayment.

Traditionally, health care providers were physicians and hospitals. Physicians saw patients in their offices and in hospitals or clinics. Managed care has introduced a large number of additional people to the health care delivery system. Many managed care organizations have begun to depend on physician assistants and nurse practitioners to provide services, especially in the areas of primary care. In the "good old days," the choice of hospital was made predominantly by the physician. In a managed care environment the choice is almost entirely made by the payor according to contractual arrangements negotiated for the entire plan. This makes the hospital a provider as well, since many of the covered benefits are provided as part of hospital services. These include home health nursing, pharmacy, physical and occupational therapy, respiratory therapy and ventilator management and dietary counseling to name a few.

To understand the cost control changes to the health care market place, we must first understand the traditional methods for managing health care costs and current managed care structures. Early managed care programs under the guidance of the professional standards review organizations (PSROs) attempted to control costs through cost sharing, education, second opinions for surgery, and incentives to use lower-cost sites of care such as ambulatory surgery. These early plans also assumed that physicians would modify their behavior based on information alone. Unfortunately, none of these early strategies controlled the continuing escalation of costs. However, the key characteristic of the most effective managed care plans was identified: control of cost and utilization. The cost, use, and appropriateness of services rendered by providers are tightly controlled. Providers are selected who are able to provide cost-effective care.

HMOs, preferred provider organizations (PPOs), and indemnity forms of insurance once were distinct products for providing health care benefits. Today the distinctions are disappearing as each product takes on characteristics of the other. Other common managed care structures include exclusive provider organizations (EPOs), independent practice associations (IPAs), and point-of-service (POS) plans. Definitions for each of these plans will be provided in an attempt to clarify this managed care alphabet soup.

HMOs are organized health care delivery systems responsible for both the financing and the delivery of health care services to an enrolled population. There are five common models of HMOs:

1. In **staff model** HMOs the physicians are employed by the HMO to provide covered services to the health plan enrollees. They are usually paid a salary with some bonus or incentive based on performance and productivity.
2. In the **group practice model** HMO the HMO contracts with a multispecialty physician group practice to provide all physician services to the HMO's members. The physician group is technically independent but depends significantly on the HMO contracts for patients. An example of this type of model is the Permanente Medical Group under the Kaiser Foundation Health Plan.
3. In a **network model** a network contracts with more than one group practice to provide physician services to the HMO's members. An example is the Health Insurance Plan (HIP) of Greater New York, which contracts with many multispecialty physician group practices in the New York City area.

4. In the **independent practice association (IPA) model** the HMO contracts with an association of physicians to provide services to its members. Physicians are members of the IPA for purposes of the HMO contract but retain their practices separately and distinctly from each other.
5. **Direct contract models** contract directly with individual physicians to provide services to their members. In direct contracting arrangements the employer contracts directly with the provider to provide health care services, thus eliminating the insurer.

An IPA is an association of individual independent physicians or small physician group practices formed for the purpose of contracting with one or more managed health care organizations. The attractiveness of an IPA structure to HMOs and other managed care organizations is the IPA's ability to provide a large panel of providers and accept payment on a capitated basis.

PPOs are entities through which employer health benefit plans and health insurance carriers contract to purchase health care services for covered beneficiaries from a selected group of participating providers. These providers may include hospitals, physicians, IPAs, or physician-hospital organizations. Most often PPOs negotiate on a basis of discounted fee-for-service charges, all-inclusive per diem rates, or payments based on DRGs. A major difference between PPOs and HMOs is the patient's ability to choose a non-PPO member for covered services, subject to a higher level of deductible and copayment.

EPOs are structured like PPOs but behave much like HMOs in their limitation of choice of providers. HMOs are carefully regulated by specific HMO statutes in the states in which they operate, whereas EPOs are insurance products subject to less rigorous insurance laws.

POS plans contain features of PPO and HMO arrangements. Under POS plans, primary care physicians are reimbursed through fixed per member–per month payments (capitation) or other performance-based reimbursement methods. The primary care provider acts as a gatekeeper for referral and institutional medical services.

Health care providers are responding to the changing market and expansion of managed care products, which place greater emphasis on value, access, and quality of care. Responses to the market include provider's developing organizations that accommodate coordinated care and shared reimbursement. For example, an integrated health care delivery system provides coordinated care that allows participating providers, using economies of scale, to increase productivity, enhance the scope and quality of services, and reduce the administrative burden associated with those services. The goal of a mature, integrated health care delivery system is to become a provider organization that is seamless in its ability to deliver a broad range of health care services. Direct contracting is another financial arrangement that is gaining in popularity in the more mature markets. In direct contracting arrangements the employer contracts directly with the provider to provide health care services, thus eliminating the insurer. The benefits to the provider in this type of arrangement are a known volume of beneficiaries and increased cash flow directly from the employer to the provider, generally on a monthly basis. The employer realizes decreased health care benefit costs and added value of working directly with the provider to realize specific services for their employee population.

RESPONSES TO MANAGED CARE

Provider responses to managed care vary from "bar the doors," to "respond only if pressured," to "let's reach out to the business community and begin strategic planning for these integrated services." The physician community appears to be most affected by the multiple changes in health care. Individual physicians have seen their autonomy and their often unique relationship with patients and families usurped by managed care companies. The individual physician in a solo practice cannot survive under either traditional managed care or any managed competition model. The cost of operating a small business is too high compared to the access to information and the discounted purchasing and discounted contracting provided by a managed care company or required by a health purchasing cooperative. Managed care places new organizational demands on physicians, such as restricted referral and hospital panels, increased bureaucratic overhead from many types of the plans, and an inability to refer out difficult patients. Many physicians view managed care with fear and loathing. Loss of autonomy is the most common fear. As more nurse practitioners are becoming providers in the managed care environment, they may also experience these feelings of loss of autonomy. However, most nurses are experiencing increased opportunities in the managed care arena. Many managed care companies are seeing nurse practitioners and nurse midwives as cost-effective providers of primary care services and are increasing their provider panels to include these health professionals.

Physicians have led attempts to reduce medical costs since the introduction of PSROs in the 1960s. But physician costs account for only about one fifth of the total health care dollar expenditure. They do, however, as gatekeepers control the expenditure of many resources such as diagnostic tests and procedures. Until recently, physician income has not been greatly affected by health care reform. As primary care providers increase their control of specialist care, however, physician income is declining. In response to the pressure to reduce overall costs, physicians have organized into managed care organizations, have worked with hospitals in the development of clinical pathways, and have supported clinical case management in both the acute and community setting.

Since the inception of DRGs in 1983, hospitals have been forced to focus on outcomes, utilization, and cost. For this reason, hospitals are better prepared than physicians for managed care. Physicians were not directly affected by DRGs because as private physicians they were reimbursed for services rendered in the hospital. Providers, such as hospitals, who accept the managed care trend as reality, take a proactive approach to managed care. HMO contracting, network development, integrated service delivery, and the formation of independent managed care organizations have proliferated across the country. Resource allocation in the areas of inpatient care, outpatient care, and continuing care services are being evaluated and analyzed by individual providers as well as by networks. The goal is to be able to deliver seamless health care to specified populations. Inpatient utilization has dramatically decreased as managed care has penetrated certain markets.

Federal and state governments have embraced the tenets of managed care and are actively promoting Medicare and Medicaid managed care programs. Under these programs, Medicare and Medicaid recipients would be enrolled in managed care programs in which they will have a primary care provider from the managed care organization or HMO. They will receive the same access, quality, and cost that other members receive. This is an attempt by the government to reduce costs associated with caring for these distinct populations. Although this may be worthwhile, some experts state that funding for these programs may actually decrease access to or eliminate such benefit services as mental-behavioral health and long-term care. Many states are also seeing managed care declared the panacea for sky rocketing worker's compensation and no-fault costs.

Although there is an impact from managed care in all operational areas of a facility, providers have seen an increase in the need for discharge planning, social services, patient education, and a medical record that will follow the patient across multiple settings in a delivery system. The clinical impact has been evidenced by increased emphasis on length of stay reductions, evaluations of medical practice patterns with the purpose of reducing variation, the development of clinical pathways, and the implementation of case management.

NURSE CASE MANAGEMENT IN A CHANGING ENVIRONMENT

Nurse case managers assist in creating and help to administer a network of services for their patients. The role of case manager was created solely to negotiate for, organize, and evaluate the necessity for using various resources for patient care. Traditionally case managers have operated between the realities of costs or covered services and the perceptions of patients' needs. The role of the case manager supports and embellishes the concepts of managed care.

Many professionals, as well as patients and families, can coordinate multiple services. The increased emphasis on discharge planning and social services highlights the need for professionals in these disciplines to coordinate these aspects of patient care in an efficient and effective manner. However, the more complicated the services become or the more unable the patient or family becomes to coordinate care, the more an official case manager may be needed.

Nurse case managers traditionally have been based in conventional care settings (hospitals, hospices, clinics), dealing with episode-based management. Case managers sequence and organize services from many departments within the organization and are accountable for good financial and clinical outcomes. Nurse case management within the managed care environment has expanded to continuum-based case management in which accountability continues for good financial and clinical outcomes. The coordination of services and resources for the individual with complex needs continues indefinitely while the individual is covered by the managed care organization. In other words, the nurse case manager maintains a relationship with the individual after the disease or episode-specific problem has been resolved. In the area of community health, nurses traditionally have practiced health promotion and disease prevention rather than cure and illness. This prevents the escalation of a person's health condition into a more serious condition. Community health nurses practice collaborative and comprehensive care rather than short-term intervention and episodic care. This integration of health services and health care delivery effects a more efficient use of health care services. Thus the community health care nurse can be an effective nurse case manager. In view of this, managed care programs have a unique opportunity to recognize the value of nursing both economically and in the provision of comprehensive care.

It is important that the nurse case manager understand the contract the managed care organization or HMO has with the provider. This information is valuable in negotiating discharge and other care options for the patient. For example, if the managed care organization has a capitated or per diem financial arrangement with the provider, the organization is more willing to support less expensive settings for care delivery, such as home care, subacute care, or nursing home. However, if the same provider has a DRG payment arrangement with the managed care organization, the organization may be less likely to support home care or a transitional care option until the patient has received inpatient services to cover the DRG prospective payment. In other words, home care may not be approved to expedite discharge, even though it is a covered benefit, until the patient has reached the DRG length of stay in the inpatient setting. In this instance the nurse case manager will need strong negotiation skills coupled with knowledge of the managed care financing system to advocate for the best quality care option for the patient.

As the nurse case manager identifies conflicts between managed care organization financing and quality of care issues, they should be brought to the attention of the provider administration. This information can be tracked and used in future contract negotiations with the managed care organization.

Nurse case managers are taking the lead in the development of clinical pathways, practice guidelines, and outcomes measurements. Their knowledge of the health care environment and complex patient needs, coupled with their education and training, have given them the opportunity to lead multidisciplinary teams to develop cost-effective models of care that achieve positive patient outcomes and increased practitioner and patient satisfaction.

There are tremendous opportunities for nurse case managers in community-based practices in which they assist individuals in managing both their health and their illnesses. Nurse case managers, who traditionally have dealt only with acute care, are now following up individuals beyond the walls of the facility into the clinic, home, and long-term care facility and assisting in coordinating services to keep them well. These practitioner-based models require sound financial and clinical judgment, as well as keen physical and psychosocial assessment skills. Some case management practices focus more on interaction with the individual by telephone rather than in person. Many managed care organizations prefer the telephone approach because of the decrease in overhead costs; however, it is impossible to measure the cost of losing the in-person interaction with the patient and family. Traditionally, nurse case managers have believed that in identifying patient needs, nothing compares with the opportunity to use all their senses in a complete face-to-face, patient or family assessment. This assessment, coupled with sound financial and resource management of the individual's health benefits, will result in the goals of managed care: high quality, accessible care at the lowest possible cost. Nurse case management should never be considered a replacement for accountability in each professional discipline at the direct care level; for complex cases, however, there is no substitute for an effective nurse case management program.

Nurse case management also provides an excellent opportunity for the profession to increase public awareness of the role and image of nursing in the health care delivery system: to educate the consumer, the provider, and the payor as to the expertise of the nurse case manager, the registered professional nurse, and the advanced practice nurse. As one looks to the future, nursing research needs to validate the positive effect of nurse case management on health care costs, access to services, quality of services, and customer satisfaction.

SUGGESTED READINGS

Blendon, R.J., et al. (1993). Physician's perspectives on caring for patients in the United States, Canada, and West Germany. *New England Journal of Medicine, 328*(9), 621-627,

Deloitte and Touche, LLP and HCIA, Inc. (1995). *The comparative performance of U.S. hospitals: The sourcebook.* Baltimore; Author.

Fuchs, V.R. (1990). The health sector's share of the gross national product. *Science, 247,* 534-538.

Kavaler, F., & Zavin, S. (1992). Health care for seamen in the port of New York. *New York State Journal of Medicine, 92*(8), 353-358.

Kongstvedt, P.R. (Ed.). (1993). *The managed health care handbook* (2nd ed.). Gaithersburg, Md: Aspen.

Kongstvedt, P.R. (Ed.). (1995). *Essentials of managed care.* Gaithersburg, Md: Aspen.

Reinhardt, U.E. (1995). Turning our gaze from bread and circus games. *Health Affairs, 14* (2),33-36.

Saward, E.W., & Fleming, S. (1980). Health maintenance organizations. *Scientific American, 243*(4),47-53.

Sonnefeld, S.T., et al. (1991, Fall). Projections of the national health expenditures through the year 2000, *Health Care Financing.*

IV

THE PLANNING PROCESS

12

ASSESSING THE SYSTEM AND CREATING AN ENVIRONMENT FOR CHANGE

▼ *CHAPTER OVERVIEW*

Successful implementation of a case management system begins with a solid, well-conceived plan. The first step in creating the plan is to assess the system in which the case management model will be implemented. Human and financial resources should be reviewed. This information helps determine the degree of change that the organization can tolerate and the chances for a successful conversion.

Implementation involves a nine-step process. Target patient populations are identified and matched to nursing units, and the design structure for the units is decided. This new structure involves a change in the staff mix. The next step is formation of interdisciplinary groups. These groups consist of the case manager, physician(s), social worker, and any other pertinent health care professionals. Benchmarks, which determine how the change will be monitored and evaluated over time, must be selected. Before implementation takes place, preimplementation data must be collected. The next step involves educating staff, physicians, and other professionals who will be affected by conversion to the case management model. At this stage training is provided for the case managers. After managers are educated on how the model works, it can be implemented. Finally, evaluation should take place at predetermined intervals. Necessary changes should be made as quickly as possible. ▲

FEASIBILITY OF THE MODEL

Converting to a case management model requires systematic planning. A solid plan that has been well thought out guarantees a higher rate of successful conversion. Without a plan, it is likely that the expected outcome of the model will be lost or that some important elements will be left out.

Administrators have always known that a plan is essential for change in any organization. This philosophy is no less true for nurses attempting to create a major change such as a conversion to a case management model. The first step in any planning process is to determine if the change is not only feasible but also worthwhile. The potential for success and the effect such a change will have on the organization must be evaluated from both a positive and negative perspective. Overall the change should lead the organization in a positive direction.

ASSESSMENT OF RESOURCES

Assessing resources requires some homework. A thorough analysis of the organization, including its structure and financial status, needs to be done. Those implementing the change need to determine if the organization is strong enough to withstand the temporary instability that will accompany the change. As with any major change, errors will be made along the way. The complete support of all top administrators and a commitment to the long haul are absolutely necessary. In the beginning the road will be a bumpy one, and everyone concerned should be aware of this and should be ready to be supportive every step of the way.

THE COST OF IMPLEMENTATION

A case management system can be implemented with few additional costs for the organization if the change is implemented carefully. For instance, good choices for the pilot program would be units that have current openings or units that have budgeted for an additional person. Such an opening can then be filled by someone qualified to be a case manager. In this way the new position will not incur any costs outside of those already budgeted. This is essential for a plan that must show success before it receives an allotment in the budget. Internal and preexisting resources can then be used for implementation.

If possible, the organization's budget should allow for certain expenditures needed for implementation. These expenditures will probably not be related to personnel costs unless the organization decides to hire a project manager. Costs may be incurred for documentation system changes or for data collection and statistical analysis necessary for measuring success.

Both administrative and financial support must be obtained before switching over to a case management system.

INTERNAL MARKETING

Obtaining the support of those in senior management is relatively easy if the administrators already have some familiarity with the model. Senior management may have heard or read about the model and already have realized the need for such a change. Conversely, they may have misconceptions or may be misinformed about the model. Senior management might also object to the change solely because it comes at an inopportune time.

National managed care infiltration has now created an environment in which most forward thinking organizations recognize that systems must be implemented that will truly and consistently control cost and quality. Infiltration may be real or anticipated. In either case, senior administrators must support a conceptual and actual shift to case management. This process is much less difficult than it was even 5 years ago. Status quo is no longer an option, and each organization must determine what changes it needs to make to support a constantly changing health-care environment.

Senior management support is a prerequisite for beginning the change process. The ways in which the change may be attained will be as diverse as the management styles of the individuals involved. Making sure that administrators are familiar with those initiating the change and that they have positive working relationships with them will be essential for success.

Furthermore, the concept of the case management system should be introduced by someone who is familiar with the administrator, the president, the executive vice president of operations, the chief financial officer, or some other executive of the organization. Use of an outside consultant to introduce the concept may provide the catalyst the organization needs for change. The individual who introduces the concept to the administrator must have the facts of implementation readily available. Estimated cost, staffing needs, and time frames must be prepared for the first meeting. Expected outcomes, goals, and long-range plans should also be presented. A review of other organizations that have implemented the concept and have had positive results will lend credibility to the proposed plan.

It may be necessary to explain the definition of case management from a nursing perspective if the administrator has no previous knowledge of the model. Emphasis should be placed on how the model will benefit all disciplines. Finally, but possibly most important, is the need to review the financial implications of such a conversion. An initiative whose goal is to reduce patient length of stay may be the best selling feature in today's financial climate. An explanation as to why a nurse may be best suited to monitor this process may take some extra effort. Many people believe that social work, utilization review, or the physicians themselves should be the facilitators and coordinators of the care plan. Other initiatives aimed at reducing length of stay may already have been attempted. The failure of these initiatives may help convince administrators to try a new approach. Do not fail to emphasize that although nursing drives the process, all disciplines must take part in achieving success. The input and participation of all health care providers is an essential component too. The keys to case management's success are its nursing and its interdisciplinary approaches.

Within the prospective payment system, length of stay can determine financial success or failure. However, in a discussion of how case management affects a reduction in length of stay, the ways in which length of stay affects quality should also be emphasized. The cost/quality ratio as it relates to case management needs to be reviewed. Any initiative that reduces length of stay without looking at quality and resources, is doomed to fail the organization and the patients.

Although length of stay continues to be the clearest and most tangible way to measure financial success, other measures may add additional credibility. If available, a cost-accounting system will help identify reductions in the use or misuse of hospital resources. Other parallel reductions must also be seen. If the length of stay is reduced but the amount of resources is simply collapsed into fewer days, then true financial savings are less likely.

In managed care reimbursement systems, shortened length of stay and overall cost reductions remain extremely important. Capitated or per diem managed care rates still require serious and consistent cost reductions.

The support of nursing administration is another vital component. Nurse managers and upper managers need to support the concept fully to achieve success. Some suspicion may initially be felt as nursing roles change. The nurse manager may feel threatened by the introduction of another individual who is also managing care on the unit. Other departments most directly involved in the change process, and from whom support is needed, include social work, utilization management, and discharge planning. Initial and on-going support is essential here.

Before the advent of the prospective payment system, flex time, increased severity levels, and technology, it was the nurse manager who carried out many of the role functions associated with case management, such as facilitation and coordination of patient care services. As the nurse manager's role expanded and became more administrative, the nurse had less time to focus on facilitating and coordinating the progression of patient care. Emphasize that the new concept will allow the nurse manager to concentrate more on administrative functions, which will in turn mean patients receive a higher quality of care. Reducing the sense of personal threat is essential to effecting a positive change.

Downsizing and restructuring in health care organizations has in many cases eliminated the assistant director of nursing position. There is often no nursing administrator between the nurse manager and the director of nursing. Elimination of this position has placed a greater administrative responsibility on the nurse manager. Add accelerated hospital stays to the equation, and the result is a less than efficient system.

Case managers, if provided with the authority and accountability necessary, can become the clinical eyes and ears for the nurse manager. Additionally, another fallout of the downsizing era has been elimination of many nurse educator positions. Perhaps among the most dangerous of reductions, removal of nurse educator positions has meant that unit-based staff development has suffered. This is particularly true for new staff nurses who need significant and consistent on-going support. Although traditionally case managers have focused on patient and family education, in downsized environments they may need to incorporate staff education. This may take the form of case conferences or unit-based inservices geared toward specific clinical issues.

STAFF INTEGRATION

If the nursing chief executive was the one who initiated the change to case management, then the staff might already accept the change. If this is the case, then conversation with this group should concentrate on explaining the case management concept thoroughly and the changes it will bring.

The need to educate and fully enlist the support of the staff nurses cannot be emphasized enough. If the organization has decided to create the case manager position as a staff position, then staff nurses must be fully aware of the role. The job expectations of the case manager should be clear. If available, the job description should be distributed and reviewed. The role of the case manager in relation to other nursing positions should be made as clear as possible.

As with the introduction of any new position, there might be some initial role blending, role conflict, or both. This can be minimized through open discussion and ongoing review of the role after implementation. Nurses should anticipate that roles and responsibilities will evolve over time. The fluid nature of the position means it can be improved and enhanced as a part of the evaluation process. Some role blending and confusion related to the changing roles of nursing and other disciplines, particularly social work and utilization management, can be expected. Job descriptions must be reviewed and amended to reflect the changing roles of all members of the health care team.

The collaborative nature of the model means that all disciplines must support it. At the top of this list are the physicians. Getting the involvement of both medical physicians and surgeons will require varying techniques, with emphasis placed on the outcomes that are achievable for their patients. Rogers says, "It is important to use nurses well known to the physicians, who have a history of solid communication, mutual trust, clinical experience, and an overall positive experiential record. This serves to gain the initial support of physicians who might otherwise be resistant."*

For the surgeon who is reimbursed on a case basis, the incentive to discharge the patient more rapidly is a financial one because the discharge of one patient allows for the admission of the next. In addition, surgeons traditionally have treated patients in a protocoled manner. In this setting the applicability of the case management approach is easily understood and appreciated. Because the surgical patient generally runs a predictable course of recovery, care can be planned in an organized way. For this reason, surgeons will probably be those most receptive to implementation of the concept.

The medical physician, however, may pose a greater challenge. Within the prospective payment system and most managed care contracts no financial incentives motivate these professionals to discharge patients more rapidly. Furthermore, it may be more difficult to predict the course of events for a particular medical diagnosis or condition.

Incentives motivating the medical physician toward an appreciation of the case management approach will probably not be based on length-of-stay improvements unless these length-of-stay reductions are tied to quality issues. For example, are significant days added to the hospital stay during which little or nothing is being done for the patient? Emphasizing that improved quality of care will result may be one way to enlist physician support. Emphasis on the role of the case manager in assuring, with the multidisciplinary action plan, that the physician's best plan is initiated and followed may also help enlist support.

In some cases other initiatives may be useful. If the institution has several medical diagnoses whose lengths of stay are beyond state or federal averages, these should be targeted for initial intervention. In these cases the chief physician may need to intervene. Essentially a practice guideline would be established that all physicians caring for a particular type of patient would be expected to follow. Whenever possible, active and positive participation is preferred.

---

*Rogers, M. (1992). Personal communication.

Chart review and research are other techniques used to sell a treatment plan for a particular medical condition. Chart review often uncovers many ways for treating a medical problem. Each plan may not be equally effective, financially appropriate concerning resource use, or equally appropriate in terms of length of stay. By using chart review, inappropriate physician and nursing treatment interventions can be enhanced. The way other institutions treat particular types of problems can be used as a resource in determination of the best possible treatment plan.

If the organization supports the notion that decreased variation in treatment will reduce costs and improve quality, then more aggressive measures may be necessary. For example, if all admitted patients are to be treated under a particular case management plan, then a mandate from the president of the organization may be necessary. In other words, if there is a case management plan available for a particular case type, all patients admitted who match that case type should be treated consistently. Regardless of whether the patient is a service or private-pay patient or of whether the attending is in full agreement, that practice plan is initiated for that patient. This sort of global support may not be possible without a decree from a top administrator who has the power to demand uniform clinical management.

Standardized treatment plans are a great resource and asset for the resident or intern house staff. In addition, the case manager serves as a skilled resource for the new physician who is rotating through a particular nursing unit and is unfamiliar with the patient's present or past condition. In addition, the case manager helps the house officer elicit quick and accurate information. Ongoing dialogue between the two helps assure that the best plan will be implemented and carried out.

Case management will not be completely successful without the support and cooperation of ancillary departments. It is doubtful that an ancillary department will have an objection to the model, although passive support is not enough to ensure success. To empower the case manager, a contact person in each department should be assigned to whom needs or concerns about patients can be referred.

Some areas will play a bigger part than others. For example, the radiology department plays a key role in some length-of-stay issues. Appropriate scheduling of tests in terms of order and timeliness is crucial to an early diagnosis and treatment. Appropriate preps also ensure that the patient's movement through the hospital is smooth.

Other ancillary departments, which play a key role in the case management model, are the admitting office, the DRG office, and the medical records department. Failure to obtain the support and commitment of these departments will create problems during implementation and evaluation of the model.

Clearly other direct care providers must be fully supportive and committed for the model to be most effective. Key areas for such support include social work, physical therapy, and nutrition. The patient problem or surgery determines the areas most vital at any particular time, but certainly each department should be fully educated and agreeable before implementation.

Most ancillary departments appreciate the opportunity to work collaboratively with other disciplines. Nursing is not the only discipline plagued by frustration because of the divergent directions taken by each group of providers.

PLANNED CHANGE

A plan for implementation will provide the foundation for successful change. Each element outlined in this chapter should be evaluated and acted upon if appropriate for the institution. Planning for implementation should be carefully thought out and choreographed. The nine-step plan for implementation outlined in the box provides the foundation for the plan and identifies subsequent changes. This nine-step process provides a structure for planning any implementation program. Each element will be reviewed, and each aspect should be covered during the planning process. The ordering of each step may vary depending on the institution, and certain steps may occur simultaneously.

Clearly the order is not as important as the actual carrying out of each step. This implementation process should be shared with everyone in the organization as the process is begun. The plan's steps for implementation, the ways in which those steps will be carried out, and the method of evaluation should be shared openly so that all those concerned have a chance to give input.

Because it will be advantageous to demonstrate some immediate success, selecting where to begin will be important. A bad choice may mean failure or the cancellation of plans for adding units or teams to the model.

Step 1: Define Target Populations for Case Management

Target patient populations should be selected on the basis of the following factors:
- ▼ Volume of discharges
- ▼ Variance from length-of-stay standards
- ▼ Variance from length-of-stay at similar institutions
- ▼ Feasibility of developing managed care plans
- ▼ Potential for control of resource consumption
- ▼ Opportunity for improvement in quality of care

If the organization's goal for implementation is to improve quality of care, this may be an additional factor to take into consideration during the selection process. This determination can be made through chart reviews of targeted populations.

NINE-STEP PLAN FOR IMPLEMENTATION

1. Define target populations for case management.
2. Define target areas.
3. Agree on design structure for areas selected.
4. Form collaborative practice groups.
5. Choose benchmarks.
6. Collect preimplementation data.
7. Provide advanced skills and knowledge.
8. Implement model.
9. Evaluate model.

Step 2: Define Target Areas

Once the selection of patient populations has been made, these patients should be matched to appropriate clinical areas. In some cases the type of patient group selected may not be found in one particular area of the hospital; therefore a *non-unit-based* case management team approach may be more appropriate.

In other cases it will be possible to gather patients from a designated geographic area. The more homogeneous the patient population on a nursing unit, the fewer the resources needed in terms of physicians and managed care plans. Thus a greater number of patients will be positively affected by the model.

Step 3: Agree on Design Structure for Areas Selected

Once the nursing unit, geographic area, or patient type has been selected, the design structure should be determined. If a *unit-based* model is being introduced, a determination must be made as to how many case managers will be on the unit. This decision will be based on the number of patient beds, the severity of the patients, the average length of stay, and the available resources. If only one position is available for conversion, this may be the deciding factor.

If a *non-unit-based* case management model is being implemented, different factors will need to be taken into consideration. Most case management teams have members from several disciplines. Therefore this type of team may require a greater number of resources for implementation. A physician, nurse, social worker, and others need to be deployed. This may mean taking them away from other jobs or assignments, thereby requiring a greater financial commitment from the organization. The disciplines represented will depend on the particular clinical type being followed by the team. For example, a diabetes team will clearly need a nutritionist and a social worker. Consultants with an affiliation to the team might include a podiatrist or an ophthalmologist.

Step 4: Form Collaborative Practice Groups

In the *unit-based* model the teams will have a fluid structure, and the members of the team will be constantly changing. The only constant member will be the unit-based case manager. The patient, physician, social worker, and so on will change as the professionals assigned to the patient change. For each new patient the case manager will need to gather a team, identify who is responsible for which aspects of the care plan, and ensure that everyone is working toward the same goals.

In the *non-unit-based* case management model the professional team members will remain constant, and the only changing member will be the patient. In this model the team members and their respective roles are clearly defined up front, so there is no need to bring the group together.

Step 5: Choose Benchmarks

As discussed in another chapter, choosing the outcome measures or benchmarks is an important step. Benchmarks must be selected as early as possible and certainly before implementation. The method of evaluation will depend on the outcome measures chosen and the resources available for tracking the data.

Step 6: Collect Preimplementation Data

Once the benchmarks have been selected, the method for data collection should be determined. The time frames should be documented in advance, and the individuals responsible for the various elements should be identified.

It may be necessary and appropriate to enlist the help of employees from other departments who have access to certain data. For example, a representative from the DRG office or the medical records department might be assigned the responsibility of monitoring and tracking the length-of-stay data.

A representative from the quality improvement department might be recruited to track quality-of-care data on a quarterly basis. In some cases, it may even be possible to use students to assist with staff and patient questionnaires. A patient representative might be another good choice of someone to help with patient satisfaction questionnaires.

Regardless of the data being evaluated, baseline data sets must be established before education or implementation of the model. If the staff is being tested via questionnaires, those questionnaires must be distributed and returned before implementation. Some of the data will be retrospective; therefore the actual time when the data is pulled together will not be as important.

Step 7: Provide Advanced Skills and Knowledge

In Chapter 12 the elements of a good educational program are reviewed and discussed. It is critical that employees from all departments understand the general concepts of a case management system. To attain such understanding, an educational program may be offered, but the extent of such a program will depend on the resources available.

The case managers should be provided with as extensive a program as possible. It cannot be assumed that an employee comes to the position with the skills and knowledge necessary to carry out the role effectively. An investment and commitment from the organization for providing advanced skills and knowledge will help develop highly effective case managers. The need for education cannot be overemphasized.

To prevent contamination of subjects, educational preparation must follow any preimplementation data collection. This maintains the integrity of the study sample.

Step 8: Implement Model

Once all the previous steps have been accomplished, the model can be effectively implemented. The date for beginning should be clearly communicated. The case management documentation system that has been selected may or may not be in place; although it is desirable, it is not essential. The case manager can begin changing the system immediately after entering the position. Having the case manager begin the changes might be the only practical way because other employees will not have the time or advanced skills necessary to make this change.

The question is often asked, "How do we begin?" The answer to this question is simple—*by beginning*. The transition phase, or the time between announced implementation and a full integration of the change, may be as long as a year or more. Therefore, after completing all pre-implementation steps, the case manager can work in the change gradually. It will take many months for all those involved to adjust to the system.

This time period will require communication with other members of the health care team, letting them know that the changeover has taken place and exactly what that means to them and to the organization. The more open and candid the communication, the more likely the change will be accepted. The beginning is when many organizations falter because they expect much of the change to have already been made. This expectation, however, is not practical. Everyone must understand in advance that the bulk of the changes will be phased in slowly.

Step 9: Evaluate Model

Evaluation of the model involves rigorous data collection and analysis. Unit VI will cover the evaluation process in detail. The time frames for analysis will be driven by the data elements themselves. It will be appropriate for some data, such as length of stay, to be collected and analyzed on a monthly basis. Other data, such as patient satisfaction, may only need to be tracked every 6 months. Annual tracking of staff satisfaction will be sufficient.

In addition to this formal data collection and analysis, an informal evaluation should be ongoing. Those responsible for the model should never forget to query practitioners who work within the model on a day-to-day basis at the patient bedside. Through discussions with the staff nurses and others, problem areas can be identified and corrective action taken. This ongoing dialogue may continue for 1 to 2 years while the change is being integrated. As the model expands, more and more employees will be affected. Barriers for successful integration will continue to appear as the model expands in sophistication and sphere of influence.

13

EDUCATING EMPLOYEES

PREPARING FOR SUCCESSFUL IMPLEMENTATION

▼ *CHAPTER OVERVIEW*

Education is an essential element in successful implementation of a case management model. This chapter reviews the two types of curricula required for implementation of a case management model. The first program, a general orientation to a case management model, is geared to a wide array of health care practitioners. The second program is a 3-day seminar designed to educate and train potential case managers. This chapter provides topical outlines and objectives for each program. ▲

CURRICULUM DEVELOPMENT

Since case management's introduction in 1985, implementation has often called for elaborate planning, meetings, time, and commitment. What has been lacking to this point is a formal means of educating the staff nurses, case managers, and other personnel who might be interacting with the case manager.

Although case management theory has been introduced into some under-graduate as well as graduate curricula, those employees already in the health care field probably have not been introduced to the concepts through formal education. Therefore, education is a key element of success. The length of the institution's educational program will depend on the time that workers can take from their units to attend classroom instruction. For the most part the concepts of case management are relatively new to most employees, so didactic methods are important.

The amount of time set aside for instruction can range from 3 to 6 or more hours. However, the longer the program, the less likely it will be that employees from other disciplines will be able to be included. Although it is crucial that all staff nurses and ancillary nursing personnel attend these introductory sessions, it is also impor-tant for members of other disciplines to participate. The number of hours that these employees can be present in the program will depend on the staffing patterns of their departments. Although other disciplines may be committed to the case management model, they may not have the financial or personnel resources to allow workers to leave their jobs for more than 1 hour. For off-peak shifts, participation may be even less possible. It may be necessary to provide different programs of varying lengths to ensure that everyone can attend. It is the material that is important here, not the length of the program.

The topical outline for an introduction to a case management program should contain the following essential elements. Development of the curriculum should reflect all elements and characteristics of the case management process (Torres & Stanton, 1982). Other topics might be added, depending on the needs of the organization. The more preparation and education provided to all members of the organization, the higher the chance for success. Even those departments not directly involved with the program should be invited to attend. Although it may not be immediately obvious, areas such as the pharmacy or the radiology department eventually will be affected by a switch to case management. At the very least, all administrators and executive management should be encouraged to attend. Those involved in operations in the hospital can provide valuable insight into elements of the successful functioning of the model. Other departments—such as medicine, social work, quality assurance, discharge planning, utilization review, the patient represen-tative department, nutrition, medical records, and admitting—are vital to the success of a case management model. Even though some individuals in these departments may be familiar with the case management concept, it is still important to educate them on how case management will be implemented in their organization. Such instruction will help prevent misunderstandings.

MULTIDISCIPLINARY EDUCATION

The content of a program geared to a broad audience must be general enough to hold the attention of a wide range of health care providers, administrators, and operations personnel. This is no easy task. Specific examples of how case management might affect some of these workers will be helpful and should be included in the program.

It is vital to begin the presentation with an overview of case management. This overview should include the evolution of nursing delivery models. This information will provide the groundwork from which to start. Next, explain the relevance of case management in light of today's health care issues. Covering such topics will answer the "Why case management?" and "Why now?" questions. An understanding of the changes in health care reimbursement, downsizing and restructuring, changes in the current patient population, and other health care issues will help explain why case management is timely and essential for the continued success of most health care organizations. This framework for discussion will enable the audience to see that case management is not just a nursing project or a nursing problem. Not only does case management need them; they also need case management.

Empowering the Case Manager

Introduction of the case manager and introduction of the case management plans are the two most essential changes to occur with the implementation of a case manage-ment model. Although many, more-subtle changes will occur, these are the two changes from which all the others will come.

Table 13-1   General orientation program content outline

OBJECTIVES	CONTENT

Define the concepts of case management.	Overview
	    A conceptual framework for case management
	    Evolution of nursing delivery models

Describe the role of the case manager.	Review
	    Job description
	    Job responsibilities
	    Daily operations
	    Relationship to other disciplines

Understand the changing roles of the health care team in case management.	Social work Discharge planning Utilization management Physicians

Explain the relationship between the prospective payment system and case management; explain the use of case management plans; review managed care reimbursement.	DRGs
	    Definition/changes in reimbursement
	    Relationship and link to case management
	    Use of managed care plans and their relationship to DRGs

Identify the case management outcomes for research.	Research outcomes
	    Improved registered nurse satisfaction
	    Decreased burnout
	    Decreased length of stay
	    Improved patient satisfaction
	    Improved quality of care

The case manager must be empowered, and one technique for empowering is ensuring that everyone in the organization knows what a case manager does and how the case manager fits into workers' daily routines. If a case manager calls to speak to the patient representative and the patient representative does not understand the case manager's role and function, problems arise.

It is also essential for other disciplines' roles to be reviewed and clearly understood. Most immediately affected will be the social workers, utilization managers, discharge planners, and physicians.

Each discipline should have an understanding and appreciation for the other's roles and responsibilities. This mutual respect and understanding will help facilitate a smoother transition as role functions and responsibilities are reallocated.

Topical Outline

A curriculum that addresses a wide audience can cover an array of topics that are relevant to all employees (see Table 13-1). The following is a list of possible topics:
- ▼ Define the concepts of case management.
- ▼ Describe the role of the case manager.

▼ Understand the changing roles of the health care team in case management.
▼ Define the relationship between the prospective payment system and case management.
▼ Review the managed care reimbursement system.
▼ Understand the use of the case management plan.
▼ Identify the case management outcomes for evaluation or research.

Defining the concepts of case management can be extensive or limited, depending on the audience. An overview should include discussion of previous nursing care delivery models, current health care crises, and health care reimbursement methods in reference to case management. An in-depth discussion of the prospective payment system and managed care reimbursements is essential.

Discussion should include the evolution of the functional, team, and primary models and how these models relate to the case management model. After all, case management combines elements of team and primary nursing models.

Because the institutions may implement either a unit-based, free-floating, or combined case management model, the subtle variations should be explored and discussed. This discussion should include the ways in which the various versions are structured, organized, and implemented.

The changing role of each member of the health care team is an important element of the discussion. Current role functions should be discussed as well as how roles will change under case management.

Finally, a general overview of the expected outcomes of the case management model should be covered. The expected outcomes provide a relevant arena from which to set the case management goals for the organization as well as for the individual workers.

A Conceptual Framework for Case Management

Any discussion of case management must take place in a context of cost and quality. Case management provides the process, structure, and outcomes that control the quality of care while reducing cost. An understanding of this framework and overall goals will provide the context for the discussions that follow. A review of how case management as a contemporary and interdisciplinary care delivery system can enhance hospital revenues is essential.

Role of the Case Manager

During implementation, many false conceptions of the role of the case manager develop, usually because of a lack of understanding. Professionals from other disciplines may draw their own conclusions as to what the case manager should or should not be doing. Although some role blending is necessary, education is the main way to avoid role confusion (Kahn, Wolfe, Quinn, Snoeck, & Rosenthal, 1964).

The case manager job description should be distributed during the educational sessions, or at the very least, it should be reviewed. This is the first step in distinguishing the roles and responsibilities of the case manager. Such steps will help ensure that other disciplines will respect the boundaries of the case manager's job description and will not expect the manager to function beyond it. It is possible that some workers may expect case managers to be less influential than their job descriptions indicate. Others may expect duties beyond the scope of their job descriptions. A clear description of the role set forth in the beginning will help minimize misunderstandings (O'Malley, 1988).

A clear way in which to define and illustrate the job functions of the case manager is through a description of daily operations, as well as a description of what the case manager's typical day might be like. It is not uncommon to be asked, *What exactly does a case manager do?* Like many jobs of this nature, the specific tasks are often invisible or intangible or both. Once again, the theoretic framework of the model and the expected outcomes should be emphasized.

Reviewing the Health Care Reimbursement Systems

Case management's basic premise is that expected outcomes of care can be achieved within appropriate time frames. A portion of the curriculum should be devoted to reviewing the present health care reimbursement systems. It is around these systems that much of case management is built (Hartley, 1986). Other points to be covered should include how DRGs work and how these predetermined lengths of stay determine reimbursement rates.

DRGs are used in case management to help determine the number of days on which to base case management plans. This relationship should be defined in detail. Other uses of case management plans should also be reviewed, including the ways in which they are used to maintain quality in an accelerated health care system. The links between quality and cost in a case management environment should be reviewed.

The effects of managed care infiltration should provide an additional context for case management. Whether the issue is capitated rates or per diem reimbursements, length of stay and resource allocation remain important. The processes applied through case management are applicable within the context of the prospective payment system or managed care. Discussion should include reviews of each.

Projected Outcomes

The projected outcomes of the model can be covered next. The general goals of any case management model and the specific goals of the organization should be covered. This section will include topics such as improved quality of care, improved caregiver satisfaction, improved patient satisfaction, decreased length of stay, and decreased resource utilization.

Once again, the length and detail of this program must be determined by the audience and the amount of time that can be allotted by the various departments.

CASE MANAGER EDUCATION

Several days should be devoted to educating the case managers. It cannot be assumed that nurses newly promoted to the role of case manager can function without training. Individual organizations will need to decide the person(s) best qualified to provide this education. In some cases, outside consultants or experts in the field may be needed to provide this service.

In a 3-day program, two of the days should be devoted to case management concepts, and one day should be devoted to leadership/management training. It is possible that nurses promoted to case management roles will have had no experience in either managing or case management.

Day 1

The differences between leadership and management should be explained during the first day (see Table 13-2). Functioning as a case manager will require the use of both skills (Holle & Blatchley, 1987).

Some topics to be covered might be the qualities of a leader, the correlation between administrative style and the nursing process, contingency management theory, and accountability versus responsibility. Although the case manager role is not identifiable as a management position in the traditional sense, it is essential that the case manager understand these concepts and be able to use them to effect the changes necessary for achieving excellent outcomes.

The case manager will, at the least, be managing patient care. This will be accomplished through the facilitation and coordination aspects of the role. Additionally the case manager will be managing the health care team by assuring that the interdisciplinary plan of care is in place and moving along in a timely fashion. These two elements of the role require excellent management skills. These management skills need to be coupled with strong leadership skills to be maximally effective.

The case manager must be empowered. A portion of this perceived empowerment must be inherent in the individual assuming the role (Bennis & Nanus, 1985). A working knowledge of the theories of power and their relationship to the role of the case manager should be included in the curriculum. Case managers should understand that their personal power sources are as related to their personal style as those found in the job description. Strategies for obtaining as well as using power should be reviewed. A positive use of power will enhance self-esteem and bring more effectiveness to the role.

Implementation of a case management model involves subtle as well as obvious changes. It has been said that change is painful, but just how painful depends on the level of organizational support as well as individual support. Understanding the stages and processes of change can help decrease the difficulties associated with change. Whether the organization is large or small, complex or simple, change is never easy and seldom goes smoothly. If the case manager understands this in advance, any difficulties can be lessened along with the possible ambiguities experienced by other workers with whom the manager comes in contact.

The specific theory of change used by the instructor is not as important as conveying the message that the conversion to case management will be bumpy and that some days will not be productive or fulfilling. Nevertheless, the case manager should understand the techniques for effecting positive change and the conditions that make change more acceptable.

Implementation will always involve some resistance. A portion of the organization will accept the change immediately; some will be resistant; and others will remain in the middle of the road reserving their judgment until they see the model in action for themselves. It will be impossible to win everyone over, and the case manager should understand this. Approaches to reducing resistance to change might be employed to help make the transition as smooth as possible.

Table 13-2 Case manager education day 1 content outline

OBJECTIVES	CONTENT

Define leadership vs. management.	Leadership vs. management
	  Definitions of leadership and management
	  Qualities of a leader
	  Difference between administrative process and nursing process
	  Contingency management (situational management)
	  Accountability vs. responsibility

Describe power and its uses for a case manager.	Definition of power
	  Definition of power
	  Five sources of power
	  Constructive and destructive uses of power
	  Strategies to obtain power

Identify the change process.	Change theory
	  Three types of change
	    Technical
	    Structural
	    People oriented
	  Lewin's Phases of Change
	    Freezing
	    Moving
	    Exploring
	    Refreezing
	    Implementation
	  Effecting positive change in management
	  Ten conditions that make change acceptable
	  Approaches to decreasing resistance to change

Relate the concepts of power and change.	Relationship between power and change
	  Empowerment
	  Change – empowerment·
	  empowerment = change

Demonstrate effective communication techniques.	Communication
	  Do's and don'ts of effective communication
	  Active listening
	  Assertive vs. aggressive behavior
	  Conflict
	    Source
	    Resolutions
	  Problem-solving strategies

Continued.

Table 13-2   Case manager education day 1 content outline—cont'd

OBJECTIVES	CONTENT

Describe the process of patient education.	Patient education
	    Adult learning principles
	    Strategies for effective teaching and
	      learning

State the legal rights of patients.	Legal rights of patients
	    Patient bill of rights
	    Health care proxy
	    Living will
	    Do-not-resuscitate (DNR) laws

Implement discharge planning process.	Discharge planning
	    Collaborative process
	    Assessment and planning
	    Referrals to provide continuity of care

Power and change are interrelated concepts. An empowered individual is in a better position to effect change. At the same time, the more change effected, the more empowered the individual becomes.

The effectiveness of any leader or manager depends on the styles of communication used. A substantial portion of the curriculum should be devoted to teaching effective communication techniques. One topic that can make a difference in the successful integration of the case manager role is the use of proper verbal and nonverbal communication styles, as well as proper techniques for listening. Active listening can result in positive communication interactions.

Integrated in this should be the technique for assertive communication versus the aggressive communication style, which has been shown to be less effective.

Finally, the case manager should be aware of the various sources of conflict that may come about as a result of the intregration of this role and of the problem-solving strategies that should be used for resolving conflict.

Patient education is one of the three main role functions of the case manager. Therefore the principles of adult learning and strategies for effective teaching and learning should be included in the curriculum. Effective inpatient teaching is an aid to successful recovery at home.

The case manager must serve as a patient advocate as she interacts on the patient's behalf with other departments and disciplines. This advocacy role is possibly more important than it has ever been. The curriculum should include a discussion of do-not-resuscitate (DNR) laws, living wills, and health care proxy laws. A lecturer with expertise in these areas should be recruited.

A portion of the curriculum should cover discharge planning, with an emphasis on collaboration. If the organization has a discharge planning department, the discharge planning process can be reviewed from this perspective. The role of the social worker is important in the discharge planning process, and a social worker should be enlisted to provide insights on how case manager and social worker roles can work together. Many disciplines share the responsibility of assessing and planning for discharge. Reaching out to the community is part of the discharge planning process. As much as possible, the case manager should be made aware of the various community resources available for varying patient problems. Some of these referral sources will come to the case manager's attention once the manager begins working in the role; nevertheless, an overview of some of the resources available should be covered.

Day 2

The second day (see Table 13-3) should provide an overview and definition of case management. The relationship between cost and quality should be reviewed as they relate to case management along with the goals of a case management model. Also included in an overview should be an in-depth historical perspective of the evolution of nursing care delivery models. This will help to put today's case management model in perspective and give it relevance.

Case management is important as it relates to the past and present health care environment. There are numerous relevant health care crises, but some of the top ones might include the nursing shortage and how it affected the evolution of case management, changes in health care reimbursement as related to the prospective payment system, an aging patient population, the AIDS epidemic, and increased technology in health care. Case management has evolved out of the current crises. Presenting case management from its historical perspective will lend relevance to the model.

The prospective payment system needs to be covered in detail because it is this system of predetermined lengths of stay as related to the DRG system that has been one of the reasons the concept of case management evolved. The system should be covered in its entirety. Differences between what the state calls an acceptable length of stay and what the federal government calls acceptable should be discussed. The case manager must understand the reimbursement system completely and must be fluent with the terms related to it. Guest lecturers who have expertise in this area or others should be invited to speak whenever possible.

Following this discussion should be one on managed care reimbursement systems. Case managers need to understand the finer points as they relate to case management in a managed care environment.

The role functions and responsibilities of the case manager should be covered, with a review of the case manager job description. The collaborative relationship between the case manager and all other disciplines should be emphasized. The specific responsibilities of the case manager can be covered during this time. These responsibilities would include education, discharge planning, and facilitation of the patient through the system.

The case management plan can be reviewed for form, content, and purpose. Possible topics to be covered in a discussion of case management plans might include design, documentation, relationship to length of stay, use as a collaborative tool, and quality-of-care monitoring. The case management plans should be reviewed in detail, as they are one of the more visible and tangible changes in case management. Methods for writing the case management plan should be reviewed. Included in this portion of the education should be the ways in which a case management plan can be used to

Table 13-3   Case manager education day 2 content outline

OBJECTIVES	CONTENT

Define the concepts of case management.	Overview of case management
	    Definition
	    Nine steps to case management
	    Goals of case management
	    Expected outcomes of case management

Identify issues affecting health care delivery in the 1990s.	Health care crisis
	    Nursing shortage
	    Changes in reimbursement
	    Aging population
	    AIDS epidemic
	    Increased technology

Explain the DRG reimbursement system.	Fiscal issues facing nursing
	    DRGs
	    Length of stay

Discuss managed care reimbursement	Managed care
	    HMOs
	    PPOs
	    Capitation

State the role of case manager and other members of the health care team.	Professional image
	    Case manager job description
	    Collaborative roles
	        Nursing
	        Physicians
	        Social work

Define case management plans.	Case management plans
	    Design
	    Documentation
	    Relationship to length of stay
	    Collaborative tool
	    Education
	    Quality of care

Document accurately the changes in case management using the case management plan.	Changes
	    Length of stay
	    Patient/practitioner variances
	    Quality of care

Identify appropriate strategies for measuring, evaluating, and assessing outcomes.	Quality assurance documentation
	    Problem-solving techniques
	    Tracking and trending: selection of population source data
	    Development of monitoring tool
	    Analysis of data
	    Evaluation and follow-up

Table 13-4   Case manager education day 4 content outline

OBJECTIVES	CONTENT

Identify role of case manager.	Role functions
	   Planning and facilitation
	   Patient/family education
	   Discharge planning
	   Utilization management

Review the roles of the case management team.	Team members
	   Social work
	   Utilization
	   Discharge planning
	   Home care

Understand the in-depth roles of the case management team.	In-depth reviews
	   Discharge planning
	   Utilization management
	   Social work
	   Home care

Review case management assessment and documentation.	Assessment
	   On admission
	   Daily
	Documentation
	   In-take assessment
	   On-going

Complete the case management plan	Review plans, practice writing

Discuss variance analysis or outcomes	Variances
	   Definition
	   Types
	   Monitoring
	Outcomes
	   Definition
	   Monitoring

Understand continuous quality improvement	Continuous quality improvement
	   Definition
	   Relationship to case management

Discuss differentiated practice	Relate differentiated practice to case management
Role play	Relate to other disciplines in case manager role

track variances in care and quality data. Tracking and trending for selected patient problems or entire disease entities can be followed concurrently or retrospectively through the case management format.

Day 3

The third day (see Table 13-4) should include a review of the roles and functions of the case manager. A "train the trainer" approach is useful during this portion of the curriculum. If someone already in the role of case manager is available, it is much more worthwhile for the new case manager to hear exactly how the role is carried out from someone who is already functioning in the role. A thorough review of how the case manager should collect data on patients should be provided. These data provide a framework from which the case manager can track the patients while they are in the hospital and after discharge. Although each case manager will individualize the data collection process, some standard methods can be reviewed. In addition, walking the case manager through the day is also helpful.

The roles of the case management team should be reviewed. If at all possible, representatives from each discipline should lecture on their role and on how their role relates to case management and to other members of the case management team. Disciplines to be included should be social work, utilization management, discharge planning, and home care. This overview should be followed by in-depth discussions on discharge planning, utilization review and management, social work, and planning for home care.

A workshop dedicated to managed care plan writing is a must for the third day. Each case manager should be given the opportunity to write a managed care plan from beginning to end. Going through the process step by step helps identify areas of confusion or uncertainty.

Variance analysis is one of the unique opportunities provided by a case management model. A retrospective analysis of what did or did not happen and looking for patterns as well as causes of the variances can be used to justify changes in care (Blaney & Hobson, 1988). The case manager should be well versed in this process. In addition to providing the rationale for changes in care plans, variance analysis will allow for future upgrading of the quality of care. It is much easier to track clinical outcomes with the variance analysis format. Methods for identifying and monitoring outcomes should be included here. Outcomes can be identified as clinical and nonclinical, diagnosis specific, and generic. Continuous quality improvement (CQI) should also be discussed in relation to case management and case management plans.

Many case management programs use some differentiated practice methods. Differentiated practice calls for the assignment of personnel based on employee level of education, experience, and expertise (AHA, 1990). An effective case management program should include a differentiated practice system so that optimal use can be made of the nurse's experience and education. One part of case management training should cover the levels of education for nurses and should include a discussion of the strengths and weaknesses associated with each of these education levels.

One part of the curriculum should be devoted to role playing. Such role playing will help case managers by walking them through some of the situations they will encounter. One of the hardest areas for some new case managers is explaining to patients, physicians, and others exactly what the case manager role encompasses. Giving out business cards to patients is equally difficult because the case managers are not familiar with such formalities. Practice with the card can address and solve these problems. This may seem rudimentary, but it is crucial that the case manager feel at ease with these tasks.

Role playing can also be used to practice ways of confronting and resolving conflicts that arise during the change process.

REFERENCES

American Hospital Association (1990). *Current issues and perspective on differentiated practice.* Chicago: American Organization of Nurse Executives.

Bennis, W., & Nanus, B. (1985). *Leaders.* New York: Harper & Row.

Blaney, D.R., & Hobson, C.J. (1988). *Cost-effective nursing practice: Guidelines for nurse managers.* New York: J.B. Lippincott Company.

Hartley, S. (1986). Effects of prospective pricing on nursing. *Nursing Economics, 4*(1), 16-18.

Holle, M.L., & Blatchley, M.E. (1987). *Introduction to leadership and management in nursing.* Boston: Jones & Bartlett.

Kahn, R.L., Wolfe, D.M., Quinn, R.P., Snoek, J.D., & Rosenthal, R.A. (1964). *Organizational stress: Studies in role conflict and ambiguity.* New York: Wiley.

O'Malley, J. (1988). Nursing care management, part II: Dimensions of the nurse case manager role. *Aspen's Advisor for Nurse Executives, 3*(7), 8-9.

Torres, G., & Stanton, M. (1982). *Curriculum process in nursing: A guide to curriculum development,* Englewood Cliffs, N.J.: Prentice-Hall.

Zander, K. (1992 Fall). Quantifying, managing, and improving quality. Part III. Using variance concurrently. *The New Definition, 7*(4), 1-4.

V

IMPLEMENTATION

14

THE CAST OF CHARACTERS

▼ *CHAPTER OVERVIEW*

Primary nursing models no longer meet the changing needs of either the health care environment or the patients. In this chapter the multidisciplinary approach is discussed in terms of its relative value to the case management model. Both this approach and case management in general are presented in response to an increasingly complex health care environment. How to form teams and how to gain the support and trust of colleagues are two of the topics discussed.   ▲

GETTING OUT OF THE PARALLEL PLAY SYNDROME

Those who began their nursing careers in the 1970s were trained and educated to function as independent, professional nurses. With the advent of the primary nursing model, *professional* meant doing everything oneself (Bakke, 1974). The team spirit and sense of esprit de corps were lost in the fight to prove nursing a worthy profession. In the attempt to show just how important nursing was to the patient, other disciplines, which also provided unique and necessary services, were neglected.

Perhaps nursing had to go through this process. Perhaps it was necessary as part of the profession's evolutionary growth. Because nurses were so used to nursing's being viewed as a second-class profession, they were riding high on the conviction that they could do it all and do it all well.

Out of this generation of parallel play came terms such as *burnout, fatigue syndrome,* and *fragmented care.* Under the primary nursing model, it was expected that the nurse would meet all the patient's needs, from the bed bath to the discharge plan. With the nursing shortage that began in 1985 and the prospective payment system that resulted in shortened lengths of stay, nurses found it almost impossible to function under the primary nursing system.

Increased complexity and technology required that registered nurses become experts in a narrower range of tasks, which meant that other tasks had to be relinquished or returned to the other disciplines. Nursing care had to become more specialized as it responded to changing patient needs both in the hospital and after discharge.

Because the hospital stay was shortened in response to the prospective payment system, the phrase "discharge them quicker, but sicker" was being quoted by both health care practitioners and patients. Members of the public were losing confidence in the health care system because they felt rushed through the process by the insurers as well as the health care providers, who now had to keep the hospital stay as short as possible.

Flexible time (flex-time) measures, which were designed to attract more people to the profession and to retain those already in the workforce, contributed to fragmented nursing care. Fragmentation was chiefly an outcome of these measures, which resulted in the advent of 10- and 12-hour shifts. Flex-time was very attractive to employees because it allowed them to have long blocks of time off to spend with their families and to continue their education.

Unfortunately, these long blocks of time created a tremendous gap in patient care. Trying to be all things to the patient for 12 hours and then not being present for 3 days was meeting the worker's needs at the patient's expense. The situation was compounded by the accelerated hospital stay. It was conceivable that patients might see a different nurse during each day of an average 4-day hospital stay. Patients complained that no one knew them or their needs, and they were unable to develop professional relationships with any of their nurses. These patients felt that no one practitioner was responsible for their care. Nursing appeared to have failed because accountability for patient care had been lost.

Although nursing departments across the country tried to keep functioning in primary nursing systems, the new environment made it impossible to do so. Primary nursing had been founded on the notion that the registered professional nurse would be responsible for all aspects of the patient's care from admission to discharge. This became unattainable with the introduction of the flex-time system. Although theoretically nurses were responsible, extended absences from the unit prevented a true continuation of their relationship with the patient or the other members of the health care team.

In addition to this, patient assignments continued, in many instances, to remain geographic, with each nurse on the shift assigned a particular geographic part of the nursing unit. If the patient was moved to some other area of the unit, it was likely that the primary nurse would no longer be caring for that patient. Such changes meant care had become extremely fragmented.

At the same time, the role of the head nurse or nurse manager was moving away from the bedside. More and more administrative responsibility was given to these middle managers as upper management positions were eliminated. In the past the nurse manager had been able to clinically monitor all the patients on the floor and still carry out managerial responsibilities. As the administrative duties increased, this became more difficult to accomplish. In addition, the average length of stay was dramatically shortened, so that patients were admitted and discharged from the unit faster than they could be followed up by a busy manager with other responsibilities.

THE EFFECTS OF A CHANGING ENVIRONMENT

It was during the 1970s that nurses and other health care providers first began to complain of stress-related problems such as chronic fatigue and burnout. In 1974 a psychologist named Freudenberger coined the clinical term *burnout*. Burnout was described as the degeneration of a once highly productive individual into a negative, exhausted one. It was seen as a direct response to work stress when the worker no longer had the resources available to deal with other people's emotional, psychological, and physical problems.

Burnout follows a particular pattern that generally begins with feelings of emotional exhaustion. Such exhaustion is a result of being emotionally overextended and exhausted by one's work with others (Maslach, 1976; 1978; 1982). This exhaustion is followed by feelings of depersonalization, which have been described as negative, unfeeling, and impersonal responses toward the recipients of one's care (Maslach). As the syndrome becomes more severe, the worker may describe feelings of reduced personal accomplishment. Personal accomplishment is characterized by feelings of competence and successful achievement in one's work with people (Maslach).

By placing registered nurses in a position that required them to be all things to the patient, the nurses experienced an incredible amount of on-the-job stress. Role overload was yet another outcome of work stress that was identified in some nurses (Cesta, 1989). Role overload is characterized by workers' subjective feelings of being unable to complete their work because of inadequate personal or environmental resources (French & Caplan, 1972; Hardy, 1976; Ritzer, 1977). These feelings have been reported to be particularly high in nurses who are in their first 2 years of employment (Cesta, 1989; Das, 1981; Maslach, 1982).

When role overload combined with feelings of burnout, the nurse's ability to deal with work began to change and gradually diminished (Cesta, 1989).

Nurses began to adjust the primary nursing system in an attempt to address changes in the health care arena. This new system eventually became known as *modified primary* and retained the theory that the nurse was accountable for all aspects of care. This did not mean, however, that the nurse retained responsibility for the patient from admission to discharge. Primary nursing responsibilities were applicable only to the day the nurse worked.

Once these modifications were made in the primary model, the stage was set for the development of a more appropriate model that addressed all the above issues (Loveridge, Cummings, and O'Malley, 1988).

Nursing responded to the changes in health care by looking for an alternative patient care delivery model. The alternative was a model that combined elements of team and primary nursing (Zander, 1985). There was really nothing new or revolutionary about the case management model for nursing care delivery. The basic premise of the model was a team or collaborative approach that allowed the case manager to function as the evaluator and coordinator of care or facilitator of the team. This new role was similar to that of the primary nurse, except that the case manager was now removed from direct patient care responsibility.

With the addition of this role, nursing moved away from attempting to be all things to the patient. Members of the profession began to admit that they could not do all things equally well, that other members of the team were needed to provide their particular areas of expertise.

Nursing was finally getting out of the parallel play syndrome and was moving toward a more dynamic and interactive modality.

FORMATION OF THE COLLABORATIVE PRACTICE GROUPS

It is perhaps easier now for nurses to reintroduce themselves to the team approach. Although social workers and physicians had functioned that way for years, nurses had been struggling to achieve independence and autonomy. Nurses now feel more confident and ready to join the team after gaining prestige among other health care providers (Farley & Stoner, 1989).

Institutions implementing case management models for the first time must explain to team members why nurses are returning to the team approach. At first, this reintroduction of the team approach may be observed with some suspicion and doubt. Without making the intentions of the team clear it will be impossible to institute collaborative practice groups.

Many physicians and other health care providers may have preconceived ideas about case management. Some of these ideas may stem from their familiarity with managed care systems that have been introduced in HMOs. Generally, these managed care systems are seen as negative by many other health care providers. They are seen as just one more way for their practices to be regulated and controlled and their services to be rationed (Schwartz & Mendelson, 1992).

Collaborative practice groups cannot be formed until all members adopt the model as their own and see its benefit for both themselves and for the patient. It should be emphasized that case management is not just a nursing care model but a way for all the disciplines to form plans of care that avoid duplication of effort, unnecessary tests and procedures, or misuse of resources.

Each discipline involved in patient care activities develops a plan that meets the objectives for that discipline as they relate to the patient. Case management provides, for the first time, the opportunity for all the disciplines to come together in an effort to use each other's expertise for maximum benefit to the patient.

Cast of Characters

Who then comprise the cast of characters, and how do they come together as a group? Formation of these interdisciplinary groups is one of the first steps for implementation, and it must take place before any real clinical changes can occur.

In a unit-based case management approach, the members of the group will be dependent upon the types of case management plans being developed. At the least each group should consist of the following members from their respective disciplines: nursing, medicine, social work, discharge planning, and nutrition. People from these areas make up the core of any group, and each one provides input related to the clinical objectives of that member's discipline. Of course, the central figures in any such team are the patient and family.

Other members are added as they relate to the particular diagnosis or procedure planned. Other disciplines that might be included are physical therapy, occupational therapy, respiratory therapy, psychiatry, and others as needed.

In some cases the groups may have already been formed as part of the implementation of a non-unit-based case management approach. In this approach, groups are formed around a particular diagnosis, and all members of the team are experts in that clinical area.

For example, a team might be formed to manage diabetic patients throughout the hospital. A diabetes case management team is often headed by a diabetologist and a nurse case manager who provide the leadership to direct the other members of the team. A cardiac case management team might be headed by a cardiologist and a cardiac nurse case manager. The members of a case management team follow the patients' cases regardless of where they might be within the hospital. Therefore the team remains constant while the patients and their locations change.

Because the case management team is developed before the arrival of the patient, these groups have already determined protocols and care methods for their specific types of patients. It is not necessary for the case manager to identify the members of the team at the time of the patient's admission to the hospital because the team is already in place.

In the unit-based case management model, however, the members of the team are determined by the patient problem. These teams are fluid and constantly changing.

After the patient's admission the attending physician, case manager, social worker, nutritionist, and others are identified, after which time the specific plan of care for the patient is formalized.

The use of internal techniques and relationships should not be underestimated in the formation of the multidisciplinary groups. If a nonthreatening, informal relationship has been developed first, it will be much easier to obtain the cooperation of some professionals. Inviting key players to lunch, meeting in the library, or just chatting on the unit can do much to gain trust and respect.

There may be occasions when a member of another discipline who is in a position of authority may be needed to intervene on the part of the case manager to obtain concurrence for collaborative practice. For example, some physicians admit large numbers of patients to the hospital every year and are therefore considered to have a great deal of power and independence in their everyday practice within the hospital. These individuals may not immediately see the advantage of joining a multidisciplinary team effort because it may not appear to benefit them, or they may view the effort to form teams as an attempt to control their practices. In a case like this, it may be necessary to have a physician administrator intervene on the behalf of the case management team. Usually, once the benefits are presented to the physicians, they give their support. Also, they may need to get their superiors' consent to participate.

Another technique to gain the support of some of the more resistant professionals is to begin working first with those who have already agreed to the model. It is sometimes more effective to begin with these individuals than try to convert the resisters right away. Perhaps, when success is proved with those who have been immediately receptive, the others will eventually give their support. Once again, support may depend on people's perceptions of what the model can do for them. There will always be a certain percentage of players who will sit on the fence, waiting to see if implementation succeeds or fails. Once success is evident, they will cross over to the case manager's side.

In both the unit- and non-unit-based case management approach the team becomes the focal point for care delivery, with each member lending information from a specific area of expertise. Most institutions rely on the case manager to be responsible for smooth operation and communication among team members. In some instances, however, social workers or physicians have been used to coordinating communication. Nurses function well in this role because they are educated to take a holistic approach to care delivery and because they are the ones who get involved in all aspects of the patient's care.

For example, it is less likely that a social worker will have the clinical skills that a registered nurse has, but most registered nurses have the basic skills required to provide discharge planning and referral services to patients after discharge. Case managers should be able to identify patients at high risk and to refer such patients to the appropriate discipline. Patients with high-risk discharge planning needs can be referred to the discharge planner or social worker, as appropriate to the organization. At the very least, the case manager should be able to work the system to the patient's advantage, knowing the appropriate members to call as needs arise. An advanced understanding of the patient's medical and nursing needs helps to make this assessment complete. The case manager can then refer the problem to the appropriate practitioner.

In the unit-based approach, it may be difficult or impossible for the complete team to meet at one time. Once again, case managers fill this gap. They provide the thread that holds all the members together. In this sense the case managers must have excellent communication skills. The information they translate between team members and to patients and families must be accurate and concise. Otherwise, the thread is broken and the team falls apart.

The team should be assembled as a group whenever possible. Dialogue and opinion can thus be shared face-to-face. It is often during meetings of this type that difficult patient problems are resolved.

The case manager may spend a good deal of time during the beginning of implementation trying to ensure that the team becomes a reality and remains on target to provide the best possible care for the patient.

The case manager role consists of three dimensions (Tahan, 1992; chapter 17): The first dimension is the clinical role, which requires collaboration with the interdisciplinary team and involves the development of protocols that list the key tasks or events that must be accomplished for handling patient problems. Case managers use these protocols to direct, monitor, and evaluate patient treatment and the outcomes or responses to treatment (Thompson, Caddick, Mathie, Newlon, & Abraham, 1991; Zander, 1988).

Case managers identify variances from the standard protocols and work with other health care team members to analyze and deal with these variances of care (Ethridge & Lamb, 1989; O'Malley, 1988b).

The second dimension is that of the managerial role, which refers to the case managers' responsibility for coordinating the care of patients during the course of hospitalization (Ethridge & Lamb, 1989; Kruger, 1989; O'Malley, 1988a; Zander, 1988). The case manager manages care by planning the nursing treatment modalities and interventions necessary for meeting the needs of the patient and the family. Goals of treatment are set at admission, and length of stay is determined as it relates to the diagnosis-related group (DRG). The discharge plan is formed as early in the hospital stay as possible (O'Malley, 1988b).

Case managers also guide the activities, nursing treatments, and interventions of other nursing staff members (Ethridge & Lamb, 1989; Kruger, 1989). They continuously evaluate the quality of care provided and outcomes of treatments and services to prevent misuse of resources (O'Malley, 1988a).

One of the informal responsibilities of the case manager is that of teacher and mentor (Cronin & Maklebust, 1989; Kruger, 1989). The case manager assesses staff development needs, especially among the less experienced practitioners, and refers them to the appropriate person or resource (Leclair, 1991). As part of the teaching responsibilities of the role, case managers conduct patient and family teaching sessions during the hospitalization period (Cronin & Maklebust, 1989; Zander, 1988).

The third dimension of the case manager role involves financial aspects. In collaboration with the physician and other health care members, case managers activate a caregiving process for each patient and use a case management plan, which is a generic tool for managing care and keeping it consistent with the predetermined financial outcomes for a defined case type (O'Malley, 1988b; Zander, 1988). The use of such clinical treatment standards helps ensure that patients do not receive inadequate care because of cost containment measures (Collard, Bergman, & Henderson, 1990).

Case managers access information related to DRGs and case types, the cost of each diagnosis, the allocated length of stay, and the treatments and procedures generally used for each diagnosis. They use this information to review resources and evaluate the efficiency of care related to the diagnosis (Cronin & Maklebust, 1989). The case manager has a great influence on the quality and price of care by helping to determine in a timely manner the most pertinent treatment for the patient (Henderson & Collard, 1988). Case managers also assess variances for each case type and act immediately to control these variances to contain costs (Crawford, 1991). They assure consistency, continuity, and coordination of care to control for duplication and fragmentation in health care delivery, which results in better resource allocation and further cost containment (Henderson & Collard, 1988; O'Malley, 1988a).

To be effective, case managers must access information on case mix index, cost of resources, and consumption and must be familiar with the prospective payment system and current third-party reimbursement procedures including managed care and capitation (Ethridge & Lamb, 1989; O'Malley, 1988b).

Case managers work closely with the utilization review department in identifying long-stay patients and planning with that department to control and prevent inappropriate hospital stays (Cronin & Maklebust, 1989).

REFERENCES

Bakke, K. (1974). Primary nursing: Perceptions of a staff nurse. *American Journal of Nursing, 74*(8), 1432-1434.

Cesta, T.G. (1989). The relationship of role overload and burnout to coping process in registered professional staff nurses newly employed in a hospital setting. Doctoral Dissertation. University Microfilms, Inc., Publication Number: 9016399.

Collard, A.F., Bergman, A., & Henderson, M. (1990). Two approaches to measuring quality in medical case management programs. *Quality Review Bulletin*, 3-8.

Crawford, J. (1991). Managed care consultant: The "house supervisor" alternative. *Nursing Management, 22*(5), 75-78.

Cronin, C.J., & Maklebust, J. (1989). Case-managed care: Capitalizing on the CNS. *Nursing Management, 20*(3), 38-47.

Das, E.B.L. (1981). Contributing factors to burnout in the nursing environment. Doctoral dissertation, Texas Woman's University. *Dissertation Abstracts International, 42*, 04B.

Ethridge, P., & Lamb, G. (1989). Professional nursing case management improves quality, access and costs. *Nursing Management, 20*(3), 30-35.

Farley, M.J., & Stoner, M.H. (1989). The nurse executive and interdisciplinary team building. *Nursing Administration Quarterly*, 24-29.

French, J.R.P., & Caplan, R.D. (1972). Organizational stress and individual strain. In A.J. Morrow (Ed.), *The failure of success* (pp.30-66). New York: AMACOM.

Freudenberger, H.J. (1974). Staff burn-out. *Journal of Social Issues, 30*, 159-165.

Hardy, M.E. (1976, Aug.). Role problems, role strain, job satisfaction, and nursing care. Paper presented at the annual meeting of the American Sociological Association, New York.

Henderson, M.G., & Collard, A. (1988). Measuring quality in medical case management programs. *Qualitiy Review Bulletin*, 33-39.

Kruger, N.R. (1989). Case management: Is it a delivery system for my organization? *Aspen's Advisor for Nurse Executives, 4*(10), 4-6.

Leclair, C. (1991). Introducing and accounting for RN case management. *Nursing Management, 22*(3), 44-49.

Loveridge, C.E., Cummings, S.H., & O'Malley, J. (1988). Developing case management in a primary nursing system. *Journal of Nursing Administration, 18*(10), 36-39.

Maslach, C. (1976). Burned-out. *Human Behavior, 5*, 17-21.

Maslach, C. (1978). Job burn-out: How people cope. *Public Welfare, 36*, 56-58.

Maslach, C. (1982). *Burnout. The cost of caring.* Englewood Cliffs, N.J.: Prentice-Hall.

O'Malley, J. (1988a). Nursing case management. I: Why look at a different model for nursing care delivery? *Aspen's Advisor for Nurse Executives, 3*(5), 5-6.

O'Malley, J. (1988b). Nursing case management, part II: Dimensions of the nurse case manager role. *Aspen's Advisor for Nurse Executives, 3*(6), 7.

Ritzer, G. (1977). *Working.* Englewood Cliffs, N.J.: Prentice-Hall.

Schwartz, W., & Mendelson, D. (1992 Summer). Why managed care cannot contain hospital cost without. *Health Affairs* 100-107.

Tahan, H.T. (1993). The nurse case manager in acute care settings: Job description and function. *Journal of Nursing Administration, 23*(10), 53-61.

Thompson, K.S., Caddick, K., Mathie, J., Newlon, B., & Abraham, T. (1991). Building a critical path for ventilator dependency. *American Journal of Nursing*, 28-31.

Zander, K. (1992 Fall). Quantifying, managing, and improving quality: III. Using variance concurrently. *The New Definition 7*(4), 1-4.

Zander, K. (1985). Second generation primary nursing: A new agenda. *Journal of Nursing Administration, 15*(3), 18-24.

Zander, K. (1988). Managed care within acute care settings: design and implementation via nursing case management. *Health Care Supervisor. 6*(2), 27-43.

15

VARIATIONS WITHIN CLINICAL SETTINGS

▼ *CHAPTER OVERVIEW*

Case management models provide an opportunity for health care institutions to provide quality, cost-effective services, regardless of the type of setting or financial resources. The model is flexible and can be adapted to meet the needs of both clinical and institutional settings.

This chapter describes the ways in which the case management model can be adapted to a variety of clinical settings, including medicine, surgery, critical care, nursing homes, clinics, and other ambulatory care settings. The way a case management model is used depends on the goals of the organization using it. The chapter also discusses the challenge facing case management in linking the inpatient and outpatient settings. ▲

FLEXIBILITY OF CASE MANAGEMENT

One of the things that makes case management models particularly appealing is that the structure is extremely flexible. A case management design can be modified to fit the needs and budgets of any clinical setting. Because the primary goals of case management are to reduce costs while maintaining quality, the model can, in many circumstances, be implemented for a minimal cost (Ethridge & Lamb, 1989).

There are probably as many variations on the case management theme as there are nursing units in the United States. There is no right or wrong way to design a case management unit. The design is not as important as the roles and functions of the unit's members. Each person's functions are what make the model unique, not the number of workers involved.* Today's health care environment calls for flexibility and creativity, and the institutions that display these features will probably be the most successful ones over the next 10 years (Armstrong & Stetler, 1991).

For an institution implementing case management for the first time, the exact design structure for the units will be determined based on an array of factors. Choosing the first units to participate is an important decision. If the first units are successful, the institution will be more likely to support continued implementation. On the other hand, if the first units are less than successful, the leaders of the

---

*This is because the team as a whole is greater than the sum of each member functioning independently.

organization may not be willing to allow the implementation process to continue. Therefore the first units should be chosen carefully.

The units selected for initial implementation should have the following characteristics:

▼ Homogeneous patient population
▼ High-volume case types
▼ Potential for improvement in length of stay
▼ A committed nurse manager
▼ A receptive physician group
▼ An interested nursing staff
▼ An open full-time equivalent (FTE) position

Of course, it may not be possible to obtain each of these elements on every nursing unit. Finding a unit with as many of these factors as possible will help ensure a positive transition to a case management model.

A homogeneous patient population is beneficial because it may mean a smaller number of professionals involved in patient care on the unit. A homogeneous population also reduces the number of case management plans that need to be written. Most units that specialize in certain diseases or surgical procedures will have a smaller physician group with which to interact. A smaller group will allow for a more rapid transition to the model and will be more helpful in formulating the case management plans because the group will probably be more likely to agree on plans of care.

A large percentage of high-volume case types will also help when generating managed care plans that will cover a wider number of patients on the unit. In general, if a unit admits more than 50% of its patients to five or fewer diagnosis-related (DRG) categories, the unit may be a good candidate for conversion to case management.

However, it is important to analyze these high-volume case types for their potential in reducing length of stay. High volume does not necessarily mean a reduction in length of stay. For example, some patient problems are on protocols that are already as brief as possible. Chemotherapy is one example. Reductions might not be attainable around the diagnosis, but other elements of hospitalization, such as preadmission blood work or prehydration therapy, may allow for reductions.

The transition to a case management system will require total commitment from those on the unit. One of the most important people in the change process is the nurse manager. The nurse manager has 24-hour responsibility and accountability and has the primary administrative responsibility for the smooth functioning of the unit. Most of the other professionals enter and exit the unit because their responsibilities take them to other areas of the hospital. The nurse manager's sole responsibility is the nursing unit. It is vital that nurse managers have a working knowledge of case management so that they can function both formally and informally as advocates for change. Nurse managers can be instrumental in obtaining the cooperation of physicians with whom they have long-standing relationships.

Most of the activities on a nursing unit revolve around nurse managers who have administrative authority for their units. Their responsibilities may include staffing, budgeting, maintaining supplies, and caring for patients. No changes in these responsibilities should be made without the nurse managers' input and support.

When selecting units for conversion to case management, at least a majority of physicians affiliated with the unit should support the change. This, of course, may not always be possible. Obtaining the support of some physicians can be enough for making a positive transition.

It is important that the chief medical officer be supportive of the conversion to case management. Chairmen of individual clinical areas should also be engaged in the change process as early as possible and should be supportive of case management.

When a case management model is implemented, it is helpful but not crucial to begin with a nursing staff that volunteered to be among the first units in the institution to convert. Often such enthusiasm came from the unit's nurse manager and filtered down to the other nurses on the unit. Again, this may be a factor that is not immediately obtainable.

Most institutions converting to a unit-based model try to do so at minimal cost to the organization. This may mean using an already existing FTE position or a budgeted position that has never been filled. It is not wise to eliminate an employee to make room for a case manager. The open FTE should be acquired through attrition whenever possible because elimination of an employee can cause ill will, resentment, and insecurity among other staff nurses on the unit.

Some organizations have had to use other creative approaches to obtaining case management positions. Some have converted existing departments or positions, such as utilization managers, discharge planners, social workers, or nurse managers. No position should be eliminated unless others in the organization are able to absorb the workload of the eliminated position(s). During this time, job descriptions should be reviewed and, if necessary, role functions reallocated. Examples might include the development of discharge planning criteria for patients that slot them into either high- or low-risk categories. Lower risk patients might remain the responsibility of the staff nurse or case manager, whereas high-risk patients are referred to the discharge planner or social worker.

It is often possible to create additional positions once some success has been shown. For these reasons it is again imperative that the initial units selected indicate a great potential for successful transition.

MEDICAL UNIT

Medical units may possibly be among the neediest in terms of case management patient needs. Medical patients are often elderly and have more complex discharge plans. These patients are often the least likely to be advocates for themselves and are likely to fall through the cracks during an extended and complicated hospital stay. They are among the most costly to hospitals and are often resource intensive.

Medical patients are also among the most difficult to plan for because their hospital course is often unpredictable. Ironically, it is for these reasons that a case manager can be a great asset to a medical unit. The medical patient whose hospital course changes daily needs someone to ensure that everything is happening as planned and that nothing is missed.

There are usually more case managers on a medical unit than on any other type of unit in the hospital. Because of the increased complexity and severity of the cases the organization should aim to have every medical patient under the authority of a case manager. The number of case managers should be based on an average case load of about 15 to 20 patients. If every patient on the medical unit cannot be followed by the case manager, then criteria must be developed for selecting those patients who will benefit the most by being followed. In general the case load of the case manager on the medical unit must be somewhat smaller than that of either a specialty unit or surgical unit. This is because these patients tend to need more resources and the number of interventions per patient will probably be greater.

Criteria for selecting patients on a general medical floor must be individually determined through a retrospective audit of those patients who seem to represent patterns of increased resource use. However, this is not the only factor that should be evaluated. Other patients who might benefit from a case manager might include those with the following:

▼ Advanced age (older than 75 years)
▼ Noncompliance with treatment
▼ Potential for falls
▼ Potential for skin breakdown
▼ Discharge placement problems/complicated plan
▼ Complicated medical plan
▼ Home care needs
▼ Complicated teaching needs

SURGICAL UNIT

Surgical cases can be as complicated as medical cases. Generally, though, the hospital course of a surgical patient is somewhat more predictable and amenable to a predetermined plan. Many surgeons practice with protocols, which manage the patient's postoperative course in the same way that the case management plan does. Although there are exceptions to every rule, the expected course can be planned around an anticipated length of stay. Surgical patients are often elected admissions, which means that there may be less potential for in-hospital complications.

For these reasons a surgical case manager may be able to carry a larger patient case load than a case manager on a medical unit. A case load of about 18 patients is probably manageable on most surgical units.

It may not be necessary to have every surgical patient under the direction of a case manager. Criteria for selecting patients should include patient need and complexity or severity of condition. Patients who are admitted for emergency surgery and who require medical clearance before surgery also might need the attention of the case manager. Patients who develop postoperative complications, which may result in a prolonged length of stay, should also be considered.

CRITICAL CARE UNIT

The critical care unit may be the last area of the hospital to convert to case management. Because this area has a lower nurse-patient ratio and a more responsive health care team, these patients are already receiving a form of case management.

Critical care can be viewed as one episode in the course of hospitalization. Case management in critical care can help with clinical management issues such as admission and discharge criteria. These criteria can support patient throughput.

The case manager and case management plans may be the only elements missing from these areas. Most intensive care units have a 2:1 or a 1:1 nurse/patient ratio. In these situations it may be possible to use the nurses, in their current positions, to function in a case management role. In this case all registered nurses working in the unit would be case managers. They would be carrying out the functions and responsibilities of the case manager in addition to providing direct patient care.

Case management plans can be developed around particular clinical problems, such as ventilator weaning, which would support and assist the staff nurses acting as case managers. Protocols for withdrawing patients from care as they improve could be incorporated into critical care case management plans.

There are problems with this system, but solutions do exist. The first problem is that continuity of care is still an issue if the unit is on flextime. Also, it may be difficult for nurses working with critically ill patients to take on the added responsibilities associated with the case manager role. They may not have the time needed to create managed care plans or to be involved in the formation of the team. They may simply be absent from the unit too much to care for patients and function as case managers.

The emergency department lends itself to the development of case management plans. Plans can be developed for the efficient treatment of specific disease entities such as asthma or for the clinical management of patient treatments such as conscious sedation. Case management plans can also be developed for beginning the "ruling-out" process, as in the treatment of abdominal pain, and the identification of tuberculosis or HIV infection.

It is possible to create this type of system in critical care areas, but the possible problems must be identified and addressed before implementation. The stress this dual role could impose on the nurses should also be considered.

NURSING HOME

The nursing home is an example of a non-acute-care facility that can financially benefit from a case management system. A case management model can ensure a higher quality of patient care with use of fewer resources. As the population ages and life expectancy increases, the needs of extended care facilities will rise proportionally. As do most other health care institutions, nursing homes struggle with increased regulations and decreased resources (Smith, 1991).

In the nursing home setting, a case manager can ensure patient outcomes. This can reduce the use of registered nurses and increase the use of ancillary personnel.

Nursing homes are required to provide plans of care and goals for their patients. Generally these plans can be carried out by personnel other than registered nurses. Regulation requires that a registered nurse be present in most instances, but this nurse could be better used as a facilitator, educator, or coordinator of services to the patient. This approach can enhance quality of life and slow deterioration of functional ability.

A team approach with the nurse manager as a case manager can be cost effective and can ensure improved quality of care. Many institutions have attempted to use the nurse manager in this facilitator role. As in the acute care setting, this dual role has become increasingly difficult in the nursing home setting. By using a case manager, in addition to a nurse manager, greater quality and more efficient clinical outcomes can be achieved.

OUTPATIENT AREA

Case management crosses all boundaries of the health care spectrum. The patient's quality of life may depend on the kind of clinical management this person receives in the primary care setting. The approach used in most clinics is a form of case management. Continuity of caregivers is often attempted for a patient's return visits. For many patients without a private family physician, these clinic visits provide their only links to the health care system. Using the team approach to manage patients enhances quality of care.

The future challenge for case management models will be to link the inpatient and outpatient settings in a way that promotes a smooth transition for the patient and ensures continuity of care once the patient returns to the community.

Development of case management plans can be based on expected outcomes for each patient visit. Such an approach can control the resources applied and the goals of care for each visit. This approach can also be used for home care visits or for clinic visits. If care is guided by the expected outcomes of care, progress can be tracked and monitored and appropriate interventions made in response to the patient's reaction to treatment.

Documentation of the patient's level of compliance after discharge from the hospital can provide valuable data as to the effect hospitalization had on the patient's quality of life. Additionally, a case manager's unique relationship with the patients, as well as follow-up visits and phone calls, can ensure patient compliance with postdischarge health care follow-up.

REFERENCES

Armstrong, D.M., & Stetler, C.B. (1991). Strategic considerations in developing a delivery model. *Nursing Economics, 9*(2), 112-115.

Ethridge, P., & Lamb, G. (1989). Professional nursing case management improves quality, access, and costs. *Nursing Management, 20*(3), 30-35.

Smith, J. (1991). Changing traditional nursing home roles to nursing case management. *Journal of Gerontological Nursing, 17*(5), 32-39.

16

BRAINSTORMING

DEVELOPMENT OF THE MULTIDISCIPLINARY ACTION PLAN
(MAP)

▼ *CHAPTER OVERVIEW*

The case management plan is the documentation that drives the case management system. Institutions implementing case management models need to determine the content of the documentation format they wish to adopt.

    This chapter reviews the evolution of case management plans and the step-by-step process of development. This chapter also discusses the links between the prospective payment system, DRGs, and the case management plan.

    Health care organizations must go beyond what the DRG suggests when designing these plans. The principal procedure or diagnosis should be used with the DRG as the underlying guide for determining the length of the plan. ▲

EVOLUTION OF THE CASE MANAGEMENT PLAN

Just as there are many ways to adapt case management models to fit the needs of a particular organization, there are multiple ways to develop a case management documentation system. Since case managements' inception, most hospitals have been using the *critical path* label on their case management plans. When introduced in 1985 by the New England Medical Center in Boston, the critical path was the first system that attempted to incorporate expected outcomes within specified time frames. The term *critical path* means that the plan defines the critical or key events expected to happen each day of a patient's hospitalization (Giuliano & Poirier, 1991; Zander, 1991; 1992).

    Since 1985, critical paths have been adapted to meet the needs of organizations implementing case management models. The paths remain an extremely flexible method of planning and documenting. In addition to *critical path* and *critical pathway*, other labels, such as *multidisciplinary plan, multidisciplinary action plan (MAP)*, and *action plan*, have been attached to these case management plans. All these terms are the same in theory. Each of the plans attempts to outline the expected outcomes of care for each discipline during each day of hospitalization. Some of these care plans place greater emphasis on the nursing plan, while some emphasize the medical plan of care. Some others, such as the MAP discussed here, incorporate all disciplines.

Some case management organizations use case management plans as one-page guides. Essentially these one-page plans are multidisciplinary protocols for the problem or diagnosis. The detail of the plan depends on the goals of the organization in which the plan is being used. In some cases, nursing documentation can be recorded directly onto the form. This format is also easily adapted to a hospital computer system. Computerization of the plan allows the case manager the flexibility of changing the plan as the patient's needs change. For those organizations without a computer system, the case management plan is still an easy, flexible tool to use.

The case management plan can also be used in place of the traditional nursing care plan. Nursing care plans have been criticized by some as useless exercises in writing. The plans are written to meet the needs of regulatory agencies but are often not used by nurses to guide or plan their day-to-day care. Once written, the plans are often never looked at again. These plans are not even written to provide a plan of care that correlates with the expected length of stay. For this reason these plans are not the preferred form for planning care in case management models.

It is no accident that the critical path or MAP format came into existence. These MAPs are the driving force behind case management models because they help determine the plan of care and arrange that plan around the expected length of stay. Unlike the nursing care plan, MAPs are multidisciplinary and take into account the unique contributions of each discipline. MAPs also link case management with the prospective payment system by using the DRG for determining the appropriate length for the plan. The most current reimbursements are consulted when any plan is started.

When developing the MAP, keep in mind that the state reimbursable length of stay may be longer or shorter than the federal length of stay. Also, it would be impractical to develop standard plans for patients with varying types of insurance coverage. Instead, these variations in reimbursable length of stay can be averaged. Another technique is to determine the length of stay the physician expects and measure it against the reimbursable length of stay. It may turn out that the stay the physician hoped for is shorter than the reimbursable length of stay. In a case like this, the physician's preference would determine the length of stay outlined in the MAP.

However, if the length of stay the physician expects is longer than the reimbursable length of stay, a compromise must be reached. The federal and state rates should be reviewed with the physician in relation to the physician's plan. Areas for reduction should be discussed to reduce the length of stay so that it matches or comes below the reimbursable length of stay. A general guideline is to design the plan so that it is shorter than the reimbursable length of stay. This allows for some margin of error in case the patient requires an additional day of hospitalization.

The case manager can control the length of stay by overseeing the movement of the patient through the system. It is difficult to implement MAPs that will be effective without the position of case manager in place. Instituting plans without a professional to drive the process is not a likely way to achieve the desired results. The staff nurse and the case manager are responsible for ensuring that the expected outcomes, as outlined on the MAP, are carried out. If the expected outcomes cannot be achieved, the case manager analyzes the patient's situation and documents the outcome that cannot be accomplished. This outcome is then documented as a variance, which is anything that does not happen at the time it is supposed to happen.

The DRG must be used as a guide for projecting the length of stay indicated on the MAP. Because the DRG categories are designed for determining hospital reimbursement rates, they are too heterogeneous to assess the effectiveness of the clinical plan at the bedside. For example, if a MAP is written to plan the care of a lumbar laminectomy patient, the discharge diagnosis of lumbar laminectomy might fall under a wide variety of DRGs, such as "medical back procedure" or "spinal procedure." Therefore, if someone wanted to look at the length of stay of all laminectomy patients within a case management system in the hospital, then asking for length of stay records for one DRG would not include the majority of laminectomy patients, who might have been classified under other DRG categories.

Other DRGs are heterogeneous in another way. For example, the DRG for chemotherapy, DRG 410, includes any and all chemotherapy protocols, whether they are for 1 day or for 5 days. The Health Care Finance Administration (HCFA) reimbursement rate for chemotherapy is 2.6 days, regardless of the type of chemotherapy being given. Once again, the DRG system will not be a suitable tool for analyzing whether the MAP decreases the length of stay, reduces resource use, or provides the most effective quality care for that problem.

If an organization wants to determine the true effectiveness of case management plans used among a specific patient group, the DRG cannot be used. Clinicians must dig deeper, using a microanalysis approach. Patients' reviews should be based on their principal procedure or diagnosis at the time of discharge. This way the plan's effectiveness can be determined. After all, there is no MAP called "medical back problem," and there cannot be one called "chemotherapy" because these would be too general. It follows, therefore, that analysis must be as specific as the level of the diagnosis.

The case management plan for chemotherapy would be specific to the type of chemotherapy being administered and the specific protocol being followed. In the interest of cost-effectiveness, several chemotherapy protocols can be combined on one MAP. At the time of admission the patient's specific protocol is identified from a menu of several possible choices on the MAP. All these plans would fall under the same DRG, even though they would be different.

The process for developing the case management plan must be based on several specific elements. The organization must first decide on the form that the plans will take. Factors that affect the form include degree of complexity, extent to which the plan will include other disciplines, and whether the form will include nursing documentation. These factors help determine the plan's design and content. Each factor must be decided before the content is developed.

Once the format has been decided and approved, the organization must decide which diagnoses or procedures are to be planned first. It is obvious that every plan cannot be developed simultaneously. Some general guidelines can be useful in making these decisions. If the model being implemented is a case management, diagnosis-specific approach, then these decisions have probably already been made. Many organizations begin with a few specific diagnoses that are easily planned. Some examples of commonly used diagnoses include "fractured hip," "open heart surgery," and "transurethral prostatectomy" (TURP). These are easily written and followed because these types of procedures are already the subjects of many protocols. It is generally easier to get the cooperation of surgeons who are managing these cases because they are already managing their patients in a protocol-oriented way. It is also easier to reduce length of stay because the chance of complication or comorbidity is slightly lower in these patient populations than in some others.

If the organization is adopting a unit-based case management model, then deciding which diagnosis to begin with is slightly more complicated, although technically it is the same as for the non-unit-based approach. One of the first factors to consider is the number of patients to include in the implementation of one plan. This involves examining the high-volume case types for the organization. Once this is done, an attempt should be made to match these high-volume case types to the units being converted to a case management model. These two factors point to the types of patient problems that should be considered first. After these determinations a match is then made to physicians who work with these patients and who are willing to help develop and adopt case management plans.

Only after all these steps have been taken can the actual process of writing begin. There will be several parts to each plan. Generally the longest of these are the nursing and medical plans. Plans for medical problems are developed from chart review, consultation with experts in the field, and literature review, all to create the "best possible plan" or ideal plan for that patient problem. To make the most of each person's time, individual brainstorming sessions between the case manager and a representative from each discipline are most effective. The case manager can make some preparation to begin the shell of the plan before meeting with anyone. The case manager can determine the approximate length of the plan, based on state and federal reimbursements, and then can begin to plan out the nursing portion of the plan, indicating the expected nursing outcomes for each day of hospitalization.

Once these pieces are complete, the case manager then arranges to meet with members of the other disciplines. The most logical person to begin with is the physician. Plans need to be physician specific, but this means that several physicians agree as a group to the same plan. Under no circumstances should a completed plan be presented to a physician until it is first made clear that the individual preferences and practice patterns of that practitioner will be taken into consideration. Plans should be individualized as much as possible.

Another technique to use is a team approach in which the members of the team physically meet as a group at specific, assigned times. The team can begin the process by developing a tool to review patient records. The tool should include demographic and clinically specific information. Clinical issues that "appear" to be affecting length of stay should be highlighted. Examples of these include progressive ambulation, timing of removal of tubes or drains, switches from intravenous to oral medications, and response time for consults. The clinical issue being studied will drive this list. Once the tool is developed, the team can begin reviewing charts. A representative number of charts should be selected randomly. For most diagnoses at least 30 charts should be reviewed. Validating the issues that "appear" to be affecting length of stay will help drive the clinical content of the plan.

Most physicians have a clear sense of their expectations or of what they would routinely order for the average patient with a particular problem. Of course, not every patient can or will fit into this projected plan exactly. Each plan must be tailored to the patient after admission. The physician should remember that the projected plan is designed for the average patient with a particular problem. This plan could be considered an aggregate of all patients the physician has treated, discounting unusual or aberrant conditions or circumstances.

On average the plan-development process can be completed in less than an hour. This hour is a small contribution compared with the amount of time it would take for the physician to individually inform all the health care providers of the care plan. Development of a MAP not only saves the physician time but also eliminates the second guessing that sometimes occurs.

One approach for developing a MAP is to simply ask the physician what would routinely be ordered for each day of hospitalization. Systematically running through each day ensures that nothing is neglected. Once all disciplines have completed this process, each should be afforded the opportunity to review the plan one last time. If a group of physicians is involved, each physician should have the chance to provide input. This content should be checked against the data collected on chart review.

The decision as to which disciplines will be represented in the plan depends on the diagnosis or procedure being planned. For some, physical therapy will be important. For others, respiratory therapy may be necessary. In most institutions, social work is a separate component but an integral part of the patient's plan, so this department should be given its own section on every plan. In other institutions some specialties such as skin care nurse may always be included. The disciplines involved will vary from institution to institution, but in general, nursing, medicine, and social work should be on every plan.

Once each representative has participated in the plan-development process, it would be beneficial to have as many of these people as possible sit down together to review the plan. This form of brainstorming may expose redundant treatments or procedures. This is another way of significantly reducing resource utilization while providing the best quality of care possible.

MAP TIMELINES

Multidisciplinary action plans can be time lined in hours, days, weeks, or months depending on the clinical area. Emergency room treatment might be mapped out in terms of hours or parts of an hour. Typical diagnoses, including common medical problems or surgeries, usually fall within a day's time frame. Weeks might be used for those diagnoses that have a longer length of stay, such as those that might be found in a neonatal intensive care unit where the length of stay is 3 or 4 months. Month time frames might be relevant in long-term care facilities, such as those for patients with chronic mental disorders, where clinical progress is extremely slow and lengths of stay are measured in years. Nursing home patients provide another example of patient goals that might be evaluated in terms of months.

Once these time frames are determined, variance time frames must be decided. In other words, when does something become a variance? In what time period should every outcome listed for a particular day be achieved? A variance is anything that does not happen at the time it is supposed to happen. The hospital must decide what kind of leeway will be allowed for achieving these outcomes. Day 1 will seldom begin at 6 AM on the day of admission because most patients are admitted later in the day. For example, emergency admissions may arrive on the unit in the late afternoon or night shift. It is clear that the beginning and end of any one day in the hospital is a loose concept. Institutions should be generous when deciding on variance time frames. If not, it is possible to set up a situation where almost everything becomes a variance. A plan lasting at least 5 days might not place something into the variance category unless it is not completed within 24 hours. The expected time frame should drive the time frames for variances. For example, if the plan is developed around 15-minute intervals, anything beyond that time period becomes a variance.

Documentation of Variances

An area designated for documenting variances should be on the plan. Each variance can be identified and categorized, if desirable. Typical variance categories include the following:

▼ Operational
▼ Health care provider
▼ Patient
▼ Unmet clinical indicators

An example of operational variances is the breakdown of a piece of equipment, which prevents the completion of a test. Another example is the inability to discharge a patient because no long-term care facilities in the area have an available bed. These are examples of operational variances that go beyond the confines of the hospital. More examples are presented in the box below.

Health care provider variances include any situations in which a health care provider is the cause of the delay in achieving an expected outcome (see the box below). Discretion must be used when documenting these variances, because some may involve a risk management issue. For example, if the resident is paged several

---

OPERATIONAL VARIANCE EXAMPLES

▼ Broken equipment
▼ Lost requisition slips causing delays
▼ Departmental delays due to staffing or other causes
▼ Interdepartmental delays
▼ Larger system delays affecting discharge, such as home care services, equipment, or insurance availability

---

HEALTH CARE PROVIDER VARIANCE EXAMPLES

▼ Deviation from plan because of physician's varying the practice pattern
▼ Change related to health care provider's practice patterns, level of expertise, or experience

times during the night because a patient has pulled out the nasogastric tube and the resident does not respond for several hours, the patient misses several doses of medication. Other variances in this category may be associated with the physician's alteration or adjustment of the traditional plan of care.

Patient variances include any patient-related delays (see the box below). The patient delay may be caused by complications of the patient's medical condition, which require a delay in completion of a test or procedure. For example, the patient may have spiked a fever and may be unable to leave the floor for magnetic resonance imaging (MRI). In other circumstances the delay may be because the patient refused to allow the test or procedure. Noncompliance frequently causes patient delays. When a patient refuses a test or procedure, the absolute need for the test or procedure should be questioned and evaluated. This sort of stringent review and follow-up is an example of how a checks-and-balances system in case management can help reduce unnecessary resource use. Tests and procedures cost the institution money not only in terms of the expense of the supplies and equipment but also in terms of the human resources needed to administer the test and evaluate the results. More timely completion of appropriate tests means a reduction in the length of stay for all patients.

Another patient variance is called *patient variance on admission.* These variances are also known as preexisting conditions or comorbidities. Case management plans are simple guidelines or expected plans for particular diagnoses or procedures. Regulatory agencies require individualization of any predetermined plans of care during patient admission. This process should be a routine part of putting any patient on a case management plan. The patient's case should be reviewed in relation to the prewritten plan. Anything different or unusual about the patient's case should yield a change in the plan to make it specific to the patient. One plan is not going to be appropriate for every patient. This process ensures that the plan meets the needs of the patient in question. For example, if the plan calls for a specific medication and the patient is allergic to that medication, the plan should be altered to adjust to that particular patient's clinical condition.

The fourth type of variance is unmet clinical quality indicators (see box on p. 174). Clinical quality indicators are developed in conjunction with the MAP. They are created by the physicians to benchmark clinical outcomes that reflect quality of care rendered. These clinical outcomes can be either intermediate or discharge patient outcomes. The box contains examples of clinical quality indicators that would be developed for asthma team patients.

Variance data are abstracted from the patient's medical record and MAP. The analysis of these data is invaluable in determining why an expected patient outcome or clinical quality indicator has not been met. In addition, these data allow for trending of patient outcomes, length of stay, and evaluation of the quality of patient care.

PATIENT VARIANCE EXAMPLES

▼ Refusal   ▼ Change in status   ▼ Unavailability

UNMET CLINICAL QUALITY INDICATORS

ASTHMA

INTERMEDIATE OUTCOMES

▼ Patient is off IV Solu-Medrol when peak flow >200

DISCHARGE OUTCOMES

▼ Peak flow measurement >250 L/sec
▼ Patient is out of bed without shortness of breath
▼ Patient is able to return demonstration of the use of metered dose inhaler (MDI) with spacer

---

Appendix 4-1 at end of Chapter 4 is an example of a MAP developed and used at the Beth Israel Medical Center in New York City. This MAP is clinically specific not DRG specific. The format illustrated is a preprinted, bound booklet that outlines the expected outcomes for care for each day of hospitalization for each discipline involved. Medicine, nursing, social work, and discharge planning are automatically included on every plan. Other departments are included as needed. Each department is given a standard place on the form, and content is filled in by members of the discipline during formation of the plan.

The length of the booklet is guided by the reimbursement for the DRGs usually associated with the diagnosis or problem. This information is correlated with what the physician expects the length of stay to be. Generally the physician will adapt to the reimbursement length of stay if this information is supplied in a positive way. If more than one DRG is involved, which is usually the case, then some judgment must be used in determining the shortest possible plan that takes into account the possibly varying reimbursable lengths of stay. In other words, it may be necessary to look at the most commonly used DRGs and follow an average or usual length of stay. Clearly, these expected lengths are "guesstimates" and will not be completely accurate every time. Each plan may be lengthened or shortened depending on patient-related variations, but some professional judgment must be used. If a plan is 7 days in length and the patient is ready to go home on the sixth day, an earlier discharge would be completed, and the documentation would be written to reflect the reasons why. A delayed discharge must be documented in the same way with variances that caused the delay being documented and explained.

During the early phases of DRG use in case management systems, the finer points of the DRG were not always synchronous with the system itself. As the system evolved into more of a financial one, clinical applications of the system needed to remain flexible, and the limitations of such uses needed to be clarified for those clinicians using the system.

Space for nursing documentation has been incorporated into the form of some MAPs. In this space, the registered nurse documents whether expected outcomes for the day were achieved and any appropriate responses of the patient. Progress notes are included only when a more elaborate or detailed form of documentation is needed, and narrative nurse's notes are eliminated unless an exception arises. This detailed list of outcomes provides the nurse with an action plan that is specific for that day and keeps the patient on track toward discharge.

For the novice nurse who is less able to project patient needs because of a lack of experience, the MAP provides a plan that is outcome-oriented and guides the new nurse through that particular day of hospitalization. Rather than correcting problems after they have happened, the MAP provides an advanced, detailed plan with tasks that can be carried out in a timely fashion.

The case manager is the driving force behind the success of the managed care plan. It is generally the case manager who checks on variances related to both cause and remedy and who is accountable for the patient's continued success in moving through the system. Using the plan as a guide, the case manager directs all other health care providers toward achieving the expected daily outcome of care.

Another responsibility of the case manager is to provide patient teaching when necessary and to find out why a test or procedure has not been done. The case manager also reviews the care plan with the physician and ensures timely outcomes. Finally, the case manager coordinates with the social worker, discharge planner, family, and patient to ensure that the best possible discharge plan has been made and that it is ready when the patient goes home. This entire process is communicated to other members of the team through the MAP format and through the case manager's documentation. All in all, the case manager views the whole picture and ensures proper and accurate progress of the patient through the hospital system.

Staff nurses work in collaboration with the case manager and other members of the health care team to ensure that the outcomes of care are achieved within the time frames specified on the MAP. The patient's outcomes are documented by the staff nurse and relate the clinical story of the patient's progress during hospitalization. Appendix 16-3 contains a sample critical path that has been adapted to the needs of a particular institution; appendixes 4-1, 5-1, and 6-1 at the ends of Chapters 4, 5, and 6 provide additional examples.

PATIENT PATHWAYS

The case management plan can be adapted for use by patients and families. The existing plans rewritten in language understandable to patients and their families can be an effective tool. It is not necessary for these adapted plans to contain as much in-depth information as the case management plans used by the health care providers. Rather, only specific information relevant to the patient's needs can be summarized from the more detailed plan.

An issue to consider in the selection of the content is the inclusion of a discussion in patient-friendly language of the general course of events patients can expect during their hospital stay. Care should be taken not to be too specific clinically because as changes are made to the medical plan, patients may become concerned that there is something wrong or that their clinical progression toward discharge is not going as planned.

Benchmarks should be outlined in the patient's version of the case management plan. These benchmarks should include milestones during the course of the hospital stay as well as discharge indicators. For example, asthmatic patients might be told that their intravenous medication will be stopped when their peak flow reading is 200 L/s. In this way the patient will clearly understand the goal of care as well as why their IV medication was switched to an oral medication. Other benchmarks should relate to the patient's clinical condition and should reflect the benchmarks or indicators outlined in the clinician's case management plan.

Another useful technique is to give the patient and family a patient version of the critical pathway. Such a document presents the discharge indicators or the factors that indicate when a particular case type is safe and ready for discharge. Again, these pathways should be written in language that is understandable to lay people and given to the patient soon after admission to the hospital. In this way the patient once again knows the indications for safe discharge and can work with the health care team toward these goals. In addition, the patient also sees that a decision to discharge is based on predetermined criteria and is not arbitrary in any way. Examples of two patient pathways are included here as Appendixes 16-1 and 16-2.

REFERENCES

Giuliano, K.K., & Poirier, C.E. (1991). Nursing case management: Critical pathways to desirable outcomes. *Nursing Management, 22* (3), 52-55.

Zander, K. (1991). Care MAPs: The core of cost/quality care. *The New Definition, 6* (3), 1-3.

Zander, K. (1992). Physicians, care MAPs, and collaboration. *The New Definition, 7* (1), 1-4.

Appendix 16-1

CHEMOTHERAPY CRITICAL PATHWAY PATIENT VERSION*

Dear Patient and Family,

This document, known as a *Critical Pathway*, has been developed to provide a plan for the hospital care of a patient receiving **chemotherapy**. Created by your doctors, nurses, health care team, and other patients, it is meant to be a kind of map of important events that are necessary in your recovery. Specially designed for patients receiving chemotherapy, your Critical Pathway allows you to participate in your care and prepares you for discharge within 3 days. The Pathway is a guideline, and *your* care may vary because of your unique needs. Your care team monitors your progress according to this plan every day. You can expect the following program of education, tests, activities, treatments, diet, medications, and discharge planning during your stay at The Long Island College Hospital. If you have any questions about this Pathway or your progress, please speak to your doctor or nurse.

---

*Created by M. Impollonia, The Long Island College Hospital, Brooklyn, New York. Reprinted with permission.

▼ PREADMISSION/DOCTOR'S OFFICE

ASSESSMENTS AND CONSULTS	You will meet with your doctor and nurse. You may wish to think about your past and present medical history and write it down in preparation for the questions you will be asked in the hospital.
LAB WORK AND TESTS	To determine your present health status you may have • blood tests • urine tests • X-rays
TREATMENTS	
ACTIVITY	Continue your normal routine unless your doctor tells you otherwise.
MEDICATIONS	Continue your regular medicines unless your doctor tells you otherwise. Discuss with your doctor any medicines that you are taking at home that you may have to bring to the hospital with you.
DIET AND NUTRITION	You may be asked to drink a lot of fluid a day or two before you are scheduled to go to the hospital and to keep a record of how much you drink.
TEACHING	You will be given information about • your disease • your chemotherapy • radiation (if necessary) • common side effects • proper nutrition You will be told to come to the hospital by 8 AM on the day you are admitted. You may wish to bring some items from home to occupy yourself while you're in the hospital (for example, battery-operated tape recorder, music tapes, reading material, crossword puzzles, knitting).
PREPARING TO GO HOME	

▼ DAY 1/ADMISSION DAY

ASSESSMENTS AND CONSULTS	Your doctor and nurse will ask you about your past and present medical history. Your temperature, pulse, respirations, and blood pressure will be taken at least once a day.
LAB WORK AND TESTS	To determine your present health status, you may have • blood tests (done at 8 AM in the admitting area or when you get to your bed) • EKG • X-ray While you are in the hospital, you may need to save your urine for a special test.
TREATMENTS	You might be given an IV (fluids flow into your veins through a tube). The staff may measure your height and weight. The nurse will measure and write down all the fluid you take in and the urine you put out.
ACTIVITY	You will be permitted to move around freely if your condition permits. Be sure to ask for help if you need it.
MEDICATIONS	If your blood work is OK, your chemotherapy will be started soon after your arrival. Depending on your treatment, you may or may not be given medicine for nausea. Try to tell the nurse when you are nauseous before it becomes too bad. You will continue to take your other medicines ordered by your doctor.
DIET AND NUTRITION	The doctor will order a diet for you. You may also receive snacks or supplements.
TEACHING	Your nurse will speak to you about • hospital routine and your plan of care • cultural considerations and preferences Your nurse will begin to speak with you about • your medication • measuring the fluids you take • your diet in and put out • preventing infection Ask questions and take notes.
PREPARING TO GO HOME	Your nurse will speak to you about • how to take care of yourself at home • whether you need more help at home • the need to have someone take you home.

▼ DAY 2

ASSESSMENTS AND CONSULTS	Your doctors and nurses will continue to check on your condition several times during the day to see how you respond to the treatment you receive.
LAB WORK AND TESTS	You may have more blood tests.
TREATMENTS	You will help your nurse measure and write down all the fluid that you take in and put out.
ACTIVITY	You will be free to move around if your condition permits. Be sure to ask for help if you need it.
MEDICATIONS	Your nurse will continue to give you your chemotherapy and other medications ordered by your doctor. Remember to tell your nurse if you feel nauseous or different in any way.
DIET AND NUTRITION	The nutritionist will visit you and obtain nutrition information. You will choose your menu. Your menu choices may have to be adjusted to match your cultural or religious considerations or your meal plan. Ask for clarification if you do not understand. You may keep some sample menus to take home.
TEACHING	Your nurse will continue to go over information about your disease, your chemotherapy and radiation (if necessary), preventing infection, and your medications. Your nurse will discuss community resources with you.
PREPARING TO GO HOME	You will be visited by a social worker or discharge planner if necessary. Professional social workers are available to discuss concerns that you or your family may have about your treatment. They can work with you to allay fears and help you cope with your illness. Also referrals can be made to support groups and other community organizations. Please ask your nurse to call for a social worker if you would like to see one. All medical services (for example, Home Health Aid, Visiting Nurse) and equipment ordered by your doctor will be discussed with you and arrangements made to have them in your home. You may be notified that you are to be discharged tomorrow. You will need to make arrangements with your family or friends to pick you up before 11 AM on the day you go home.

▼ DAY 3/DISCHARGE DAY

ASSESSMENTS AND CONSULTS	Your doctors and nurses will continue to check on your condition several times during the day to see how you respond to the treatment you receive.
LAB WORK AND TESTS	You may have more blood tests.
TREATMENTS	You will help your nurse measure and write down all the fluid that you take in and put out.
ACTIVITY	You will be permitted to move around freely if your condition permits. Be sure to ask for help if you need it.
MEDICATIONS	Your chemotherapy is finished and your IV is discontinued. You will continue to take your other medications as ordered by your doctor.
DIET AND NUTRITION	You may go home with a special diet that you should follow.
TEACHING	Your nurse will reinforce all previous teaching. You should ask your nurse any questions you still might have or about anything you are unsure of. Your nurse will tell you which symptoms you might expect and which need to be reported to your doctor immediately.
PREPARING TO GO HOME	You are ready to go home. Your nurse will review discharge instructions with you. Your doctor may give you other instructions. You will be given an appointment to visit your doctor.

Notes

_____   _____

_____   _____

_____   _____

_____   _____

_____   _____

_____   _____

_____   _____

_____   _____

_____   _____

_____   _____

_____   _____

_____   _____

_____   _____

_____   _____

_____   _____

Appendix 16-2

DIABETIC CRITICAL PATHWAY PATIENT VERSION*

Dear Patient and Family,

   This document, known as a *Critical Pathway*, has been developed to provide a plan for the hospital care of a patient with **diabetes.** Created by your doctors, nurses, health care team, and other patients, it is meant to be a kind of map of important events that are necessary in your recovery. Specially designed for patients with diabetes, your Critical Pathway allows you to participate in your care and prepares you for discharge within 6 days. The Pathway is a guideline, and *your* care may vary because of your unique needs. Your care team monitors your progress according to this plan every day. You can expect the following program of education, tests, activities, treatments, diet, medications, and discharge planning during your stay at The Long Island College Hospital. If you have any questions about this Pathway or your progress, please speak to your doctor or nurse.

---

*Created by M. Impollonia, The Long Island College Hospital, Brooklyn, New York. Reprinted with permission.

▼ DAY 1/ADMISSION DAY

ASSESSMENTS AND CONSULTS	Your doctor and nurse will ask you questions about your diet, your blood sugar, and what kind of insulin or medication you take. Your temperature, pulse, respirations, and blood pressure will be taken at least once a day.
LAB WORK AND TESTS	To determine your present health status, you may have • blood tests • EKG • X-ray
TREATMENTS	To determine the amount of insulin you need, your nurse will prick your finger to test for the sugar in your blood during the day (usually before meals). You might be given an IV (fluid flows into your veins through a tube). Staff may measure your height and weight.
ACTIVITY	You will be permitted to move around freely if your condition permits. Be sure to ask for help if you need it.
MEDICATIONS	To lower the sugar in your blood, your nurse might give you insulin injections or a pill. Your insulin regimen may be different from your regimen at home, and your treatment may change as your condition does.
DIET AND NUTRITION	You will be given a low-calorie diet. Snacks will be provided if indicated. A nutritionist will speak with you during your hospital stay to give you special instructions. Ask for clarification if you do not understand.
TEACHING	Your nurse will speak to you about • hospital routine and your plan of care • cultural considerations and personal preferences Your nurse will begin to speak with you about • your medications • your diet • preventing infection • measuring the fluid you take in and put out Watch the Patient Education channel. Ask questions and take notes.
PREPARING TO GO HOME	Your nurse will speak to you about • how to take care of yourself at home • whether you will need more help at home • the need to have someone take you home.

▼ DAY 2

ASSESSMENTS AND CONSULTS	Your doctors and nurses will continue to check on your condition every day to see how you respond to the treatment you receive. Some of your treatment may need to be adjusted or changed. For example, the amount of insulin you need may vary.
LAB WORK AND TESTS	You may have more blood tests. You may be asked to save all your urine for 24 hours for a special test.
TREATMENTS	Your nurse will show you how to measure and write down all the fluid you take in and urine you put out. You might continue to do this for a few days. Your nurse will prick your finger to test the sugar in your blood.
ACTIVITY	You will be encouraged to move around freely if your condition permits. Remember to ask for help if you need it.
MEDICATIONS	Your nurse may continue to give you insulin or pills or both to control the sugar in your blood. Your doctor may change your medications as your condition changes. Your nurse may give you other medications if the doctor orders them.
DIET AND NUTRITION	The nutritionist will visit you to discuss your past and present diet. A meal pattern will be developed for you. You will receive a menu. Your menu choices may need to be adjusted to match your meal plan or cultural or religious considerations.
TEACHING	Your nurse will continue to go over information about diabetes, your medication, diet, and preventing infection. She will teach you how to prepare insulin for injection.
PREPARING TO GO HOME	You will be visited by a social worker or discharge planner if necessary. Professional social workers are available to discuss concerns that you or your family may have about your treatment. They can work with you to allay your fears and help you cope with your illness. Also, referrals can be made to support groups and other community organizations. Please ask your nurse to call for a social worker if you would like to see one.

▼ DAY 3

ASSESSMENTS AND CONSULTS	Your doctors and nurses will continue to check on your condition every day to see how you respond to the treatment you receive. Some of your treatment may need to be adjusted or changed. For example, the amount of insulin you need may vary.
LAB WORK AND TESTS	You may have more blood tests.
TREATMENTS	You will continue to measure and write down all the fluid that you take in and put out. Your nurse will continue to prick your finger to test for the sugar in your blood. You will begin to write down and track the amount of sugar in your blood.
ACTIVITY	You will continue to be encouraged to move around freely if your condition permits. Remember to ask for help if you need it.
MEDICATIONS	Your nurse may continue to give you insulin or pills or both to control the sugar in your blood. Your doctor may change your medications as your condition changes. Your nurse may give you other medications if the doctor orders them.
DIET AND NUTRITION	The nutritionist will discuss meal planning with you. Nutrition information will be given to you during your hospital stay. You will continue to choose your own menu. You may wish to keep some sample menus to take home.
TEACHING	Your nurse will continue to go over information about diabetes, your medication, diet, and preventing infection. You will show her how you prepare insulin for injection after you practice and are ready. She will begin to teach you how to give yourself an insulin injection.
PREPARING TO GO HOME	All medical services and equipment ordered by your doctor will be discussed with you.

▼ DAY 4

ASSESSMENTS AND CONSULTS	Your doctors and nurses will continue to check on your condition every day to see how you respond to the treatment you receive. Some of your treatment may have to be adjusted or changed. For example, the amount of insulin you need may vary.
LAB WORK AND TESTS	You may have more blood tests.
TREATMENTS	You will continue to measure and write down all the fluid that you take in and put out. Your nurse will continue to prick your finger to test for the sugar in your blood. You will continue to write down and track the amount of sugar in your blood.
ACTIVITY	You will continue to be encouraged to move around freely if your condition permits. Remember to ask for help if you need it.
MEDICATIONS	Your nurse may continue to give you insulin or pills or both to control the sugar in your blood. Your doctor may change your medications as your condition changes. Your nurse may give you other medications if the doctor orders them.
DIET AND NUTRITION	You will choose your own menu.
TEACHING	Your nurse will continue to go over information about diabetes, your medication, diet, and preventing infection. She will reinforce all previous teaching and begin to teach you how to manage yourself at home on a "sick day." After practice and when you are ready, you will begin to show her how you give yourself an insulin injection.
PREPARING TO GO HOME	All medical services and equipment ordered by your doctor will be discussed with you and arrangements made to have them in your home.

▼ DAY 5

ASSESSMENTS AND CONSULTS	Your doctors and nurses will continue to check on your condition every day to see how you respond to the treatment you receive. Some of your treatment may need to be adjusted or changed. For example, the amount of insulin you need may vary.
LAB WORK AND TESTS	You may have more blood tests.
TREATMENTS	You will continue to measure and write down all the fluid that you take in and put out. Your nurse will continue to prick your finger to test for the sugar in your blood. You will continue to write down and track the amount of sugar in your blood. You may prick your own finger and test for the sugar in your blood.
ACTIVITY	You will continue to be encouraged to move around freely if your condition permits. Remember to ask for help if you need it.
MEDICATIONS	Your nurse may continue to give you insulin or pills or both to control the sugar in your blood. Your doctor may change your medications as your condition changes. Your nurse may give you other medications if the doctor orders them.
DIET AND NUTRITION	The nutritionist will discuss meal planning with you. Nutrition information will be given to you during your hospital stay. You will continue to choose your own menu. You may wish to keep some sample menus to take home.
TEACHING	Your nurse will reinforce all previous teaching. You will be able to show her how you prick your finger to test your blood for sugar, how you prepare your insulin, and how you give yourself the injection. Your nurse will discuss community resources with you.
PREPARING TO GO HOME	Plans are complete for all the services and equipment you will need at home. You may be notified that you are to be discharged tomorrow. You will need to make arrangements with your family or friends to pick you up before 11 AM on the day you go home.

▼ DAY 6/DISCHARGE DAY

ASSESSMENTS AND CONSULTS	Your doctors and nurses will continue to check on your condition every day to see how you respond to the treatment you receive. Some of your treatment may need to be adjusted or changed. For example, the amount of insulin you need may vary.
LAB WORK AND TESTS	You may have more blood tests.
TREATMENTS	You will continue to measure and write down all the fluid that you take in and put out. Your nurse will continue to prick your finger to test for the sugar in your blood. You will continue to write down and track the amount of sugar in your blood. You may prick your own finger to test your blood for sugar.
ACTIVITY	You can continue to move around freely if your condition permits. Remember to ask for help if needed.
MEDICATIONS	Your nurse may continue to give you insulin or pills or both to control the sugar in your blood. Your doctor may change your medications as your condition changes. Your nurse may give you other medications if the doctor orders them.
DIET AND NUTRITION	The nutritionist will discuss meal planning with you. Nutrition information will be given to you during your hospital stay. You will continue to choose your own menu. You may keep some sample menus to take home. You will go home with a special diet to follow.
TEACHING	Your nurse will reinforce all previous teaching. You will be able to show her how you prick your finger to test your blood for sugar, how you prepare your insulin, and how you give yourself the injection. Your nurse will discuss community resources with you. You should ask your nurse any questions you still might have or about anything you are unsure of. Your nurse will tell you which symptoms you might expect and which need to be reported to your doctor immediately.
PREPARING TO GO HOME	You are ready to go home. Your nurse will review discharge instructions with you. Your doctor may give you other instructions. You will be given an appointment to visit your doctor.

Notes

_____   _____

_____   _____

_____   _____

_____   _____

_____   _____

_____   _____

_____   _____

_____   _____

_____   _____

_____   _____

_____   _____

_____   _____

_____   _____

_____   _____

_____   _____

APPENDIX 16-3

ST. MICHAEL HOSPITAL
MILWAUKEE, WISCONSIN

Uncomplicated MI Critical Path

DRG: _____

HCFA LOS: _____   Exp. LOS: _____

Physician: _____

Date Reviewed by Physician/RN: _____

Day/Date

	DAY 1 ED	DAY 1 CCU	DAY 2	DAY 3	DAY 4
Floor:				Transfer to MCU	
Consults:			Cardiac Rehab PT and OT – – – → Dietitian		
Tests:	CBC EKG Lytes Glucose BUN Creatinine CXR Cardiac enzymes	CCU Standing Orders – – – → EKG – – – → Assess Need: CPK Isoenzymes x 3 (total) per protocol Chem profile & electrolytes – – → 	EKG – – – → Electrolytes in AM	EKG – – – → Stress test/cath ordered Day 7 or 8	EKG
Activity:	Bedrest – – – →	→	Bed rest c commode PRN	Up in chair & progress – – – → Progression of self-care ADL – – – →	
Treatments:	IV D₅W Ko – – → Cardiovascular Assessment & VS q 10-15 min & PRN – – → Monitor – – →	Daily weights I&O – – → VS q 4° & PRN	Heplock VI	VS q 8° & PRN	

Continued.

Day/Date

	DAY 1 ED	DAY 1 CCU	DAY 2	DAY 3 Transfer to MCU	DAY 4
Floor:					
Medications:	Nitrates – – – O₂ 2-4 PNC – Analgesics – Lidocaine	→ → – – – – → → Stool softener Beta blockers Calcium channel blockers	O₂ PRN →		
Diet:		Low cholesterol			
Discharge Planning:	Complete ED data base	Complete data base. Assessment of home situation	Mutual goal setting – – – → *Multidisciplinary Staffing (T or F) Assessment of IP & OP plans of care. (*Inpatient Cardiac Rehab only)		Assess D/C needs & date Contact SW/HC prn

Key Nursing Diagnosis/Interventions:	-Orientation to ED, staff & equipment. *Assess & monitor:* -Head-to-toe assessment x 1 -Hemodynamic & cardiovascular stability (4) *Instruct:* -Pain scale 1-10 (1) -Preparation for adm. to CCU(2) [ ] brochure given [ ] family/sig. other notified -Offer emotional support	-Orientation to CCU routine, equipment, CCTV, & care delivery system. -Assess pain q 30" until under control (1) -Reinforce use of pain scale (1) -Position for comfort q 2° or prn (1) *Assess & Monitor:* -Head-to-toe assessment q 4° or prn -Activity restriction (3) -Hemodynamic & cardiovascular stability (4) -Arrhythmatic disturbances (4)	Position for comfort q 2° or prn (1) -Pt. booklet given (2) -Orient to CCTV, channels 3 & 11 (2) Review basic medication instruction c̄ adm. of routine doses (2) *Instruct:* -ID risk factors specific c̄ pt (2) -Diet modification (2) -Gradual progression of activity (3) – –	Assess pt. readiness to learn, observe verbal/non-verbal cues, & pt's. condition (2) *Instruct:* Stress Reduction (2) -stress management relaxation techniques – – → -time management -ID support systems & resources – – →	→
Key Patient Activities/Outcomes:	-Pt &/or sig. other verbalizes fears & anxiety -Pt rates pain & intensity on 1-10 scale (1) – → -Pt. &/or sig. other verbalizes reason for hospitalization (2)	-Pt. demonstrates use of call light – → Pt's. behavior indicates pain reduction or elimination (1) Pt. verbalizes that pain is decreased, alleviated, or under control (1)	-Pt. verbalizes understanding of diagnosis (2) -Pt. voices specific concerns related to coping with illness (2) -Pt. watches CCTV (2)	-Pt. behavior shows progress toward acceptance of illness (2) -Pt. able to identify own learning needs (2) -Pt. demonstrates readiness to learn (2) -Pt. verbalizes own risk factors (2) -Pt. demonstrates gradual progression of energy using energy conservation techniques (3&4)	Behavior shows signs of: -stress management (2) -relaxation techniques (2) Pt. verbalizes time management skills (2&4) Pt. verbalizes support system & resources (2)

Continued.

Day/Date

	DAY 5	DAY 6	DAY 7-8	
Floor:	Transfer to 2N with telemetry			
Consults:		Assess Need OP Cardiac Rehab		
Tests:			Stress Test/Cath	
Activity:	Ambulate BID	Up ad lib		
Treatments:	VS q 8° & prn I&O	VS BID or q shift D/C I&O	D/C Heplock	
Medications:				
Diet:	Low cholesterol →			
Discharge Planning:		D/C orders D/C meds Follow-up MD appointment		
Key Nursing Diagnosis/Interventions:	Review previous learning (2)	Review Home Program (2) -Post MI status -Diet -Meds a) schedule b) indications/side effects c) med sheet given -Follow-up with MD -Program given by pt.	OP Cardiac Rehab Post list	**Possible Nursing Diagnoses** 1) Pain 2) Knowledge deficit (Learning needs with diagnosis of MI) 3) Activity in tolerance 4) Decreased cardiac output *Nursing Care Guide available

| Key Patient Activities/ Outcomes: | Pt. verbalizes understanding of cardiac disease and/or MI (2) | Pt. plans activity progression and after D/C (home, work, sexuality, social) using energy conservation/work simplification techniques (2, 3, 4) | Pt. describes home med schedule with indications/side effects (reference med sheet) (2)

Pt. verbalizes follow-up MD, early warning signs, and emergency plan (2) | **WIPRO Criteria →**
All Met and Documented before Discharge
72 Hours a D/C
  No evidence of EKG changes.

48 Hours a D/C
  No change in type/dosage of antiarrhythmic drug(s).
  Chest pain controlled with anti-anginal drugs.
  Vital signs WNL for pt.

24 Hours a D/C
  Lab values WNL for pt. (lytes, BUN, enzymes)
  Oral temp <99° s antipyretic.
  Invasive monitoring devices removed.
  Activity/mobility/amb. documented as improved/stabilized.
  Improved clinical status (e.g., chest clear, rales & wheezing, absence of friction rub & S, gallop).
  If DC'd to self care, document completion of pt. education.
  D/C plan documented.

If hospital stay < 3 days for R/O MI, no evidence of EKG changes or enzyme rise. |

Definitions
1. DECREASED CARDIAC OUTPUT: A state in which the blood pumped by the individual's heart is sufficiently reduced that it is inadequate to meet the needs of the body's tissues. **2. PAIN:** A state in which an individual experiences and reports the presence of severe discomfort or an uncomfortable sensation. **3. ACTIVITY INTOLERANCE:** A state in which an individual has insufficient physiological or psychological energy to endure or complete required or desired daily activities.

4/91 © St. Michael Hospital

17

THE ROLE OF THE NURSE CASE MANAGER

HUSSEIN A. TAHAN

▼ *CHAPTER OVERVIEW*

There is no standardization in the job description of the nurse case manager. Each institution implementing case management systems has established its own version of the role. This chapter, however, presents a thorough description of the roles, responsibilities, and functions of the case manager. It delineates the clinical, managerial, and financial aspects of the role. It also discusses why nurses are, among all health care professionals, best fit to become case managers. In addition, it describes the skills and selection criteria required for the role. A special section of this chapter is designated for the various functions assumed by case managers while delivering patient care. Among these functions are change agent, clinician, consultant, coordinator and facilitator of care, educator, negotiator, manager, patient and family advocate, quality improvement coordinator, researcher, and risk manager.

▲

Over the past decade, nurses have played a crucial role in the success of case management as a patient care delivery system. This is evidenced through the drastic changes such delivery systems have undergone. In the early 1980s case management models were implemented by nursing executives as nursing efforts to meet the demands and challenges of the ever changing health care system: cost containment and higher quality care. Today, however, these models are being implemented in a broader perspective as patient care delivery systems that are interdisciplinary, surpassing the boundaries of nursing care.

Despite the fact that for over a decade case management models have been successful in improving quality of patient care and containing the incurred costs, the literature regarding the nurse case manager's role description and functions is limited. Nurse case managers are introduced as integral members of interdisciplinary health care teams every time a health care institution implements a case management system for patient care delivery. The presence and achievements of case managers in such institutions are important for the success of the case management system. Regardless of the patient care setting in which these systems are implemented, the institutions rely heavily on the nurse case manager, who acts as the gatekeeper of the interdisciplinary health care team and as the coordinator and facilitator of care. The case manager in most institutions is a registered professional nurse who assumes an advanced nursing role.

There is no standardization in the role of the nurse case manager. The institutions that have implemented case management systems have created their own case manager's role in a way that correlates with their organizational chart and operations, policies and procedures, and financial status. Regardless of the type of health care institution, there is some common ground in the role of nurse case managers. A summary of these commonalities is based on three dimensions (Cohen & Cesta, 1993; Tahan, 1993) related to the clinical, managerial, and financial or business aspects of the role.

THE NURSE CASE MANAGER'S ROLE DIMENSIONS

Generally the nurse case manager is responsible for

> coordinating the care delivered to a group of patients (case load/case mix) that begins at the time of admission and extends beyond discharge. This is carried out through applying the nursing process (assessment, diagnosis, planning, implementation, and evaluation). . . . The nurse case manager ensures the delivery of cost-effective, outcome-oriented quality care, . . .and access to health care. . . . The nurse case manager is accountable for applying nursing case management successfully to the daily activities of patient care [Tahan, 1993, pp. 55-56].

The three role dimensions allow nurse case managers to make sound decisions that reflect what is best for the patient and family, interdisciplinary team, and the organization.

The Clinical Role Dimension

Nurse case managers are responsible for the assessment of patients and families every time a patient presents with a problem. They identify the existing or potential health problems by evaluating the patient's physical, psychosocial, and spiritual condition. They then, in collaboration with other members of the interdisciplinary health care team, develop a plan of care that meets the patient's needs (Bower, 1989; Ethridge & Lamb, 1989; Giuliano & Poirier, 1991; Tahan, 1993; Zander, 1988a). The plan of care is usually the outcome of individualizing a preexisting care protocol. It lists the key tasks or events that must be accomplished for handling patient problems and meeting the care goals, the patient and family teaching activities based on the identified health needs, and the discharge plan that assures a timely and appropriate discharge back into the community. Case managers use these protocols to direct, monitor, and evaluate patient treatments and nursing interventions, and the outcomes or responses to treatments (Cohen & Cesta, 1993; Tahan, 1993; Thompson, Caddick, Mathie, Newlon, & Abrahams, 1991; Zander 1988a).

Nurse case managers, when caring for patients, follow a holistic approach to care and spend a considerable amount of time discussing preventive services. They may or may not provide direct patient care activities. They assess the patient's and family's coping abilities and social support systems and intervene if a problem is identified. Case managers are also responsible for facilitating the patient's progress through the health care system, arranging for consultation with specialists or specialized services, and assuring that transfers to more appropriate care areas are made when needed (Brockopp, Porter, Kinnard, & Silberman, 1992; Henderson & Collard, 1988; Leclair, 1991; Zander, 1988b).

As to case management plans, case managers are responsible for their development. They participate in an interdisciplinary health care team for that purpose. When these plans are implemented for guiding patient care, nurse case managers identify any variances from the standards and work with other team members to analyze and, when possible, resolve these variances (Cohen & Cesta, 1993; Ethridge & Lamb, 1989; O'Malley, 1988a; Tahan & Cesta, 1995).

The Managerial Role Dimension

The managerial role dimension refers to the case manager's responsibility for facilitating and coordinating the care of patients during the course of their illness (Cohen & Cesta, 1993; Ethridge & Lamb, 1989; Kruger, 1989; O'Malley, 1988a; Zander 1988a). The nurse case managers manage care by planning the treatment modalities and interventions necessary for meeting the needs of patients and families. They determine, in collaboration with the interdisciplinary team, the goals of treatment and the projected length of stay and initiate the discharge plan at the time of admission. This is important because it provides a clear time frame for accomplishing the care activities needed (O'Malley, 1988b; Tahan, 1993).

Case managers also guide the patient care activities, nursing treatments, and interventions to be carried out by nurses and other staff members. They continuously evaluate the quality of care provided and the outcomes of treatments and services to prevent misuse of resources (Ethridge & Lamb, 1989; Kruger, 1989; Loveridge, Cummings, & O'Malley, 1988; O'Malley, 1988b; Tahan, 1993; Zander, 1988a). They also conduct retrospective and concurrent chart reviews to evaluate the efficacy and efficiency of care and to identify any quality improvement opportunities (Cohen & Cesta, 1993; Tahan, 1993).

Nurse case managers act as gatekeepers of the interdisciplinary care team. They facilitate communication among the various members and disciplines involved in the care of patients internally (e.g., medicine, nursing, rehabilitation, occupational therapy, social services, pharmacy, medical records, nutrition, and radiology) and externally (e.g., managed care organizations, home care agencies, nursing homes, and durable medical equipment companies).

One of the informal responsibilities of case managers is that of teacher and mentor. The case manager assesses staff development needs, especially among less experienced practitioners, and refers them to the appropriate person or resource (Brockopp et al., 1992; Cronin & Maklebust, 1989; Kruger, 1989; Leclair, 1991; Tahan, 1993).

The Financial/Business Role Dimension

In collaboration with physicians and other health care team members, case managers initiate case management plans to assure that patients do not receive inadequate care while trying to maintain appropriate resource allocation and length of stay and to contain cost (Collard, Bergman, & Henderson, 1990; Tahan, 1993).

Case managers access information related to diagnosis-related groups (DRGs), the allocated cost for each diagnosis, the predetermined length of stay, and the treatments and procedures generally used for each diagnosis. They use this information to review resources and evaluate the efficiency of care related to the diagnosis. They exert a great influence on the quality and cost of care by determining, in a timely manner, the most important treatment for the patient. Case managers also assess variances for each DRG and act immediately to control these variances to contain costs (Cohen & Cesta, 1993; Crawford, 1991; Tahan & Cesta, 1995; Tahan, 1993). They assure consistency, continuity, facilitation, and coordination of care activities to control any duplication or fragmentation in health care delivery, resulting in better allocation and consumption of resources and further cost containment (Henderson & Collard, 1988; O'Malley, 1988a).

To be effective, nurse case managers must access information on case mix indexes, cost and consumption of resources, and practice patterns and must be familiar with the prospective payment system, current third-party reimbursement procedures, and the operations of managed care organizations in today's health care environment of managed competition (Ethridge & Lamb, 1989; Kruger, 1989; Loveridge, Cummings, & O'Malley, 1988; McKenzie, Trokelson, & Holt, 1989; O'Malley, 1988b).

Case managers may work closely with utilization review nurses or may assume utilization review responsibilities, particularly in institutions that dissolved utilization review departments, in identifying long-stay patients, and in planning to control and prevent inappropriate hospital stays (Cohen & Cesta, 1993; McKenzie et al., 1989; Tahan, 1993).

THE NURSE CASE MANAGER'S SKILLS

To be successful in their role, nurse case managers need to have certain skills that make them capable of carrying out their clinical, managerial, and business responsibilities. These skills transcend the issues of where or by whom case managers are employed. These skills are needed by case managers regardless of the care setting.

As to their clinical skills, case managers need to be clinically astute and competent in all related tests and procedures. They are considered role models and clinical experts for nursing and other staff. They should be skilled in coordinating patient's discharge and patient and family teaching and should be particularly knowledgeable in adult learning theory and the health belief model. Nurse case managers should also be able to function as mentors for less experienced staff.

Since they function as members of interdisciplinary health care teams, nurse case managers should be highly skilled in communication, negotiation, contracting, teamwork, delegation, and conducting meetings. They also should be capable of making sound decisions and resolving conflicts. To do this successfully, they should acquire critical thinking and problem solving skills. Because of their managerial responsibilities, case managers are required to write progress reports and quality improvement and length of stay reports, to speak publicly, and possibly to write for publication.

Looking at the business responsibilities embedded in the role of nurse case managers, one can see it is crucial that they have skills in financial analysis, contracting procedures of managed care organizations, financial reimbursement procedures, marketing, and customer relations. These skills are important, since nurse case managers are pressured to improve quality of care and reduce length of stay, hence contain cost.

SELECTION OF NURSE CASE MANAGERS

Health care administrators and policy makers have always struggled and still struggle with deciding who is best qualified to become the case manager. The question focuses on the following:

1. Should the case manager be a nurse-clinician or a paraprofessional staff member?
2. Are nurses the ideal candidates or are other professionals such as social workers and utilization reviewers equally effective in the role?
3. What is the financial implication of such a decision? Can the institution absorb the incurred cost?
4. Who best fits the institutional policies, procedures, and systems?

To respond to these issues, it is necessary to evaluate the case management system to be implemented and the proposed scope of practice and extent of responsibilities of case managers. Schwartz, Goldman, and Churgin (1982) argue that case managers should be clinicians because case management activities require substantial clinical knowledge, decision making, and skills. Grau (1984) describes case management as a set of clinically based functions that require a clinician to obtain the optimum benefit for the client. This definition also stresses that the background of the case manager is important because it influences the kind of direct and indirect care activities to be provided and other aspects of care delivery and monitoring.

Mundinger (1984) and Cohen and Cesta (1993) support the argument that nurses are best fit for case management roles because they can provide most services that other professionals offer to clients. Professionals, other than nurses, are neither prepared for nor capable of providing the direct care activities nurses are responsible for, which makes it more difficult for them to assume case management roles. Bower (1992) recommends nurses for case management roles because of their clinical abilities and skills that prepare them for better coordination of services to meet the total needs and concerns presented by patients and their families. Bower also argues that "nurses have skills and knowledge that extend beyond the biophysical and pathological aspects of care, bringing a holistic perspective and knowledge base to the care of case-managed clients" (p. 15). This strengthens the argument that nurses are the best prepared professionals for this role.

According to Zander (1990a), nurses are born for the role of case managers, because they are "the generalists; they are the detail people, and they excel in managing care. They are at the juncture of cost and quality, and they know the human implications of trade offs such as early discharge, patient education in groups, or the use of new technology" (p. 201). Case management responsibilities are an extension of the traditional role of nurses. These new functions advance the role, promote professionalism, and bring nursing to a higher level of professional standards among the other health care professions.

One might say that physicians are the case managers of their patients. This may not work well in case management systems, since physicians' care basically is centered around the medical management of the disease. The patients need professionals who can attend to all their other needs, however, not just the medical ones. Nurses can fill this need. They are prepared to address the total picture of patient care, the actual and potential problems their patients may experience. Nurses in the case manager role act as facilitators and coordinators of care, a role which compliments that of the physician. Because of their educational preparedness and clinical experience, nurses bring a wholeness approach to the total management of patient care. Such an approach complements the physician's role and the medical plan.

The literature is clear that nurses should be selected to assume the case manager role. But the question regarding the criteria that make the best nurse case manager remains to be answered. These criteria, as considered by most institutions implementing case management systems, are related to the educational preparation of nurses, communication skills, leadership skills, and clinical knowledge and experience. The personality traits of nurse case managers are important to their success as interdisciplinary team players, negotiators of care, and patient and family advocates.

Tahan, in 1993, examined the selection criteria for nurse case managers. In this study, 26 nursing administrators of case management systems were surveyed on their preferences and perceptions of the criteria that make a successful case manager. It was found that

▼ 40% of the nursing administrators recommended a BSN as the minimum requirement for the role.

▼ 48% recommended 4 to 6 years of nursing experience, and 38% recommended 2 to 4 years.

▼ 38% did not approve of the clinical ladder as a requirement for the role.

▼ 61.9% did not have any preference for generalized versus specialized nursing experience; 28.6% preferred specialized practice.

▼ communication skills and certification in area of practice or specialty were recommended as prerequisites for the role.

Most institutions use registered nurses in the role of case managers. Some of them require a BSN degree as the minimum educational level, however; others use a combination of BSN and associate degree–prepared nurses. Bower (1992), in her book *Case Management by Nurses*, recommends a BSN degree as an entry level for nurse case managers. Loveridge et al. (1988) suggest that nurses with a BSN degree can assume case management responsibilities on a professional level, that is, no direct care activities, and that those with associate degrees can act as case associates, that is, function on a technical level or be responsible for direct care activities.

Zander (1990b), on the other hand, suggests that other skills and experiences may be as important as the education level. These areas should be looked at when screening nurses for case management roles. Examples of such skills and experiences are (1) knowledge of the nursing process, (2) skills in collaborative practice and interdisciplinary teams, (3) managerial and leadership characteristics, and (4) communication skills.

CHARACTERISTICS OF THE ROLES OF NURSE CASE MANAGERS

Nurses who assume case management roles are given the opportunity to demonstrate effectiveness and efficiency in patient care. It is imperative that nurse case managers be able to assure that the benefits of providing case-managed care exceed the incurred costs while maintaining or improving quality. The wide scope of functions, characteristics, and activities provided for nurse case managers illustrate many of the opportunities, challenges, and threats faced by nurses who are a part of any case management system. As a result, when delivering care, they tend to activate more than one role function or characteristic simultaneously. The nurse case manager's role characteristics and functions are best described in the following general categories.

Change Agent

Successful implementation of any case management system relies heavily on the change agents in the institution. Nurse case managers are integral to this change process (Cohen & Cesta, 1993). They are important in selling the new patient care delivery system to others in the institution, such as physicians, staff nurses, social workers, and personnel in the ancillary departments who are affected by the change. Nurse case managers act as role models and experts when promoting this change. They play a crucial role in teaching all health care personnel about case management systems and answer their questions and concerns. Nurse case managers act to spearhead change by encouraging health care personnel in their efforts to adapt to a new way of delivering care and by encouraging patients in their attempts to quit smoking or to abstain from alcohol, or in other healthful lifestyle changes.

Implementation of case management systems is not an easy process. Some resistance (Cohen & Cesta, 1993; Tahan, 1993), mainly from those most affected by the change, may be encountered. Nurse case managers are prepared to meet this challenge before assuming their new role. They understand that resistance is one way some people might choose to deal with the change. But helping people go smoothly through the process is the case managers' number 1 challenge. They are well educated in how to conquer resistance and are empowered by administration to employ any approaches deemed appropriate for dealing with resistance and helping make the transition as easy and smooth as possible.

Clinician

Nurse case managers use their clinical expertise in assessing the patient's and family's current status and in identifying their actual and potential problems. They depend on their clinical knowledge and previous experiences when implementing the approaches to care that will help resolve these problems. Keeping abreast of the current advances in medical technology and the latest strategies in patient care is crucial to their meeting the client's needs across the health care continuum.

It is important for nurse case managers to be astute in the nursing process (Bower, 1992), that is, to have assessment skills that enable them to identify the patient's actual and potential health problems and to be able to implement the interventions required to successfully resolve these problems and to evaluate the outcomes of care and responses to treatments.

The clinical skills enable nurse case managers to assess their clients as biopsychosocial beings and to plan the treatments to meet the clients' needs as a whole system and not just the disease. These skills allow them to establish more effective treatment goals and deliver better coordinated and timely care that helps the case-managed patients recover in a timely fashion.

Nurse case managers are also popular for their role modeling and clinical expert functions. Because of their extensive clinical background, they act as a resource for less experienced practitioners, some of whom may be from disciplines other than nursing.

Consultant

Nurse case managers guide the interdisciplinary team through the case management process of patient care. They act as consultants for physicians, house staff, fellow nurses, and other providers (Green & Malkemes, 1991; Meisler & Midyette, 1994). Because of their knowledge of institutional policies and procedures, operations, and systems, they provide the interdisciplinary team with a better understanding of the standards of care and practice and facilitate the coordination of tests and procedures, hence the provision of care. They play an important role in identifying the practices that best support efficient and effective care.

They also act as consultants on clinical and administrative issues regarding the delivery of care. Nurse case managers coordinate the needs for consultants, especially for those patients with multiple, complicated needs, and assure that consultations are obtained in a timely fashion. They are involved, as consultants, in comparing and evaluating medical products that provide the best patient outcomes in the most cost-effective manner (Meisler & Midyette, 1994).

Some nurse case managers may provide consultation services for patients and families via the telephone. This is best accomplished if case managers function in ambulatory care settings such as the emergency department, outpatient clinic, or home care or in the managed care organization setting when a client contacts the case manager for guidance or approval regarding care.

Coordinator and Facilitator of Care

As patient care coordinators, nurse case managers collaborate with the interdisciplinary team members to meet the patient's needs and the goals of treatments that are set at the time of admission. They are held responsible for coordinating and facilitating the provision of care on a day-to-day basis, the discharge plan, and the patient and family teaching efforts. They also coordinate the required tests and procedures as specified in the case management plan to facilitate a timely delivery of care and patients' movement through the complex health care system, to reduce fragmentation or duplication of care, and to promote a collaborative practice atmosphere among the various care providers.

Nurse case managers consult and collaborate on an on-going basis with other team members every time a problem regarding the provision of care arises or the patient's condition changes. This aspect of the role is important because it permits immediate intervention and change in the plan of care, timely communication with the appropriate personnel, and better decision making regarding patient care. As coordinator and facilitator the nurse case manager also prevents any delays in patients' discharge and helps control length of stay and resources, and hence, costs. This role responsibility makes nurse case managers important in the institution because they acquire the reputation of being "able to get things done." Health care providers then seek them out every time a problem arises or a certain care activity is not getting done.

It is easier for nurse case managers to assume responsibility for patient care coordination and facilitation because of their understanding of the operations of the institution, the existing systems, and the policies and procedures but mainly because of the power implicit in their role as granted to them by the organization's administration.

Educator

Patient and family education and staff development are other aspects of the nurse case manager's role (Cohen & Cesta, 1993; Meisler & Midyette, 1994; Smith, Danforth, & Owens, 1994; Tahan, 1993). Nurse case managers assess the patient's and family's educational needs at the time of the patient's admission to the hospital and ensure that a teaching plan to meet these needs is put together to guide the nursing staff in the process of patient teaching. They may or may not be directly involved in conducting the actual teaching sessions. Case managers are responsible for making sure that patient and family teaching is completed, however, as indicated by the assessed needs. They also may act as members of institutional patient teaching committees responsible for developing patient and family teaching materials and overseeing the patient teaching process. Nurse case managers in most institutions play a great role in assuring compliance with the standards of regulatory and accreditation agencies associated with patient and family teaching and in promoting any institutional policies and procedures.

Regarding staff development, nurse case managers help the clinical staff in professional growth and development by enhancing and disseminating new knowledge and skills. They assess the teaching needs of the nursing and support staff and plan educational sessions to meet these needs or make referrals to the training and development or continuing education departments. They also act as mentors and preceptors for junior and less experienced staff. In reference to case management systems, nurse case managers play a crucial role in disseminating knowledge regarding case management models, case management plans, and the role of case managers with all health care providers. This is done either formally through prescheduled classes or informally whenever the opportunities arise.

Manager

The manager aspect of the nurse case manager's role entails managing patient care and allocation of resources. As gatekeepers of care, nurse case managers assure the completion of patient care activities in a timely fashion and that the use of resources is appropriate and based on the needs of patients. As managers of care, they ensure that the plan of care or the case management plan reflects the patient's needs. They also direct and supervise the provision of care and optimize positive financial outcomes.

Nurse case managers conduct a review of current and past medical records to evaluate the cost of resources and quality of care. This review is important because it provides data regarding inefficient use of resources, medically unnecessary services, and the incurred costs. It also provides administrators with feedback regarding organizational performance.

Negotiator

Nurse case managers play an important role in negotiating the plan of care of patients—the length of stay, the required services, and the time in which patient care activities should be completed—with members of the interdisciplinary team and more importantly with the patient and family. They are popular for their negotiation skills in getting tests and procedures scheduled with ancillary departments in a timely manner and even in expediting reporting of results. Nurse case managers also play the role of gatekeeper of the interdisciplinary team, a role that requires a tremendous amount of negotiation. Using these skills, they improve the productivity of the team and assure successful completion of its goals.

Nurse case managers are also responsible for working closely with managed care organizations and insurance companies. They negotiate the approval (certification) of patient care services before the patient's hospitalization and the length of stay as determined by the patient's condition. This task is done before and on a regular basis during hospitalization. They exchange information with the representatives of the managed care organizations regarding patient care and the continued need for medical attention.

Nurse case managers also negotiate the need for community services or nursing home placement with the physician and the patient and family. They then negotiate with appropriate agencies the approval of such services.

Patient and Family Advocate

Patient and family advocacy is an integral component of the case manager's role. This role is important in case management systems because nurse case managers are responsible for assuring that the needs of patients and families are met. They always inform their clients of their treatment plans and of their progress and support them while they are struggling with decision making regarding the available options of care. Nurse case managers may act as spokespersons for their patients with other health care team members or managed care organizations.

Nurse case managers convey the care options to the patients, which may include the appropriate treatment plan, medications, tests and procedures, expected length of stay, and whether there is a need for any community services after discharge. They answer those questions raised by the patient or family that they can and seek those answers they do not know. The role of nurse case managers as patient and family educator is an excellent example of advocacy.

Quality Improvement Coordinator

Nurse case managers are responsible for assuring that quality of patient care is maintained or improved at all times. With the current increased pressure on the health care system for cost containment, case managers are given the authority to ensure that quality of care is not compromised at the expense of reducing length of stay and costs. They act as quality improvement coordinators through their assigned responsibility of collecting and analyzing patient care–related data.

Case managers usually evaluate the provision of care by monitoring delays in patient care and deviations (variances) from the preestablished case management plans. They are proactive in improving patient care quality through developing, in collaboration with an interdisciplinary team of care providers, case management plans that reflect the ideal or best practice and delineate the patient care activities including time frames for completion.

They also participate in continuous quality improvement teams as active members for monitoring patient care activities, system problems, care quality, patient satisfaction, length of stay reduction, and so forth. They provide feedback on improvement efforts to all those involved in patient care on a unit level as well as administrative level. By virtue of their roles as case managers, they are always sought by health care providers, physicians and nonphysicians, to resolve delays in care processes and to investigate any patient care problems arising.

Nurse case managers generate monthly variance reports that summarize patient care delays, omissions, and changes from the established case management plans. Such reports are an analysis and trending of the data collected. On the basis of these reports, case managers usually make recommendations to administration for improving the institution's way of operating. They also suggest to the interdisciplinary teams any necessary revisions to be made in the case management plans to improve patient care and reduce delays or variances.

Researcher

In most institutions, research is considered an integral component of the role of nurse case manager. Case managers are encouraged to write grant and research proposals for studying patient care. They are active members of committees researching development, dissemination, and utilization of nursing knowledge. They evaluate patient care through research and make recommendations for changes in care standards, policies, and procedures on the basis of research results. They help bridge the gap between theory and practice by applying research in the clinical setting.

Nurse case managers are the best supporters of research related to product-line quality, health care issues, accessibility to care, professional issues, cost, system problems, and effectiveness of case management plans. Such research is important in the evaluation of the effectiveness of case management systems as patient care delivery models. Since they are at the forefront of patient care, case managers are the best people for data collection in such research efforts.

Risk Manager

Risk management is scrutinized in all health care institutions. Nurse case managers play an important role in identifying patient care issues that present legal risk. As coordinators, facilitators, and managers of patient care, they pay close attention to patient care outcomes and ensure that these outcomes meet the preestablished patient care goals and that care is delivered in compliance with

▼ The institutional policies, procedures, and standards of care and practice

▼ The requirements and standards of managed care organizations

▼ Regulatory and accreditation agencies on the state and federal level

It is important that there be a complete description of the case management system to be implemented and a clear definition of the nurse case manager's role. Most institutions expect case managers to

▼ Develop case management plans that presumably will improve quality of care

▼ Select the treatment that is best for the patient

▼ Manage the patient's total care to ensure optimum outcomes.

It is through these role functions that case managers reduce the medical liabilities an institution may face. They work closely with the legal or risk management department to prevent any patient care problems from escalating into a medical liability. In their role as patient and family advocate and in their proactive approach to patient care, they are influential in preventing and reducing legal risk and potential law suits. Case managers may also minimize liability through

▼ Immediate investigation and solving of patient care problems

▼ Constant review and revision of hospital policies and procedures and standards of care and practice

▼ Knowledge of managed care contracts and assuring that care is precertified and provided in compliance with these contracts

▼ Supervision of appropriate allocation and utilization of resources.

•   •   •

With the constant and rapid changes of health care delivery models the role of nurse case managers has become more important than ever before. The popularity and success of case management systems have made these changes desirable. Nurse case managers have been empowered to function in advanced roles and to prove that their presence in such roles is crucial whenever any efforts are made to improve patient care quality and reduce cost and to help institutions maintain their financial stability, survival, and marketability.

REFERENCES

Bower, K. A. (1989). Managed care: Controlling costs, guaranteeing outcomes. *Definition: The Center for Case Management, 3*(4), 3.

Bower, K. A. (1992). Case management by nurses (2nd ed.; pp. 13-15). Kansas City, Mo: American Nurses Association.

Brockopp, D. Y., Porter, M., Kinnard, S., & Silberman, S. (1992). Fiscal and clinical evaluation of patient care: A case management model for the future. *Journal of Nursing Administration, 22*(9), 23-27.

Cohen, E. L., & Cesta. T. G. (1993). Nursing case management: From concept to evaluation. St. Louis, Mo: Mosby.

Collard, A. F., Bergman, A., & Henderson, M. (1990). Two approaches to measuring quality in medical case management programs. *Quality Review Bulletin, 16*(1), 3-8.

Crawford, J. (1991). Managed care consultation: The "house supervisor" alternative. *Nursing Management, 22*(5), 75-78.

Cronin, C. J., & Maklebust, J. (1989). Case-managed care: Capitalizing on the CNS. *Nursing Management, 20*(3), 38-47.

Ethridge, P., & Lamb, G. (1989). Professional nursing case management improves quality, access and costs. *Nursing Management, 20*(3), 30-35.

Grau, L. (1984). Case management and the nurse. *Geriatric Nursing, 5*(8), 372-375.

Green, S. L., & Malkemes, L. C. (1991). Concepts of designing new delivery models. *Jour-*

nal of the Society for Health Systems, 2(3), 14-24.

Giuliano, K. K., & Poirier, C. E. (1991). Nursing case management: Critical pathways to describe outcomes. *Nursing Management, 22*(3), 52-55.

Henderson, M. G., & Collard, A. (1988). Measuring quality in medical case management program. *Quality Review Bulletin, 14*(2), 33-39.

Kruger, N. R. (1989). Case management: Is it a delivery model system for my organization? *Aspen's Advisor for Nurse Executives, 4*(10), 4-6.

Leclair, C. (1991). Introducing and accounting for RN case management. *Nursing Management, 22*(3), 44-49.

Loveridge, C. E., Cummings, S. H., & O'Malley, J. (1988). Developing case management in a primary nursing system. *Journal of Nursing Administration, 18*(10), 36-39.

McKenzie, C. B., Trokelson, N. G., & Holt, M. A. (1989). Nursing case management improves both. *Nursing Management, 20*(10), 30-34.

Meisler, N., & Midyette, P. (1994). CNS to case manager: Broadening the scope. *Nursing Management, 25*(11), 44-46.

Mundinger, M. (1984). Community-based care: Who will be the case managers? *Nursing Outlook, 323*(6), 294-295.

O'Malley, J. (1988a). Nursing case management. 1: Why look at a different model of nursing care delivery. *Aspen's Advisor for Nurse Executives, 3*(5), 5-6.

O'Malley, J. (1988b). Nursing case management. 2: Dimensions of the nurse case manager role. *Aspen's Advisor for Nurse Executives, 3*(6), 7.

Schwartz, S., Goldman, H., & Churgin, S. (1982). Case management for the chronic mentally ill: Models and dimensions. *Hospitals and Community Psychiatry, 33*(12), 1006-1009.

Smith, G. B., Danforth, D. A., & Owens, P. J. (1994). Role restructuring: Nurse, case manager, and educator. *Nursing Administration Quarterly, 19*(1), 21-32.

Tahan, H. T. (1993). The nurse case manager in acute care settings: Job description and function. *Journal of Nursing Administration, 23*(10), 53-61.

Tahan, H. T., & Cesta, T. G. (1995). Evaluating the effectiveness of case management plans. *Journal of Nursing administration, 25*(9), 58-63.

Thompson, K. S., Caddick, K., Mathie, J., Newlon, B., & Abrahams, T. (1991). Building a critical path for ventilator dependency. *American Journal of Nursing, 91*(7), 28-31.

Zander, K. (1988a). Nursing group practice: "The cadillac" in continuity. *Definition: The Center for Case Management, 3*(2), 1-3.

Zander, K. (1988b). Why managed care works. *Definition: The Center for Nursing Case Management, 3*(4), 3.

Zander, K. (1990a). Case management: A golden opportunity for whom? In J. C. McCloskey & H. K. Grace (Eds.), *Current issues in nursing* (3rd ed.; p. 201). St. Louis, Mo: Mosby.

Zander, K. (1990b). Managed care and nursing case management. In G. G. Mayer, M. J. Madden, & E. Lawrenz (Eds.), *Patient care delivery models* (pp. 37-61). Rockville, Md: Aspen Publishers.

VI

METHODS OF EVALUATION

18

THE IMPORTANCE OF RESEARCH IN THE EVALUATION PROCESS

▼ *CHAPTER OVERVIEW*

Implementation of a case management model should include establishment of a nursing research methodology. Nursing research data provide the framework for evaluating and justifying the efficacy of the overall model.

This chapter explores methods for designing the research and provides samples for data analysis including patients, staff, and length of stay for selected DRGs. Each organization must determine its own research design based on its goals for the model, but some sort of research base is recommended to provide a framework for evaluation. ▲

DATA TALKS

Someone once said, "In God we trust. When all else fails, use data." Creating change in any organization is never an easy task. Obtaining the support and cooperation of hospital administration is necessary for complete integration of a nursing case management model. With such support the model can be viewed as both a nursing and a multidisciplinary model.

Perhaps the best way to obtain the support of the institution as a whole is through the use of data. This includes collecting, analyzing, and disseminating the results of a statistical data analysis as well as any anecdotal data collected. Some data will already exist and be available in the organization. Other data will need to be collected.

Obtaining the administration's support is only part of what is needed as the change to case management proceeds. A sound, valid evaluation process must be implemented to provide ongoing support as the model continues to develop and become part of the institution. It is imperative therefore that the elements to be monitored and evaluated be determined before any changes are implemented (Jennings & Rogers, 1986).

Case management provides an opportunity for nursing to conduct research, as well as to quantify the case management model. Research, broadly defined, is an attempt to find the solution to a problem so that it may be predicted or explained

213

(Treece & Treece, 1973). Research has also been described as a formal method for carrying on the scientific method of analysis, which, in turn, involves the use of several problem-solving steps. These include problem identification, hypothesis formation, observation, analysis, and conclusion (Polit & Hungler, 1983).

These basic elements are no less important in the analysis of a case management model, and all the changes that come about as a result of the integration of this system (Jennings & Rogers, 1986). Generally, research is divided into two categories. The first is basic research, the goal of which is to obtain knowledge for the sake of knowledge. The second category is applied research, which takes this process one step further as it seeks to apply the research to everyday situations (Nachmias & Nachmias, 1981). Case management research is applied research in its truest sense. Everyday questions concerning the efficacy of the model are asked, answered, and applied as the case management research data are collected and analyzed.

The methodology used for case management analysis can take several forms and can encompass several different elements. It need not be limited to one particular process but can include several steps and processes. Nursing research includes the clinical elements of the nursing profession, such as the steps of the nursing process: assessment, diagnosis, outcome identification, planning, implementation, and evaluation. Nursing research also involves the preparation and evaluation of practitioners and studies the systems in which nurses work and apply the steps of the nursing process (Corner, 1991).

EVALUATION VERSUS EXPERIMENTAL RESEARCH

Research involving case management can be approached as evaluation research. It can also be designed as an experiment or quasi-experiment. In evaluation research, data are collected and analyzed to evaluate or assess the effects of some project or change. This type of research helps to evaluate how well implementation of the program is going.

Experimental research tests the relationships between the variables being manipulated. A control group and an experimental group are used in classic experimental research. The control group symbolizes a normal representation of subjects, and the experimental group consists of those subjects for whom at least one variable has been altered.

In case management research it is difficult to devise a classic experimental design. If patients are compared, the researcher must be sure that the cases are similar enough to justify comparison. Some examples of factors to be controlled when choosing subjects are severity of illness, concurrent problems, gender, and age. In addition, random assignment to each group must be conducted. This process involves the admitting office, which ensures that certain, previously evaluated patients are placed on particular units.

If nurses on nursing units are being studied for job satisfaction, for example, it would be impossible to separate those nurses who had been affected by the model from those who had not. Comparing nurses between nursing units can lead to some of the same methodology questions that arise when comparing some patients with others (Schaefer, 1989). The registered nurses could only be matched if differences were controlled in some way.

Even comparing one nursing unit with another is difficult. There are few institutions in which nursing-unit patient populations are so similar, and yet so randomized, that nurses' and patients' experiences could be said to be similar from one to the next. It is more likely that comparing one nursing unit with another is like comparing apples with oranges. Nursing units are often designated by specialty, and physicians will usually, whether formally or informally, prefer that patients be sent to a particular nursing unit because the physicians believe that unit is most suited to meeting their patient's nursing needs.

The Quasi-Experimental Approach

Because of the difficulties in matching subjects for control and experimental groups, it becomes practical to use each nursing unit as its own control. Once this takes place, the methodology becomes quasi-experimental. Unit data, including staff satisfaction, length of stay, and so on, are compared before and after implementation. Additional postimplementation data are collected and analyzed at predetermined intervals. A longitudinal approach of this kind cannot guarantee that the same staff members will be compared from one time frame to the next (Kenneth & Stiesmeyer, 1991). Whenever possible, the same nurses and staff members should be compared from one time period to the next. For those staff members who come and go during the study, global score comparisons can be made.

Certain intrinsic factors affecting internal validity are impossible to control (Lederman, 1991). One such intrinsic factor that always affects longitudinal studies is maturation. The nurses tested may have either an increase or a decrease in job satisfaction solely because of the passage of time. For some workers the passage of time provides a certain comfort that increases job satisfaction and sense of accomplishment. For others, longevity can lead to exhaustion, disillusionment, and decreased job satisfaction. In either case, these elements associated with maturation can probably not be controlled.

Another intrinsic factor is that of experimental mortality. One of the goals of case management is to decrease turnover rates among registered nurses, but there will always be a certain amount of turnover among any group of employees, no matter how happy they are with their work. Some may leave because they cannot deal with the changes accompanying the introduction of case management. In either case, it is clear that the researcher will not have the same sample at each stage of data collection. Dropouts from the study can prejudice the results. Unfortunately this factor cannot be controlled.

One way to account for the issue of experimental mortality or dropouts is to statistically analyze the entire sample size as a global unit, then match subjects from a previous data collection period with those in the current period and study this group separately.

Subjects serve as their own controls in a pretest-posttest design (Nachmias & Nachmias, 1981). The advantage to this design is that the variable is measured both before and after the intervention. In other words, the variable is compared to itself.

As the first step in either process, preimplementation data and continuous data are obtained as the model goes forward. The provision of a solid nursing research base for evaluation provides credibility to the model for those evaluating it in 6 months, 1 year, 2 years, or longer. (Rogers, 1992).

Typically when changes are made in nursing, very little data collection occurs during the implementation phase (Acton, Irvin, & Hopkins, 1991). This lack of data makes validation of results difficult, which in turn makes it difficult to maintain the momentum and support needed for change to progress.

To determine what to measure, the organization must first decide what it hopes to achieve by implementing the case management model. After identifying the goal of implementation it will be easier to formulate the questions that should be asked. Based on these questions the researcher can begin to form a hypothesis. The hypothesis indicates what the researcher believes to be the cause and effect of a given situation, and it states the relationship between the variables.

Basic research questions will not be affected by the type of methodology used, regardless of whether an evaluation or experimental methodology is chosen. These research questions are prospective and based on hoped-for outcomes. The outcomes will fall into several categories. Data collection will be longitudinal because it will probably be collected at predetermined intervals over a long period of time. The changes attempted in case management will take years to take hold, so choosing an evaluation time period that is too short may make it appear as if implementation has failed to achieve the desired outcomes. On the other hand, some measure of changing trends will need to be shown within the first year of implementation to prove that things are moving in the desired direction.

The areas affected by the implementation of a case management model are diverse and complicated. They range from patients to staff to finance. Many of the changes are obtuse, intangible, and anecdotal, but others can be validated through stringent data collection and statistical analysis. Those changes to be measured must be determined in advance so that baseline data can be collected. These data will provide the foundation for comparison.

If a case management model is being implemented, the focus of evaluation must be on patients, finance, length of stay, and quality of care.

A non-unit-based case management model is broadly focused, and it may be difficult to prove a relationship between implementation of the model and the level of staff satisfaction. Therefore this might not be a variable worth trying to measure.

In the unit-based case management model, certain changes affect particular nursing staff members in specific ways (Swanson, Albright, Steirn, Schaffner, & Costa, 1992). The response of these individuals can be measured and evaluated in terms of job satisfaction, turnover rates, absenteeism, and vacancy rates.

One of the most difficult but essential elements to measure in a case management model is quality of care. The basic tenet of case management is to move the patient through the hospital system as quickly and efficiently as possible. Because the hospital stay is being accelerated, some controls must be put in place to guarantee that quality care is not being compromised.

Accrediting institutions, such as the JCAHO, are struggling with questions regarding the measurement of quality. These issues will undoubtedly continue into the next century (Williams, 1991).

Perhaps the most tangible measure, and possibly the most important in terms of hospital viability, is the length of stay. Decreases in the length of stay have come to be associated directly with case management. It is difficult to address case management without also addressing the issues of hospital reimbursement and patient length of stay.

The Prospective Payment System provided the first and most potent incentive to hospitals to move toward reducing length of stay. Now with the rapid infiltration of managed care, other financial incentives are in the health care arena. These include capitation and negotiated per diem rates under managed care. These payment schemes provide for the same need to control cost and reduce length of stay as the prospective payment system did in the 1980s. These incentives are strictly financial. Shorter hospital stays mean increased profits. It is only a matter of time before every institution in the United States will be looking at measures for reducing length of stay as well as controlling other costs.

Caution should be taken when studying and reporting length of stay statistics. The Prospective Payment System and diagnosis-related groups (DRGs) were designed to be used only as financial tools for determining reimbursement.

Because of a lack of other ways to tap into this information the DRG has become the basis for studying length of stay and related clinical interventions. A serious analysis of many DRGs will reveal that the DRG is usually too broad and too heterogeneous to be used as a determinant of the effect of a particular clinical intervention.

To report this information with the utmost accuracy, it is more advantageous and appropriate to analyze the situation at a microlevel. For example, there is one DRG for chemotherapy, despite the fact that there are 1-day, 2-day, and 5-day chemotherapy protocols. The reimbursable length of stay is 2.6 days, no matter what the protocol. If a managed care plan is applied to a particular case for a specific chemotherapy protocol in order to determine the effectiveness of the plan, the researcher would have to identify more than just the DRG. If the plan is a 5-day plan, clearly the reimbursable rate is inadequate. But having this information would allow the investigator to determine, for example, whether the length of stay could have been shortened or whether quality care was provided.

Elements of Data Collection

One form of data collection is the questionnaire. Using questionnaires that have been previously determined to be valid and reliable can reduce or eliminate many of the problems associated with this technique. The content of the questions determines their ability to control bias, which could influence a respondent's answer in a particular way.

One way to test the staff nurses is to compile packets of various questionnaires, including one on demographics, that the researcher can use to describe the sample itself. The questionnaires should take no longer than 15 to 20 minutes to complete (Kenneth & Stiesmeyer, 1991).

DATA COLLECTION MONITORS

1. Improved staff satisfaction
   Outcome indicators:
   a. Registered nurse job satisfaction
   b. Physician job satisfaction
   c. Nursing assistant job satisfaction
   d. Decreased registered nurse burnout scores
   e. Decreased absenteeism
   f. Decreased turnover rate
   g. Increased recruitment
2. Improved patient satisfaction
   Outcome indicators:
   a. Patient satisfaction
   b. Family satisfaction
3. Improved quality care
   Outcome measures:
   a. Quality assurance data
   b. Patient satisfaction
   c. Readmission rate
   d. Uniform treatment of all cases
   e. Frequency and type of patient education
   f. Outcome indicators
   g. Variance analysis
4. Decreased length of stay
   Outcome measure: reduction in length of stay
5. Improved communication or collaboration among disciplines
   Outcome measures:
   a. Development of collaborative practice groups
   b. Opened lines of communication between all disciplines
   c. Development of managed care plans
6. Decreased costs
   Outcome measures:
   a. Improved resource use (both product and personnel)
   b. Decreased absenteeism, turnover, and vacancy rates
   c. Decreased delays in waiting for tests and procedures
   d. Uniform treatment within physician groups
   e. Alteration of registered nurse and ancillary staff mix

The consent form should clearly indicate that participation in the study will in no way affect the respondent's employment in the institution.

When questioning patients, nurses must ensure that patient care is not being disturbed. The researcher must also determine whether the patient is able to understand, read, and respond to the questionnaire appropriately. One way to do this is to provide questions on the demographic questionnaire that address the respondent's highest level of education, age, and ability to speak and understand English.

The box on page 218 presents some of the broad categories that an organization converting to a case management model might want to address when collecting data for determining success or failure of implementation. The list in the box is certainly not exhaustive. An organization on the brink of implementing case management may choose to study any or all of these questions. Questions may involve a multitude of benchmarks or only a few. There may be areas for study that are not listed in the box but that are still important to the organization in question. Each organization must decide for itself what is most important to measure and how it will be measured. The tools for measuring each of these expected outcomes are determined by the nurse researcher involved in the case management analysis. Valid and reliable tools exist to measure most of the variables, but others will have to be obtained from already-existing hospital information systems, DRG information, and managed care and hospital billing records. The areas from which to obtain the data vary from institution to institution. The finance department, the DRG office, and the managed care departments can be of great assistance to the nurse researcher evaluating a case management system. Each unit of analysis will require the use of the nurse researcher's expertise for selecting the most appropriate data with which to answer the research questions.

REFERENCES

Acton, G.J., Irvin, B.L., & Hopkins, B.A. (1991). Theory-testing research: Building the science. *Advances in Nursing Science, 14*(1), 52-61.

Corner, J. (1991). In search of more complete answers to research questions. Quantitative versus qualitative research methods: Is there a way forward? *Journal of Advanced Nursing, 16,* 718-727.

Jennings, B.M., & Rogers, S. (1986). Using research to change nursing practice. *Critical Care Nurse, 9*(5), 76-84.

Kenneth, H.K., & Stiesmeyer, J.K. (1991). Strategies for involving staff in nursing research. *Dimensions of Critical Care Nursing, 10*(2), 103-107.

Lederman, R.P. (1991). Quantitative and qualitative research methods: Advantages of complementary usage. *The American Journal of Maternal/Child Nursing, 16,* 43.

Nachmias, D., & Nachmias, C. (1981). *Research* methods in the social sciences. New York: St. Martin's Press.

Polit, D., & Hungler, B. (1983). *Nursing research.* Philadelphia: J.B. Lippincott Company.

Rogers, B. (1992). Research utilization, *AAOHN, 40*(1), 41.

Schaefer, K.M. (1989). Clinical research: Gaining access to patients. *Dimensions of Critical Care Nursing, 8*(4), 236-242.

Swanson, J.M., Albright, J., Steirn, C., Schaffner, A., & Costa, L. (1992). Program efforts for creating a research environment in a clinical setting. *Western Journal of Nursing Research, 14*(2), 241-245.

Treece, E.W., & Treece, J.W. (1973). *Elements of research in nursing.* St. Louis: The C.V. Mosby Company.

Williams, A.D. (1991). Development and application of clinical indicators for nursing. *Journal of Nursing Care Quality, 6*(1), 1-5.

19

DOCUMENTATION OF QUALITY CARE

▼ CHAPTER OVERVIEW

For health care organizations to improve delivery of services, they must first determine their definition of quality. Recently, quality issues have moved from an organizational perspective to a consumer-oriented one, in which the needs and concerns of the customer count.

Among the elements measured in defining quality is patient satisfaction. Patients can be questioned directly through focus groups or indirectly through written questionnaires.

Each organization must determine its measures in relation to the incorporated case management documentation system. Patient, health care provider, and operational variances can be used to continuously improve quality. The case manager serves an important role in this process.

▲

WHAT IS QUALITY?

The meaning of quality takes on a new twist when introduced as a concept relevant to health care. Quality may be seen in terms of its effect on the health care delivery system or on specific dimensions of the system (Institute of Medicine, 1976).

On the larger scale of the entire health care system, quality may include the availability and accessibility of health care services, credentialing requirements and standards of the providers, comprehensive assessment and documentation, collaborative and informed relationships with the patient and family, minimal injuries or complications in hospitalized patients, evaluation of new technology and resources, and effective management of health care resources (McCarthy, 1987).

The advent of the Prospective Payment System forced health care institutions to focus on health care as a business. Leaving good quality care to chance did not work and ultimately did not make good business sense. As organizations, regulatory agencies, and patient needs became more complicated, it became obvious that health care was no less a business than any other and that the product of the business was patient care. Increasingly, the value of that care became dependent on the matching of cost and quality. Before they could determine the value of the product, organizations had to know what the expected quality comprised.

Manufacturers, small-business owners, and large corporations have known for years that to provide quality, the organization or business must first determine its definition of quality (Davis, 1990). Discovering what attributes the organization wants to attain is one way to arrive at such a definition.

Health care organizations have already begun to realize that a change in the definition and measurement of quality is needed (Jones, 1991). The products of health care are often intangible items that are difficult to identify and measure. Quality assurance measures in the past have attempted to identify errors and then place blame on the individual who made the error. However, one could argue that counting the number of bedsores or medication errors does not help define quality health care. It also did not provide a mechanism for monitoring and then *improving* quality.

Consumer Focus

As in business, it became obvious that one useful technique for defining quality health care was to ask the recipients of that care how they defined quality care. This technique of asking consumers what they want often highlights issues to which the health care practitioner is blind. In the past, our definition of quality was to count the number of patient falls. If the organization came in below the desired threshold, it was providing quality care. However, the patient's definition of quality care was care given by a competent, pleasant employee who was familiar with the patient and the patient's needs.

Of course, the issue of falls is an important one in terms of assuring quality, and patients will surely consider this equally important if they have ever fallen. The point is, that once the customer's needs have been queried and identified, an entirely new area can be addressed. Invariably the necessary dimensions of quality that the consumer identifies focus on the business end of health care. This area has been ignored in the past. Organizations believed they knew what patients needed and supplied it to them within the constraints and needs of the organization. The patient had to conform to the organization. There are occasions when this approach is truly necessary. But remaining forever in this mind set eliminates the possibility of ever going beyond providing basic services, and it certainly does not allow for an atmosphere of continual improvement.

By determining what constitutes quality, it can be measured. Once measured, it can be managed. Managing care allows for a process of continual improvement toward excellence, and excellence is the definition of quality.

PATIENT SATISFACTION

With a renewed focus on patient needs, the issue of how to measure patient satisfaction has never been more important. Patient satisfaction is quickly becoming the benchmark for measuring quality health care. Customer needs not only are identified but also are the basis on which quality improvements are made. Within the mission statement of most health care organizations is a clause that cites patient satisfaction as a goal. Although the health care industry has always identified itself as a service industry, clearly this was a self-serving need. In most instances the attitude of health care providers was that the patient was lucky to be getting what they were getting.

How often have nurses used the following phrases in defense of a system that was obviously failing the patients and customers?

"You had to wait 5 days for a CAT scan? Well, Mrs. Jones had to wait 6 days. Aren't you lucky?"

"You haven't seen your surgeon since the operation? That is something you are going to have to accept if you want to have the best surgeon in this field."

The patients were certainly not lucky to be sick, to be in the hospital, or to be having surgery. When even minimal expectations are not being met, something is terribly wrong with the system.

Customer service will be what defines quality in the next century. Health care organizations that provide service to all customers, from physicians to patients to the community, will be the most successful. The focus must shift away from a purely organizational approach to one that blends consumer and organizational needs (Strasen, 1991).

Depending on the philosophy, resources, and goals of the organization, the approach for measuring patient satisfaction can be made in a number of ways.

Generally a questionnaire is used to gauge the level of patient satisfaction. Such a survey can be administered while the patient is in the hospital or after discharge (Steiber & Krowinski, 1990). Generally an attempt is made to administer the questionnaire 24 to 48 hours before discharge. However, some patients may be intimidated by a questionnaire that is filled out while they are still in the hospital, fearing that if a bad report is given, one of the health care providers may retaliate with less than optimal care.

On the other hand, patients' memories of their hospital stays will be most vivid if recorded while still in the hospital. Positive and negative impressions will be fresh in their minds, and these impressions can provide valuable information.

However, patients who are queried after discharge, in the safety and comfort of their homes, may be more likely to provide honest information because they have no fear of retribution. Unfortunately, positive and negative experiences can be quickly forgotten once the patient is home, which means valuable information can be lost if patients are questioned in this manner.

The pros and cons of each method must be evaluated by each organization. There is no perfect way, and it is possible that some form of patient satisfaction questioning is already in place. These data can be used both as preimplementation data and for ongoing studies.

If the questionnaires are administered to patients while they are in the hospital, someone who is not directly involved in the care of the patient should administer the survey to the patient. This method will help to diminish potential for bias.

Because people who are ill or who have been ill recently are being questioned, care should be taken to select a questionnaire that has short, understandable questions. The focus of each question should be clear to the patient. Patients who are questioned while still in the hospital are more likely to be experiencing increased anxiety or other physical conditions that may affect their ability to participate.

It is best to select instruments that have been identified previously as valid and reliable. Most instruments use closed-ended questions in which a series of possible choices are given. This format is easiest to score and analyze statistically. Open-ended questions provide the investigator with less control of response content and are more difficult to analyze. Even so, the open-ended format may provide the most meaningful information. It may be beneficial to design an instrument that combines both closed-ended as well as open-ended questions. This allows for some control over responses and the opportunity to elicit useful anecdotal information.

The focus of the survey also may depend on the philosophy and goals of implementing the case management system. Many patient satisfaction surveys focus on hygiene needs, such as food, room comfort, noise, and so on. Although these factors are important, they may not be capturing the elements that a case management system is attempting to change. Therefore it may be necessary to find a questionnaire that focuses more on the professional care provided. In some cases the institution may have to develop its own instrument that clearly questions the patients in regard to this unique switch to case management.

Developing an instrument can be difficult. The decision to develop a unique questionnaire should not be taken lightly. If the organization is looking for immediately valid and reliable results, the use of a pilot instrument is not the best route to take. The use of more than one instrument is one way to address this dual need so that the needs of both the organization and the researcher can be met. Previously established questionnaires allow for a rapid compilation of information with which to measure implementation. In the long run, however, a new questionnaire, aimed at determining specific effects of the case management system on the patient, will contribute a great deal to the validation of the model's efficacy. In addition the questionnaire can be used by other organizations that implement case management systems.

Another technique is the qualitative method. Qualitative assessment is used to compile data that can be used later in a self-report or paper-and-pencil questionnaire. Patient-focused groups and interviews provide data for development of written questions. Qualitative approaches allow the researcher to see the situation through the experience of the patient. The perceptions of the patient are used to compile information that is later categorized. These categories are then transformed into specific questions.

The qualitative method is time consuming. Personal interviews or focus groups last from 1 to 2 hours, but the researcher has to devote even more time to use this form of data collection. However, the information gained can be invaluable.

Determining which patients to question is really a matter of good research technique. The sample should be as heterogeneous as possible to allow for the greatest deal of generalizability. Random sampling will provide this.

Every health care organization compiles statistics that are fed back to regulatory agencies. This information is generally used to determine accreditation and licensing and to analyze mistakes, untoward effects, and outcomes. Information categorizing the number and type of falls, infections, and medication administration errors has been tracked for years. Analysis of these data helps identify patterns or frequent offenders. Such a system has been referred to as the "bad apple" approach. If a health care practitioner makes a mistake, that person is counseled. If the practitioner makes the same kind of mistake repeatedly, more serious intervention on the part of the employer might take place. This system does not take into account possible system issues that may contribute to the problem. Instead, one person is seen as the cause of the problem as well as the means for fixing it.

This approach not only looks for the bad apple but also lies in wait for the accident or error. The approach does not provide a mechanism for addressing the larger elements of the problem, and it does nothing to control the recurrence of this problem.

Nevertheless, most institutions evaluating case management systems have turned to the bad-apple approach in an attempt to improve quality patient care. A reduction in patient falls or patient infections might be reported as a result of the introduction of a case management model. In reality, the factors leading to a fall or an infection go beyond a managed care plan or a case manager.

If the goal of data analysis is to improve the quality of care, a method other than the bad-apple approach must be selected. Patient care is simply too multidimensional to be analyzed effectively by this method. Identifying more appropriate data to measure will come as a direct result of establishing a definition of quality. Case management data is positive outcome data because it focuses on the expected outcomes of the interventions in which we participate as health care providers. The case management plan provides all the expected outcomes of care during hospitalization, from patient teaching expectations to expected resource use to expected length of stay. It also provides for the expected clinical outcomes of care.

These expected outcomes provide the foundation for determining quality care. By delineating these outcomes, each discipline is identifying the quality issues around a particular diagnosis or procedure.

Additional indexes of patients' perceptions of quality can be identified. These indicators should be incorporated into any measure of quality. Until the organization has converted to a case management system or until the new case management plans are in place, it may be necessary to continue to report the quality assurance data to obtain baseline indexes of quality. Ultimately this format can be abandoned or combined with other quality indicators.

CRITERIA FOR MEASURING OUTCOMES

Some of the outcomes identified on the case management plan can be tracked during hospitalization. These outcomes are the day-to-day clinical, psychosocial, and teaching interventions identified on the plan. The case manager addresses these on a daily basis and ensures that the patient is moving along the continuum of health care in a timely fashion. If any outcome is not achieved, the case manager is responsible for determining why and correcting the problem or changing the plan.

The unit of analysis within the case management plan will vary depending upon the increments in which the hospital stay is measured. For example, while most case management plans are developed on the basis of the 24-hour day, others may have longer or shorter units of analysis. In the neonatal intensive care unit, where the expected length of stay can run from 1 to 3 months, daily measures are not appropriate. In this case the managed care plans are "time-lined" in 1-week intervals, during which the expected outcomes should be achieved.

In some cases, such as an emergency room setting, the time frames may be short. In these cases the case management plan time frames are set at 15-minute or 30-minute intervals. During these shorter time periods, specific outcomes are expected. Whatever the time frame, it should realistically correlate to the clinical situation being planned. Once a unit of analysis or time period is chosen, analysis can begin.

In case management anything that does not happen when it is supposed to happen is called a variance. Variances alert practitioners to changes in the patient's condition, or they highlight problems in the health care delivery system itself. Any variances that occur are identified daily as well as retrospectively. Every expected outcome on the plan is a potential variance, and, unless the outcome is achieved within a predetermined time period, it falls into the variance category. As outlined in Chapter 16, there are four causes for variances: the patient, the health care provider, operations, or unmet clinical indicators.

There are two types of patient variances. The first is a patient variance, comorbidity, or a condition identified on admission. These conditions may or may not require an alteration in the usual plan for that diagnosis or procedure. For example, a patient allergy identified at the time of admission might mean that a drug usually considered standard for that diagnosis or procedure cannot be administered. As a result, the plan of care must be discussed with the physician, who decides either to refrain from using the drug or to replace it with a suitable alternative.

In some cases the variance is noted, but no change is made to the plan at that time. An example of this is a patient who has diabetes. The person admitting this patient reviews the plan and notes that no changes are needed. The patient's condition still needs to be noted in the Patient Variance on Admission section of the case management plan. This section may also be labeled as preexisting conditions or comorbidities. This alerts all health care providers that the patient has diabetes. It also indicates that the plan was individualized at the time of admission.

The other type of patient variance is one that the patient causes. In other words, this type involves situations in which an expected outcome cannot be achieved because of the patient's condition or noncompliance.

For example, a tuberculosis case management plan might call for collection of sputum specimens on the first, second, and third days of hospitalization. If the patient is unable to produce sputum on the second day, that outcome cannot be achieved within the anticipated time frame. In such a case, specimen collection is moved to the third and fourth days.

An example of a patient variance caused by noncompliance might occur on the second postoperative day, when the plan calls for the patient to dangle his legs over the edge of the bed. Because of pain, the patient refuses. Despite pain medication, the patient continues to refuse. This refusal results in an inability to achieve the desired outcome, and the patient's plan has to be adjusted accordingly.

By reviewing the patient's progress throughout the day and anticipating the course of recovery for the entire hospital stay, the case manager can adjust the plan so that the variance does not change the length of stay. If the patient refuses to ambulate, the "dangling" and "out-of-bed-to-the-bathroom" goals can be combined into expected outcomes for the following day, when the patient is feeling better. Another possibility might be to try the dangling step again on the next shift, when the pain medication is more effective.

Regardless of the reason for the variance, the case manager and the staff nurse should be aware of the recovery protocol and should attempt to get the patient back on track as soon as possible. This method helps avoid unnecessary delays and makes the patient's progress and expected plan well known and easily tracked. This in turn means that potential problems will be less likely to continue for several days without being noticed.

A health care provider variance is caused by an omission or error made by a health care practitioner. Institutions have unique regulations regarding documentation, and employees must acquaint themselves with these policies. However, mistakes are bound to occur.

An example of a health care provider variance might involve a transcription error. If a physician order for a medication is not transcribed by the nurse but the error is detected on the next shift, the patient might have missed a dose of the medication. Other health care provider variances involve changes in practice patterns that alter the patient's predetermined case management plan.

Operational variances are probably the most common variances. Operational variances include those that happen within the confines of the hospital as well as some caused by a condition outside the hospital.

A large-system variance, one that occurs because of something outside the hospital, might involve discharge placement. These types of variance would fall within the operational category. Sometimes a patient is assessed as appropriate for nursing home placement, so all the paper work is completed, and the patient is clinically ready for discharge, but no nursing home beds are available. As a result, the patient remains in the hospital until a bed becomes available, and the extended stay is classified as a large-system variance.

The most typical large-system variances are postdischarge problems in which a proper discharge location is not available. This type of variance is difficult to control. The best prevention is for the case manager to attempt to identify those patients who will need placement as early in the hospital stay as possible and begin to prepare the necessary paperwork so that delays can be avoided.

Other operational variances can occur because of the institution's infrastructure. Most health care institutions are large, complex places. Systems have developed over time, often without planning. Once these systems are in place, most workers are too busy to correct the operational problems. Instead, informal mechanisms are developed to work around the flaw in the system. Such operational problems can delay the patient's progress toward discharge. An inadequate patient-scheduling system may mean that the nursing unit is unaware of a scheduled procedure, and the patient is not correctly prepped. Thus the procedure cannot be performed, which may increase the length of stay.

Other operational variances occur when equipment breaks. One such operational variance is an inability to complete a CT scan because the machine is not functioning. Any equipment malfunction results in a delay, which in turn takes the patient off the case management schedule. Clinical quality indicators are those expected clinical indicators identified by the physician that may include intermediate and discharge outcomes. These indicators are used to assess clinical progress and quality of care. See Chapter 16 for more information on variances.

Any of these variances require the input of the case manager, whose responsibility it is to identify the variance and intervene to correct it. The goal is to minimize the effect the variance will have on the patient's length of stay.

The other responsibility of the case manager is to document the variance. Retrospective analysis of operational variances results in the identification of frequently occurring, but rectifiable, problems. It is important that variances also be documented for the purposes of utilization review and reimbursement.

REFERENCES

Davis, W.W. (1990). Quality care and cost control? *The Case Manager, 1*(3), 24-29.

Institute of Medicine. (1976). Assessing quality in health care: An evaluation. (DHEW Publication No. 282-75-0437 PM). Washington, D.C.: National Academy of Sciences.

Jones, K.R. (1991). Maintaining quality in a changing environment. *Nursing Economics, 9*(3), 159-164.

McCarthy, C. (1987 Feb.). Quarterly health care inches closer to precise definition. *Hospital Peer Review,* 19-20.

Steiber, S.R., & Krowinski, W.J. (1990). *Measuring and managing patient satisfaction.* Chicago: American Hospital Publishing.

Strasen, L. (1991). Redesigning hospitals around patients and technology. *Nursing Economics, 9*(4), 233-238.

20

THE LINK BETWEEN CONTINUOUS QUALITY IMPROVEMENT AND CASE MANAGEMENT

▼ CHAPTER OVERVIEW

The continuous quality improvement (CQI) process has gradually been adapted to the health care setting to improve quality without increasing costs. In traditional quality assurance models, quality is measured by the number of accidents or errors occurring. No provision is made for improving the conditions under which the errors occurred.

However, continuous quality improvement focuses on the processes used to achieve a goal. These processes may be clinical, financial, or operational issues. Each step in the process is analyzed; then a plan for improvement is tested and refined.

The three leaders in the CQI process are Deming, Juran, and Crosby. Each has made unique contributions toward improving the quality of work performed in the industrial setting. Now their concepts are being applied in the health care arena.

Case management and CQI are linked in philosophy and process. The steps of the CQI process can be applied to managed care plans from both clinical and financial perspectives.

▲

INTRODUCTION TO CONTINUOUS QUALITY IMPROVEMENT (CQI)

The CQI process was officially introduced in 1991 as a more effective approach to improving the quality of health care. In that year the JCAHO announced that it would be introducing new standards requiring all chief executive officers of hospitals to be educated on CQI methods (*Hospitals, 1991*). This mandate went into effect for accreditation surveys as of January 1, 1992.

This seemingly abrupt switch from traditional quality assurance methods to an approach that had had tremendous success in the business arena was timely. Quality had become the promotional tool for many health care organizations as they adopted a more consumer-oriented approach (Naisbitt, 1982).

At the same time, the prospective payment system had changed the speed and scope of health care delivery. Techniques that had been successful in the past were no longer financially feasible. Change, once considered something to be avoided, was hailed as the way to financial viability for the industry (Kanter, 1983). The changes included new and more effective management styles, which could provide quality under a cost-containment umbrella.

Another force driving the need for change was an emerging consumerism (Naisbitt, 1982). The average person had become an educated health care consumer who expected quality care. Consumers wanted to be involved in their care, which included participation in decisions involving treatment, cost, and self-care (O'Connor, 1984).

Continuous quality improvement falls in the realm of total quality management, a concept originated by W. Edward Deming (*Hospital Peer Review*, 1988). Quality improvement involves an analysis, understanding, and improvement of the processes of care. In the case of the health care industry, these processes include the hospital system, the personnel, the clinical management, and financial structure that surround each patient case.

In this format, quality is defined as the meeting or exceeding of customer requirements (Marszalek-Gaucher & Coffey, 1990). In other words, the customer defines quality. Suppliers and customers are involved in each of the above mentioned processes. The supplier is the one who passes on the patient, information, or equipment, and the customer is the one who receives the patient, information, or equipment.

One of the first steps in CQI is the identification and study of the individual steps that make up each of the processes of health care. This CQI extends beyond individual departments because the exchanges between departments are usually the areas that yield difficulties. Each process can be broken down into its working parts in a variety of ways. One way is with the use of a flow chart. The flow chart pictorially describes each step and is useful in helping to identify where bottlenecks or overuse of resources is occurring. Fig. 20-1 is a simplified example of how a computed tomography (CT) scan scheduling process is broken down into its major steps.

Root causes of problems are identified through the flow chart. Once the root causes have been determined, more data can be gathered, and the team can begin selecting solutions. It is necessary to pick the root cause that may result in the greatest initial improvement of the process. Additional causes can then be addressed, after one solution has been tried. At this point, more data should be collected to evaluate whether the solution was given enough time to take hold and whether it was effective.

TRADITIONAL QUALITY ASSURANCE

The health care industry has been crippled by waste and misuse of resources (Marszalek-Gaucher & Coffey, 1990). Within this wasteful environment, quality care has always been difficult to measure (Goldfield & Nash, 1989). Compounding this difficulty is the unabated growth of industry inspection, which has resulted in an adversarial relationship between health care organizations and inspection agencies. Sanctions mandating quality as defined by agencies, such as the Peer Review Organizations (PRO), the JCAHO, the state licensing agencies, and others, have resulted in measures designed to ensure minimum expectations rather than continuous improvement (Laffel & Blumenthal, 1989).

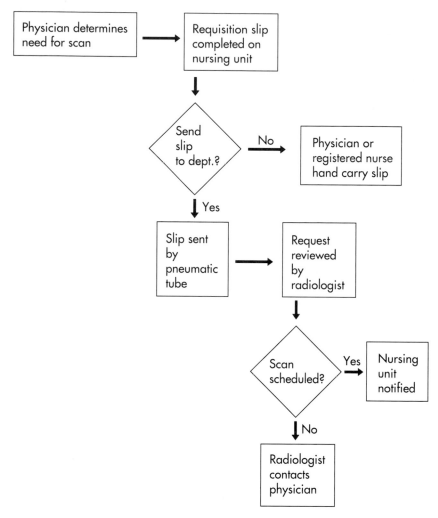

Fig. 20-1 Flow diagram of CT scan scheduling process.

Relatively arbitrary thresholds have been established within organizations. These thresholds define minimum expectations and identify bad apples but do not provide any mechanism for finding causes or suggestions for improvements. These techniques for assuring quality do not address health care's increasing need for improvement in all processes of the industry (Donabedian, 1980). It is clear that while quality has to be maintained, systems have to be designed for improving business at all levels.

The traditional quality assurance process provides a system for identifying opportunities to improve care or problems. These opportunities are based on the collection of information on incidents or errors that have surpassed a predetermined

---

QUALITY ASSURANCE MONITORING AND EVALUATION

The 10-Step Process

1. Assign responsibility for monitoring and evaluating activities.
2. Delineate the scope of care provided by the organization.
3. Identify the most important aspects of care provided by the organization.
4. Identify indicators (and appropriate clinical criteria) for monitoring the important aspects of care.
5. Establish thresholds (levels, patterns, trends) for the indicators that trigger evaluation of the care.
6. Monitor the important aspects of care by collecting and organizing the data for each indicator.
7. Evaluate care when thresholds are reached in order to identify either opportunities to improve care or problems.
8. Take actions to improve care or to correct identified problems.
9. Assess the effectiveness of the actions and document the improvement in care.
10. Communicate the results of the monitoring and evaluation process to relevant individuals, departments, or services, and to the organization-wide quality assurance program.

---

threshold (see the box above). Factors affecting the occurrence of the incidents, the systems affecting the errors, or processes for improvement are not identified.

In addition, errors or incidents are identified through individual finger-pointing based on the mistake of one person. Therefore, each quality issue appears to be the fault of one particular person, acting independently. This focus removes all accountability from the organization or the systems within which the individual practitioner is working.

THE NEW HEALTH CARE AGENDA

Quality has become paramount on the health care agenda. Industrial models of quality improvement have been adopted and used successfully in the health care arena. Industry's goals, the reduction of costs and the improvement in the quality of the product, match those of health care. More than a decade ago, industrial leaders realized that to compete and survive in a world economy, quality improvement techniques were needed, which would yield significant operational improvements (Drucker, 1991; Hickman & Silva, 1984; Naisbitt & Aburdene, 1985; Tichy & Devanna, 1986).

The three individuals most closely associated with these processes are Philip B. Crosby, W. Edwards Deming, and Joseph M. Juran.

Crosby is probably the best known of the three quality experts. His approach is based on his *14 steps* for the quality improvement process (QIP) (Crosby, 1979):

1. Management commitment
2. Quality improvement team
3. Measurement
4. Cost of quality
5. Quality awareness
6. Corrective action
7. Zero defects planning
8. Employee education
9. Zero defects
10. Goal setting
11. Error cause removal
12. Recognition
13. Quality councils
14. Do it all over again

Crosby (1979) explains that his efforts are different from those of Juran or Deming in that these *14 steps* provide a complete process. This process, says Crosby, provides a methodology for improving quality, not just a series of quality improvement techniques.

W. Edward Deming is the leading figure in quality improvement. It was Deming who, working with Japanese manufacturers in the 1950s, was responsible for the tremendous improvements made in Japanese manufacturing. To make improvements, Deming relies on technical expertise as well as statistical analysis. His work helped place the Japanese in a completely different class of manufacturing.

Deming's (1986) approach places emphasis on 14 points, which have been used in the transformation of American industry:

1. Create constancy of purpose for improvement of product service.
2. Adopt a new philosophy.
3. Cease dependence on inspection to achieve quality.
4. End the practice of awarding business on the basis of price tag alone. Instead, minimize total cost by working with a single supplier.
5. Improve constantly every process for planning, production, and service.
6. Institute training on the job.
7. Adopt and institute leadership.
8. Drive out fear.
9. Break down barriers between staff areas.
10. Eliminate slogans, expectations, and targets for the work force.
11. Eliminate numerical quotas for the work force and numerical goals for management.
12. Remove barriers that rob people of pride of workmanship. Eliminate the annual rating or merit system.
13. Institute a vigorous program of education and self-improvement for everyone.
14. Put everybody in the company to work to accomplish the transformation.

Deming (1986) may be best known for his work in involving the employee in the quality improvement system. Concepts such as the "quality circle" or the "QC

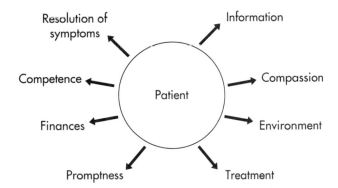

Fig. 20-2   Patient care concerns. (Courtesy A. Ron and M. Holtz, Beth Israel Medical Center, 1992.)

circle" grew out of the development of these processes, which involved groups of employees in problem identification and solving. Perhaps most relevant in adapting Deming's work to the health care industry is its focus on implementing intervention strategies to improve quality and reduce cost. Other aspects applicable to health care are the continuous improvement in quality and the use of employee teams trained in problem-solving techniques (Deming, 1986).

Juran was with Deming in the 1950s in Japan and had previously worked with Deming in the 1920s at the Hawthorne Western Electric Plant in Chicago. Juran, like Deming, is considered a pioneer and an expert in quality improvement technology. Best known for his *quality trilogy* (Juran, 1987; 1988), Juran broadened the quality approach to a wider operational or managerial perspective:

▼ **Quality planning:** The process of developing the products and processes required to meet customer needs.

▼ **Quality control:** The regulating process through which actual performance is measured and compared to standards and the difference is acted upon.

▼ **Quality improvement:** The organized creation of beneficial change.

The structure, process, and outcome approaches of these quality issues can be operationalized and evaluated for continuous improvement. With the patient as focus, quality is identified as those factors most important to patient and family. If asked, the patient might identify many of the factors outlined in Fig. 20-2 as important to his or her care.

THE LINK TO CASE MANAGEMENT

Data for analysis in traditional quality assurance methods have focused on "unquality" or "disquality," such as infections, falls, medication errors, returns to the operating room, and deaths.

Some of these elements focus on the institution, such as global indicators of quality within the hospital. Examples of global indicators include morbidity and mortality rates and generic risk-management indicators. The focus of these elements has been on those identified as outliers.

Another traditional data base has been financial data and analysis, which tracks the cost of specific procedures or diagnosis-related groups (DRGs). The finance department uses this information to determine case mix index, which in turn helps determine the reimbursement rate.

Data related to individual practitioners have been more loosely followed. Utilization review evaluators and other quality management departments have focused on specific practice patterns.

Within case management, each of these elements can be followed more comprehensively. The data, once collected, are linked to continuous quality improvement methods. The first step in a CQI process such as this is to identify problems that appear to be more than isolated events and to identify all of the issues that may be affecting the outcome. These issues might be linked to a DRG cost analysis as well as to individual practice patterns. In a case management framework, all practitioners are monitored for quality, use of resources, and length of stay.

The case management plan is the foundation for this kind of data collection and analysis. The case management plan provides a guideline for administering care to a particular patient type. These plans take into consideration not only length of stay but also resource use. During the development of the case management plan the optimal treatment plan, one that streamlines care without compromising quality, is identified.

If planned correctly, these collaborative guidelines are agreed on by the group of practitioners for whom the guidelines are relevant. These plans, in essence, describe the one best treatment plan for a particular patient problem. By following these guidelines, quality issues are easily tracked. The case management plan provides the collection and evaluation of variances or complications or both. These data may or may not reveal the need to alter the plan to improve quality (Deming, 1986).

For example, a plan for the treatment of pneumonia may indicate that more than 50% of the patients managed by this plan develop some complication on the third or fourth day. This pattern is seen when retrospectively analyzing the variances documented on the case management plan. A review of this information may indicate the need for a change in the protocol. This may mean providing some element of the plan either earlier or later in the hospital stay.

The cost of the hospital stay can also be followed through the use of the case management plans. Performance within a particular DRG can be tracked financially or through a quality perspective. Comparing case-managed patients to similar patients who are not case managed is one way to do this tracking. Another method is to compare physicians' practice patterns and any deviations from the care plan. This information then can be evaluated for both quality and cost.

Monitoring length of stay or cost before and after implementation of the case management system allows particular nursing units to be their own controls.

If nursing documentation is a part of the managed care plan, the documentation is reviewed for completeness. The registered nurse documents against each expected outcome as it appears on the plan. Thus the documentation more accurately reflects the plan of care and the expected outcomes.

In any case, the processes surrounding the quality issue become the main focus when a CQI approach is taken. Theoretically this process makes continuous analysis and improvement possible because it pinpoints every imperfection in the process and opens the door for change (Berwick, 1989).

THE COST OF QUALITY

Poor quality is costly (Marszalek-Gaucher & Coffey, 1990) and can be assessed by the following:

▼ Cost associated with giving wrong medications or treatments
▼ Increased costs related to misuse of personnel or product resources
▼ Cost of delays
▼ Loss of sales because of dissatisfied patients or physicians

Crosby stresses a "cost of quality" determination as part of the quality improvement process (Quest for Quality, 1989). His outline parallels actions used when developing a managed care plan. However, the development of the managed care plan takes Crosby's process one step further, because it adresses issues and incorporates solutions into the plan of care:

▼ Audit medical records to determine medically unnecessary tests, treatments, or procedures and other factors contributing to increased cost or length of stay.
▼ Meet with a quality assurance or utilization review representative and review incident reports to determine opportunities for improvement.
▼ Interview key members of the organization to identify barriers to the smooth operation and coordination of care.
▼ Interview the medical staff to identify areas for improvement.
▼ Review and analyze patient records to identify costs that can be eliminated.
▼ Evaluate current reporting procedures, information related to operations, and data related to patient satisfaction.

The cost-of-quality analysis identifies a number of potential opportunities for quality improvement. From a case management perspective the information may lay the foundation for managed care plans by taking into account the best, most cost-effective method available.

THE CQI PROCESS

The CQI process consists of a number of specific steps. Although it is not necessary to follow the steps in a precise sequence, all steps should be evaluated and addressed (Marszalek-Gaucher & Coffey, 1990). The achievement of quality care and cost savings is the foundation of both case management and CQI. The process is a cycle that continuously repeats itself.

As with the case management implementation process, the first major step in the CQI process is that of planning and preparing to improve; the second step is to implement; the third step is to innovate.

Preparing to improve involves seven essential steps (Marszalek-Gaucher & Coffey, 1990). Once again, it is not necessary to follow them in precise order, but each should be addressed in some manner:

1. **Find a process.** The first step is to find a process that needs quality improvement,

cost control, or both. These processes may be within a clinical, operations, or financial setting from admitting, to medication distribution, to billing.

2. **Assemble a team that knows the process.** It has been said that those who know the process best are those working the front line or those who work within the process on a day-to-day basis. Therefore a large percentage of the team should be those directly involved in health care delivery. Management should also be included because this division can remove obstacles and facilitate change and improvement. The members of the team should know the process they are evaluating.

3. **Identify the customers and the process outputs and measure the customer expectations of these outputs.** Quality has been defined as meeting or exceeding customer expectations (*Hospital Peer Review*, 1988). Because of the complexity of health care, each process may be made up of several smaller processes. The first thing the team should do is identify its customers, the outputs of each process, and customer expectations regarding these outputs. In some cases, such as clinical settings, the expectations may not be those of individuals but of the profession as a whole. These expectations may be based on professionwide standards for the practice of nursing and medicine.

4. **Document the process.** Each process consists of a series of steps or inputs, each of which is working toward a particular output. Each step can usually be broken down into substeps, which are hierarchical. A fundamental knowledge of the process is necessary to identify each of the steps accurately, and this is why the input of the front-line worker is so important. A process cannot be managed or improved without this fundamental knowledge.

5. **Generate output and process specifications.** Specifications are measurable, explicit attributes expected of the process and the output. Output specifications may involve the expectations of the customers, which are considered expectations external to the process. However, process specifications are the key internal process factors.

   Each of the specifications must be measurable. When these specifications are achieved, quality is achieved. Quality is maintained by conforming to these specifications, which is precisely what the managed care plan facilitates. The expected outcomes, if met, ensure quality care has been delivered for that particular problem. As these processes and outputs are evaluated, the process is adjusted to continuously improve it.

6. **Eliminate inappropriate variation.** The sixth step involves implementation. Each specification denotes a measurement point, which is evaluated. One major goal is to prevent quality failures or variations. Two types of variations will occur. The first is random variation. These variations result from factors inherent in the process, and they occur each time the process is played out. The other form of variation is the specific variation, which is a variation that occurs because of one specific component within the process. Once the processes for improvement are implemented, specific variation frequency should be reduced.

   The goal of the CQI process is to eliminate as many specific variations as possible (Deming, 1986). This results in consistently high-quality output.

   Within case management the managed care plans allow for the documentation

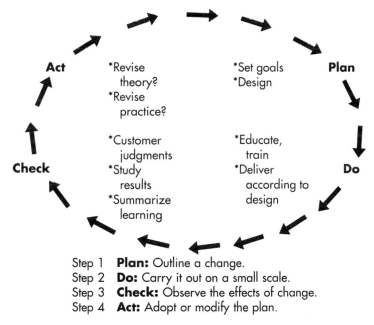

Act	**Plan**
*Revise theory? *Revise practice?	*Set goals *Design
*Customer judgments *Study results *Summarize learning	*Educate, train *Deliver according to design
Check	**Do**

Step 1 **Plan:** Outline a change.
Step 2 **Do:** Carry it out on a small scale.
Step 3 **Check:** Observe the effects of change.
Step 4 **Act:** Adopt or modify the plan.

Fig. 20-3   The Shewhart cycle.

of variations in clinical practice. By working as a team, the health care professionals can differentiate between random variation and specific variation. The elimination of inappropriate variations results in an approach to health care delivery in which only random variations occur.

Random variations are inherent within every process because every patient is different, and every response to treatment is slightly different. These "noises" in the system occur for every process and affect every output.

7. **Document continuous improvement.** This is the final process and the one that makes continuous improvement possible. Once the opportunities for specific or nonrandom variations have been reduced or eliminated, improvements or innovations are introduced.

Team members can make changes that result in improved quality or increased productivity. Because the opportunity for variation has been reduced, it is easier to evaluate the impact of the innovation. After such evaluation the change either becomes permanent, or the team discontinues its use.

Walter A. Shewhart described this method of using a stable process to test innovations as the *plan-do-check-act cycle* (PDCA) (Deming, 1986). First developed in the 1930s, this process has become known as the Shewhart cycle. See Fig. 20-3 (Deming, 1986).

The PDCA cycle is applied to the process used in case management for addressing and improving health care delivery for particular patient types. Planning involves the identification of specific clinical areas for improvement. As discussed earlier, these areas are either patients in a specific DRG or nurses in a particular unit chosen to undertake the switch to case management.

The **plan** step involves determining the best case management plan. The **do** step involves implementation of the case management approach. The third step, **check,** involves the analysis of variances that hinder efficient use of the plan. The effects of such variances can be observed by changes in length of stay, patient satisfaction, staff satisfaction, or costs. In some cases the plan might need further revisions until these tangible results are noted.

The **act** step is for modifications if needed. Minimal case management variances indicate that the plan is usable and can be adopted at that point as the standard. If the variances are not minimal, the process begins again with the plan changed, tested, checked, and finally adopted.

The aim of the team is to continuously improve the process. In health care the process may never be brought to a conclusion because of the evolutionary nature of the treatment of disease. Changing technology, an aging patient population, and economic considerations, all have a prolonged effect on the delivery of health care. Therefore the process probably will remain open ended and continuous.

In any case, each process should be seen as one that unremittingly moves forward because today's goals may be tomorrow's standard.

REFERENCES

Berwick, D.M. (1989, January 5). Sounding board. *The New England Journal of Medicine,* 53-56.

Bryce, G.R. (1991, February). Quality management theories and their application. *Quality,* 23-26.

Crosby, P. B. (1979). *Quality is free: The art of making quality certain.* New York: McGraw-Hill.

Deming, W.E. (1986). *Out of the crisis.* Cambridge: Center for Advanced Engineering Study, Massachusetts Institute of Technology.

Donabedian, A. (1980). *Explorations in quality assessment and monitoring. Vol 1: The definition of quality and approaches to its assessment.* Ann Arbor, MI: Health Administration Press.

Drucker, P. (1991, November-December). The new productivity challenge. *Harvard Business Review,* 67-79.

Goldfield, N., & Nash, D.B. (Eds.). (1989). *Providing quality care.* Philadelphia: American College of Physicians.

Hickman, C.R., & Silva, M.A. (1984). *Creating excellence: Managing corporate culture, strategy, and change.* Ontario, NY: New American Library.

Hospital Peer Review. (1988). Deming's philosophy improves quality. *13*(10), 12-24.

Hospitals. (1991, August 5). New JCAHO standards emphasize continuous quality improvement (pp. 41-44).

Joint Commission on Accreditation of Hospitals. (1990). *Quality assessment and improvement proposed revised standards.* Chicago: Author.

Juran, J.M. (1987). *Juran on quality leadership: How to go from here to there.* Wilton, CT: Juran Institute.

Juran, J.M. (1988). *Juran on planning for quality.* New York: Free Press.

Kanter, R.M. (1983). *The change masters: Innovations for productivity in the American corporation.* New York: Simon & Schuster.

Laffel, G., & Blumenthal, D. (1989). The case for using industrial quality management science in health care organizations. *Journal of the American Medical Association, 262*(20), 2869-2873.

Marszalek-Gaucher, E., & Coffey, R.J. (1990). *Transforming healthcare organizations.* San Francisco: Jossey-Bass.

Naisbitt, J. (1982). *Megatrends: Ten new directions transforming our lives.* New York; Warner Books.

Naisbitt, J., & Aburdene, P. (1985). *Reinventing the corporation.* New York: Warner Books.

O'Connor, P. (1984). Healthcare financing policy: Impact on nursing. *Nursing Administration Quarterly, 8*(4):10-20.

Quest for quality and productivity in health services. (1989, September). Excerpts from the 1989 Conference Proceedings. Washington, D.C.

Tichy, N. M., & Devanna, M. A. (1986, July). The transformational leader. *Training and Development Journal,* pp. 27-32.

21

JOB SATISFACTION

▼ *CHAPTER OVERVIEW*

Many variables affect job satisfaction in the workplace. Among these variables, autonomy, professional status, and socialization are consistently and positively related to increases in job satisfaction for registered nurses. Job satisfaction has also been positively related to retention of nurses.

Case management models integrate many of the elements associated with greater job satisfaction, including autonomy, a feeling of connectedness on the job, and professional status.

Two case studies show the relationship between a case management model and job satisfaction. The Nursing Initiatives Program at Long Island Jewish Medical Center in New York demonstrated that the introduction of the case manager role on three pilot units increased job satisfaction and reduced vacancy rates for registered nurses.

This study was replicated at Beth Israel Medical Center in New York City. Data on three pilot units were collected before start-up and at 9 months. Outcomes demonstrated improved job satisfaction for staff registered nurses and case managers and reductions in vacancy and turnover rates.
▲

JOB SATISFACTION AS A VARIABLE

Among the variables affected by the implementation of a case management model is staff job satisfaction. The introduction of a case manager to a nursing unit can improve the work environment and thus the job satisfaction of nurses working there.

The case manager plans and organizes the care of patients who have the most complex cases, assists with patient teaching, and follows through with discharge planning. In an era when many nurses complain that they spend more time documenting patient care, meeting regulatory documentation requirements, filling out requisitions, or making telephone calls than they do with patients, this model lets nurses remain at the bedside while ensuring that all peripheral patient needs are met. Because the case manager relieves staff nurses of some of the indirect nursing functions related to their patients' care, many staff nurses report that they are able to spend more time in direct contact with their patients.

Clearly the case management model builds in a support system to help busy practitioners meet complex patient needs. The model promotes independent practice in those nurses providing the direct patient care. But it does not expect these same nurses to function in a vacuum without the proper support systems to meet all their patients' needs in a rapid paced, complicated health care environment.

Job satisfaction has been related to nurses' job-turnover rates (Curry, Wakefield, Price, Mueller, & McCloskey, 1985; Reich, 1984; Slavitt, Stamps, Piedmont, & Haase, 1978). Choi, Jameson, Brekke, Anderson, and Podratz (1989) demonstrated that nurses' overall dissatisfaction with their work was the strongest predictor of intent to leave the place of employment or current position. Job satisfaction has been directly related to nurse retention and turnover (Hinshaw & Atwood, 1982; Weisman, Alexander, & Chase, 1981). Therefore the importance of this variable should not be overlooked when a new nursing care delivery system is being designed or evaluated.

A case management model affects the staff nurses providing direct patient care as well as the case managers. The model takes a team approach to care. The team consists of the patient, the family, the physician, the case manager, the direct nursing care provider, the social worker, and others as needed. The model brings all members of the team together with a common focus. Whereas primary nursing led to feelings of isolation and separation for the direct care providers, the case management model does just the opposite. The model's structure works to bring everyone together. Each member supplies information relevant to the care of the patient, and value is placed on every member's input.

As a highly socialized model, case management allows for combined work units organized around a common goal: good patient care. Communication and conflict resolution become needed skills for each team member. If the members of the team cannot function as a group, the outcomes of care will not be achieved in a timely and efficient manner. Because these are among the primary goals of case management, group dynamics play a significant part in the success or failure of the model.

The case manager role, which fosters teamwork, also provides the nurse with an autonomous job that requires independent thought and action. The support provided by the case manager to the other nurse providers reinforces similar feelings of autonomy and independence in them (Alexander, Weisman, & Chase, 1982). It does this by positioning the direct-care provider in a strategic position. A team must rely on the information provided by each of its members, and it is the nurse responsible for direct patient care who provides the information that determines the clinical course of treatment, the teaching needs, and the discharge plan.

This enhanced role for nurses builds feelings of professionalism and self-esteem because nursing's input is valued and deemed important to the patient's progress. In the past, communication was of a hierarchical nature, with the physician dictating to the other members. In the case management model the nurse case manager serves as the thread that links all members of the team. Each member's input is needed so that appropriate and timely outcomes of care are achieved. In this system the staff nurse providing direct care at the bedside supplies the case manager and the rest of the team with valuable information.

As discussed in Chapter 27, clinical career ladders help organizations reward both experience and education. A case manager position allows clinically expert, educated, experienced nurses to take on increased responsibility while remaining close to the patient. The position provides for a new set of job responsibilities and a new wage scale that takes into account all these factors.

The case management model incorporates those elements that have been correlated to increased job satisfaction and decreased turnover. These elements include autonomy, a feeling of connectedness on the job, and salary (Johnston, 1991; McCloskey, 1990; Pooyan, Eberhardt, & Szigeti, 1990).

Some institutions have attempted to measure the satisfaction of their nurses when implementing a case management tool. Although it may be said that other factors can affect the nurses' feelings of satisfaction or dissatisfaction with their work—such as the physical work environment, the presence of a computerized clinical information system, the hours of work, or the fringe benefits—some of these other variables can be controlled by testing the same nurses before and after implementation.

CASE STUDIES

In 1988 as part of the United Hospital Fund's Nursing Initiatives Program, five hospitals—The Brooklyn Hospital Center, Long Island Jewish Medical Center, The Neurological Institute of the Presbyterian Hospital, The New York Hospital, and New York University Medical Center—were selected to orchestrate innovative methods for addressing the nursing shortage. Four of the sites proposed and tested new methods of structuring nursing care providers' work, with the goals of increasing nursing productivity, satisfaction, and retention. The fifth site, New York University Medical Center, introduced a stress reduction program with similar goals (Gould & Mezey, 1991).

Long Island Jewish Medical Center, New York

At Long Island Jewish Medical Center a new nursing position was created as part of the United Hospital Fund's program. The new position was titled patient care manager and became part of a case management delivery model. The position was designed specifically to match the nurse's expertise with the patient's needs and the severity of the illness. One of the reasons for the new position was to keep nurses at the bedside. The position provided the patient care manager with a challenging and rewarding role (Gould and Mezey, 1991).

Three data collection points were used to gauge nurses' job satisfaction. The first point was before implementation, the second at 1 year, and the third at about 18 months into the project. Job satisfaction was measured by the Nursing Job Satisfaction Scale (Atwood and Hinshaw, 1981; 1984). The instrument, which has been tested for validity and reliability, was given to all nurses on all shifts at each collection point (Ake et al, 1991).

The medical center's implementation strategies were
▼ Selecting expert registered nurses as patient care managers
▼ Assigning patient care managers to coordinate care
▼ Decentralizing unit decision making to registered nurses and physicians
▼ Upgrading nursing attendant tasks
▼ Establishing walking rounds

Registered nurse vacancy rates and registered nurse hours per patient were evaluated in addition to tracking nurse job satisfaction.

Nurses were chosen as patient care managers based on their clinical expertise and willingness to participate in what was, at that time, an experimental role.

The three units participating in the project were a 39-bed medical unit, a 32-bed surgical unit, and a 40-bed neonatal intensive care unit (NICU). At the end of the first 18 months of implementation, 20% of the registered nurses on each unit involved were patient care managers. They managed the care provided for one to three patients in addition to their regular direct care functions.

After about 1 year the patient care managers on the medical unit reported that this dual role was too difficult and stressful. At that time, one patient care manager was recruited to take on the role full time and was removed from direct nursing-role functions. This individual functioned in a truly autonomous and independent case management role.

Average nursing hours per patient remained relatively consistent throughout the project. However, the number of registered nurse hours per patient and the number of registered nurses on the unit decreased from 119.8 full-time equivalents (FTEs) at the start to 113.7 FTEs at 18 months, indicating an increase in productivity.

The registered nurse vacancy rate also improved during the 18-month period. On the medical unit the rate decreased from 8% to zero; on the surgical unit the vacancy rate decreased from 23% to zero; and in the NICU it remained constant at zero.

Among the most dramatic findings was the improvement in nursing job satisfaction, particularly comparing start-up scores to those at 18 months for nurses functioning as patient care managers and those working as staff nurses on the units (see Table 21-1).

Beth Israel Medical Center, New York, New York

The findings of the Nursing Initiatives Program at Long Island Jewish Medical Center pointed to a relationship between nurse roles and responsibilities and job satisfaction. The study was replicated at Beth Israel Medical Center in New York City to determine if the case manager role did indeed play an important part in the job satisfaction of registered nurses.

At the time of implementation of the three pilot units at the Beth Israel Medical Center in January of 1991, all patient care managers were employed on a full-time basis, carrying a case load of 15 to 20 patients. Three pilot units were chosen for the study. These units included a 38-bed neurosurgical unit, a 12-bed AIDS unit, and a 45-bed medical/surgical unit for the chemically dependent. One case manager was employed on each unit on a full-time basis, meaning that all three were removed from direct care responsibilities.

Indirect care responsibilities included coordination and facilitation of services to the patient, multidisciplinary care planning, patient and family teaching, and discharge planning.

It was anticipated that the introduction of a case management model would increase employee job satisfaction. The case managers, working as staff nurses,

Table 21-1   Registered nurse satisfaction by service and by title on case-managed pilot units at Long Island Jewish Medical Center 1988-1990

	AT START-UP (1988)		AT 12 MONTHS (1989)		AT 18 MONTHS (1990)	
	N	AVERAGE SCORE	N	AVERAGE SCORE	N	AVERAGE SCORE
UNIT						
Medicine	20	87	26	90	19	94
Surgery	13	92	16	98	15	97
NICU	79	103	69	105	59	105
Total	112		111		93	
TITLE						
Staff PCMs	26	99	17	104	15	110*
Other RNs	86	99	94	100	78	100
Total	112		111		93	

Patient care managers (PCMs) include all full-time and part-time PCMs.
$p = .008$
Lowest possible score: 23
Highest possible score: 115
(Gould & Mezey, 1991)

remained close to the bedside. Relieved of any administrative responsibilities or direct nursing functions, the case managers were better able to provide not only indirect care to the patients but also assistance to other staff nurses.

The case manager was the only staff nurse working a 5-day-a-week schedule. The case manager was able to fill the information gaps caused by flextime schedules, which were fragmenting care. This built-in continuity factor allowed the staff nurse to spend more time in direct patient contact, rather than in reviewing reports or trying to catch up on what happened to the patient in the nurse's absence.

It was also hypothesized that a case management documentation system would enhance registered nurse job satisfaction. With the new system, involving the use of multidisciplinary action plans (MAPs), the nurse could anticipate care needs on a daily basis. In addition, nursing documentation was collapsed onto the form itself, eliminating the need for long, narrative notes. Instead of paragraph notation, the nurse responded to a series of implementation strategies designed to achieve the goals outlined on the plan. Each 24-hour period was attended to separately, and enough room was provided so that all nurses caring for the patient within that period could document patient progress and outcomes.

The management of patient care provides a structure that addresses length of stay as well as quality of care. Because the case manager is not geographically bound within the nursing unit, this person is the primary caretaker for the patient and family from admission to discharge from the unit. The case manager's lack of geographic constraints and the 5-day-a-week schedule provide for continuity of care for the patient and family.

Table 21-2   Registered nurse satisfaction by unit and by title on case-managed pilot units at Beth Israel Medical Center New York, New York

	AT START-UP (12/90)		AT 9 MONTHS (9/91)	
	N	AVERAGE SCORE	N	AVERAGE SCORE
UNIT				
Neurosurgery	11	82	11	82
AIDS	9	88	9	91
Medical-surgical for chemical dependency	10	84	10	90
Total	30		30	
TITLE*				
Patient care managers	3	78	3	86
Other RNs	27	84	27	89
Total	30		30	

T = 2.57, *df* = 29, *p* = 0.0157.
Not significant at the .05 level.
Lowest possible score: 23
Highest possible score: 115
*Data at both points.

The case management system, which improves communication between staff members, leads to a greater feeling of teamwork and collegiality. In addition, the enhanced information base from which nurses function provides a greater level of autonomy in their practices.

All registered nurses working on the pilot units were tested for job satisfaction via the Nursing Job Satisfaction Scale (Atwood & Hinshaw, 1981; 1984). Testing took place before implementation and about 9 months after implementation of the case management model. Thirty registered nurses, or 70% of all nurses filling out questionnaires, completed the questionnaire at both data collection points. Of those 30, three were case managers and 27 were staff nurses. All three shifts were represented in the sample.

Job satisfaction scores before start-up and after 9 months indicate that there was a statistically significant increase in satisfaction for those nurses working on case-managed care units who were there for both data collection periods (Table 21-2). Comparisons of case managers to other staff nurses at both collection points indicated an increase for both groups (Table 21-2).

For all three units, both registered nurse vacancy rates and turnover rates decreased over the period of the pilot project (Table 21-3).

On neurosurgery the vacancy rate decreased from 17.33% at start-up to 6% at the end of 9 months. The turnover rate decreased from 21% to 12.5%. On the AIDS unit the vacancy rate went from 11% at start-up to 7% at the end of 9 months, and the

Table 21-3 Registered nurse vacancy and turnover rates at Beth Israel Medical Center before and after case management introduced

UNIT	TIME	VACANCY RATE	TURNOVER RATE
Neurosurgery	Start-up	17.33%	21%
	9 Months	6%	12.5%
AIDS	Start-up	11%	9%
	9 Months	7%	7%
Medical/surgical for chemical dependency	Start-up	9%	17.6%
	9 Months	0	12%

turnover rate went from 9% to 7%. The medical/surgical unit for chemically dependent patients achieved a reduction in the vacancy rate from 9% to zero and a drop in turnover from 17% to 12% at the end of 9 months.

REFERENCES

Ake, J.M., Bowar-Ferris, S., Cesta, T., Gould, D., Greenfield, J., Hayes, P., Maislin, G., and Mezey M. (1991). The nursing initiatives program: Practice based models for care in hospitals. In *Differentiating nursing practice: Into the twenty-first century*. Kansas City, MO: American Academy of Nursing.

Alexander, C.S., Weisman, C.S., & Chase, G.A. (1982). Determinants of staff nurses' perceptions of autonomy within different clinical contexts. *Nursing Research, 31*(1), 48-52.

Atwood, J., & Hinshaw, A. (1981). Job stress: Instrument development program results. *Western Journal of Nursing Research, 3*(3), 48.

Atwood, J., & Hinshaw, A. (1984). Nursing job satisfaction: A program of development and testing. *Research in Nursing and Health.*

Choi, T., Jameson, H., Brekke, M.L., Anderson, J.G., & Podratz, R.O. (1989). Schedule-related effects on nurse retention. *Western Journal of Nursing Research, 11*(1):92-107.

Curry, J., Wakefield, D., Price, J., Mueller, C., & McCloskey, J. (1985). Determinants of turnover among nursing department employees. *Research in Nursing and Health, 8*, 397-411.

Gould, D.A., & Mezey, M.D. (1991). *At the Bedside: Innovations in Hospital Nursing.* New York: The United Hospital Fund of New York.

Hinshaw, A.S., & Atwood, J.R. (1982). Anticipated turnover: A preventive approach. *Western Journal of Nursing Research, 4*, 54-55.

Johnston, C.L. (1991). Sources of work satisfaction/dissatisfaction for hospital registered nurses. *Western Journal of Nursing Research, 13*(4), 503-513.

McCloskey, J.C. (1990). Two requirements for job contentment: Autonomy and social integration. *Image, 22*(3) 140-143.

Pooyan, A., Eberhardt, B., & Szigeti, E. (1990). Work-related variables and turnover intention among registered nurses. *Nursing and Health Care, 11*(5), 255-258.

Reich, P.A. (1984). *The relationship between Jungian personality type and choice of functional specialty in nursing.* Unpublished master's thesis. Adelphi University, Garden City, N.Y.

Slavitt, D.B., Stamps, P.L., Piedmont, E.B., & Haase, A.M. (1978). Nurses satisfaction with their work situation. *Nursing Research, 27*, 114-120.

Weisman, C.S., Alexander, C.S., & Chase, G.A. (1981). Determinants of hospital staff nurse turnover. *Medical Care, 19*, 431-443.

22

MEASURING COST-EFFECTIVENESS

▼ *CHAPTER OVERVIEW*

Measuring cost-effectiveness is one of the most important tasks in the evaluation of nursing case management models. This chapter reviews a variety of strategies for measuring cost savings in a case management system and provides examples of case studies using these approaches. In addition, suggestions for using these methods in further research are reviewed.
▲

EFFECT OF CASE MANAGEMENT ON VARIANCES OF LENGTH OF STAY AND RESOURCE UTILIZATION

In a study done by the American Hospital Association titled *1990 Report of the Hospital Nursing Personnel Survey* (AHA, 1990), the case management model represented the largest increase of nursing care delivery systems most frequently used in the acute care setting. In light of this study and others, it is important to present some of the methods of evaluating the cost-effectiveness of nursing case management. The studies presented in this chapter represent some of the groundbreaking work done in measuring cost-effectiveness of nursing case management and health care delivery approaches. In general, case management has been associated with reduced total costs per patient case, decreased patient length of hospital stay, increased patient turnover, and potential increase in hospital-generated revenues.

In a program instituted at Long Regional Hospital in Utah, cost savings were achieved through the use of a bedside-centered case management model (Bair, Griswold, & Head, 1989). With this approach the registered nurse controls the use of patient care resources, guides the outcomes of this care within acute care and community-based settings, and, as a member of a multidisciplinary care coordination team, monitors and evaluates the costs and quality components of hospitalization for patients within defined diagnosis-related group (DRG) categories.

The registered nurse was given the responsibility and accountability for assessing the inpatient and discharge care requirements and for developing and implementing the plan of care related to the prescribed length of stay and amount of patient care resources used. To determine actual costs, focus was placed on the clinical management of defined groups of patients within 10 DRGs or service lines. Each of these groups was analyzed with special emphasis placed on patient care services, length of hospitalization, treatment and educational outcomes, discharge and postdischarge care planning, and outpatient and community-based services. Some of the DRGs that were investigated included major joint procedures, angina, heart failure, chest pain, circulatory disorders, acute myocardial infarction, and pneumonia.

A cost containment study that focused on reducing the average loss per DRG case type was implemented. A comparison was made of the actual cost per case and the average reimbursement for 10 DRGs. It was demonstrated that bedside case management resulted in cost savings associated with a decrease in length of stay of 0.4 day, an average hospital savings of $284 per case and overall cost savings of $94,572.

Additional savings were realized through strategic planning and better use of patient care resources as evidenced by a reduction in admissions to the intensive care unit by 0.7 day and through the accurate assessment and classification of Medicare reimbursement criteria related to inpatient and outpatient group status.

An investigation done by McKenzie, Torkelson, and Holt (1989) showed that interventions associated with nursing case management had a significant effect on patient resource consumption and expenditures.

Case management plans and critical paths were developed for specific high-volume DRGs associated with diseases and disorders of the circulatory system, coronary artery bypass, and catheterization. This study demonstrated an average cost saving per case that was equivalent to $350 for laboratory charges, $180 for radiology charges, and $766 for pharmaceutical charges for nursing case-managed patients. The average length of stay was also reduced by 1.1 days. Within a 1-year period, close to $1 million was saved by using the case management system of care.

Stillwaggon (1989) demonstrated the effect of a nurse model on the cost of nursing care and staff satisfaction. This study was conducted at Saint Francis Hospital and Medical Center in Hartford, Connecticut. An approach to the delivery of patient care called *managed nursing care* was developed and implemented. This model promoted collaborative practice arrangements, encouraged care based on individualized patient assessment and need, eliminated routine and nonnursing tasks, and established nursing practice guided by professional standards of care. In addition, the professional nurse was able to contract for services and care needed by the patient. This contracting eliminated the need for the traditional work schedule.

The study sample consisted of 100 cases of normal, spontaneous delivery without complication or comorbidity. Comparisons were made between the traditional nursing care delivery system and the new approach to patient care under the nurse managed care model. An assessment was made of the nursing care hours actually delivered and the staff's satisfaction with the nurse managed care model.

Results showed a reduction of 5 hours spent delivering nursing services and a $61.71 decrease in cost of care per case. Additional findings indicated a high level of nursing staff and patient satisfaction with the nurse managed care delivery system.

In another study, Cohen (1991) incorporated a cost-accounting methodology with a combined team nursing–case management model to investigate personnel factors and variable cost components such as pharmaceuticals and supplies under the nursing case management model. The purpose of this study was to substantiate the financial benefit of using the nursing case management model within the acute care setting.

It was predicted that cesarean section patients who received care under the nursing case management model would have a shorter length of stay than those patients who received care under the existing practices. It was also predicted that the nursing case management system of care would result in an overall decrease in hospital costs and expenditures associated with the cesarean section patient (Cohen, 1991).

The study used a quasi-experimental design on the experimental and control units. The cesarean section case types, DRGs 370 and 371, were selected for study because of the high volume and long length of stay associated with these DRGs. The study sample consisted of 128 cesarean section patients who made up 768 total patient days in 1988. A nonrandom selection was used.

Because randomization was not used, homogeneity controlled for individual extraneous variables that may have affected patient length of stay. Restricting the patient sample to cesarean section helped to control for patient gender, type of diagnosis, and surgical operation.

The data needed for the study required the development and implementation of the nursing case management delivery system. Use of the case management model required thorough orientation for the nursing staff. This orientation period introduced nurses in the experimental group to care under a case management model and helped the case managers assume their roles. Those who were in the experimental group included registered nurses, licensed practical nurses, and nursing assistants. Critical paths and nursing case management care plans were also used.

Demographic data, length of stay, and comorbidity information were received and compiled from the patient subject group. An evaluation was made of professional staff mix as well as the amount of time spent by nurses in delivering patient care (Cohen, 1990; 1991).

Nursing staff members were expected to cooperate with the investigator of this hospital-based administrative research project. The implementation of the nursing case management model included the following guidelines:

1. The case manager (registered nurse) became responsible for the patient when she was admitted to the unit.
2. Case associates (co-case managers or primary registered nurses) and case assistants (licensed practical nurses and nursing assistants) were given responsibility for ensuring continuity of care and accountability throughout the patient's length of stay. Each of the co-case managers was assigned different schedules to avoid overlapping days on the unit. Each patient was designated one case manager whose case load was covered by the co-case manager on the case manager's days off.
3. Each case manager was to collaborate with the attending physician in assessing and evaluating the outcomes of patient care and individualizing the case management plan and critical path.
4. Each case manager was trained to use the case management care plan and critical path to facilitate patient care.
5. The critical path was used for the change-of-shift report.
6. Variance from the case management care plan or the critical path required

discussion with the attending physician and a nursing case management consultant.

7. The nursing case manager and physician were to communicate at least twice during the patient's length of stay.

8. The nurse case manager and the patient care coordinator (head nurse) were to collaborate on a daily basis to negotiate assignment planning that would optimize the use of nursing resources.

9. Daily documentation was to reflect the monitoring of patient progress and evaluation of outcomes specified in the case management care plan or variances on the critical path, or both (Cohen, 1990).

COST ACCOUNTING METHOD

One of the primary objectives of the nursing case management system is to develop a cost management information system that validates the patient's use of clinical resources and services and confirms the financial benefits of case management to the institution. In this investigative project a nursing case management concept was established with the cesarean section case type that incorporated the following fiscal priorities:

▼ To maximize control over patient hospital stay by implementing definable and attainable patient goals within a short period of time.

▼ To decrease service-related costs and enhance DRG reimbursement by reducing patient length of stay through anticipatory planning, early intervention, and the coordination and arrangement of services.

The cost accounting process used in this study involved the following four procedural steps:

Step I: Establishment of a Resource Use Profile on the Typical Cesarean Section Patient. A historical patient profile that was reflective of conventional practice patterns was developed from the hospital's management information system. This procedure involved a review of detailed charges based on the hospital's charge description and general ledger code reports. These charges were summarized and then compressed from 272 service codes into 14 major clinical use and expense categories. Those categories were then separated by sample group. The categories included routine care, delivery room, operating room, anesthesia, recovery room, laboratory or blood, radiology, respiratory physiology, general pharmacy, antibiotics, IV (intravenous therapy), other pharmacy, routine treatment, and other.

A 2-month sample from 1988 medical records and bills was accessed so that clinical information, financial data, volume of tests and services, posted charge rates for room and board, and ancillary services could be analyzed. An average of the accumulated costs was obtained to arrive at the cost of a unit of service (i.e., patient day, tests, procedures, pharmaceuticals) for all clinically related resources used.

Step II: Establishment of a Resource Use Profile for the Cesarean Section Patient Based on the Nursing Case Management Concept. The historical data obtained from the patient profiles were used to develop a patient profile adjusted for nursing case management outcome standards. The major nursing, medical, and ancillary outcome indicators of care were derived from the cesarean section patients' critical paths and were used to assess the nursing case management model's efficacy and productivity. Cost standards were set by reducing patient length of stay by 2 days (from 6 to 4 days), streamlining tests and procedures, and initiating patient teaching early in the hospital stay.

Step III: Comparison of the Charge and Resource Use Associated with Comparable Cesarean Section Cases. A charge and clinical resource use comparison was made between the experimental (case management) and control (conventional practice) groups. The comparison involved correlating the average unit of service for both the experimental and control groups to establish the average clinical resource use for the cesarean section patient. For example, the following was identified: average number of tests incurred, average number of supplies used, average number of pharmaceuticals given, average number of nursing care hours provided, and average length of stay. This comparison established a mechanism for monitoring the change in resource use after switching from conventional practices to case management. Such monitoring helped ensure that efficient use of services was maintained. The results of this comparison substantiated the efficacy of the case management model.

Step IV: Determination of the Total Average Cost for the Nursing Case Management Model. The above analysis provided the total room and board charges. However, to more effectively determine the average cost of the nursing case management model as well as the required nursing care resources, the following methodology was used: (1) The total direct nursing care costs were computed for both sample groups; (2) nursing care was segregated from total room and board costs; and (3) the ratio of cost to charge (RCC) factor was applied. The comparisons in step III were then categorized by skill mix to determine the number of direct nursing care hours required under each system for the care of the cesarean section patient.

To determine the total direct nursing care costs associated with both the experimental and control groups, the following computation was completed:

Average base salary per skill mix by sample group ÷ 1,950 hours (the number of hours worked in a year by an employee) = Average hourly wage rate

Average hourly wage rate × Sum total of direct nursing care hours provided by skill mix (from the Nursing Case Management Activity form) × 1.25 (average fringe benefits) = Total average costs of direct nursing care for the cesarean section patient.

The direct nursing care costs were then segregated from the total expenditures to arrive at the remaining room and board costs.

The method used for determining costs was the departmental RCC, which is the cost-accounting methodology most widely used by health care institutions. The RCC is delineated from the Institutional Cost Report, which is a cost statement used by the Medicare program for various reimbursement processes. This report contains revenue, cost, and clinical service use information by department.

The method involved taking the RCC for each major clinical use and expense category and applying it against the total charges to arrive at an approximate

Table 22-1   Beth Israel Medical Center case managed incremental revenue for

DIAGNOSIS		DRGs	ALOS 1990*
Laminectomy		4/755/756/577/ 758/214/215	10.0
Endocarditis		126	14.4
Soft tissue infection		278	9.1
Pneumonia		89	11.06
Orthopedics		209/211/233/234/218/ 219/220/221/223/224	1/91-6/91 9.0
Diabetes team	Principal diagnosis	294/295/296/297/566	9.9
	Secondary diagnosis	—	11.8
	High-risk obstetrics	383	—

*Average length of stay data compiled from an MIS download from the Charms systems.

determination of the total cost per case. This provided the final pieces of data needed to establish the total average costs for the nursing case management model (Cohen, 1990; 1991).

Findings indicated that a significant reduction in patient length of stay was achieved. Length of stay declined by 1.16 days, or 19%, between the experimental and control groups ($p \leq .0001$). Expenditure and cost analysis showed an increase in direct patient-centered nursing care hours and intensification in use of inpatient services and treatments. This intensification of nursing time and resource use led to the reduction in patient length of stay and a decrease in total overall costs.

The analysis further demonstrated a savings of $930.40 per patient case and a general decrease in hospital costs and expenditures associated with the cesarean section patient. This profit was made possible because of the increase in patient turnover and the availability of additional patient beds. Potential savings and revenues of more than $1 million were identified for the hospital (Cohen, 1991; Health Care Advisory Board, 1990).

Although an analysis of the demographic data showed comparability between the experimental and control groups, the rigor of this investigation can be strengthened by using matched sampling to decrease the likelihood of extraneous variance and by using randomized assignment of the sample groups.

At Beth Israel Medical Center in New York City the case management model is used as a vehicle for reducing patient length of stay. Coupled with other initiatives such as CQI, reductions in the length of stay for selected diagnoses were realized in the first year of implementing the case management model (Table 22-1).

selected diagnoses

NO. CASES 1990	ALOS 1991*	NO. CASES 1991	INCREMENTAL REVENUE†
260	9.08	213	$238,000
94	8.7	58	$900,000
189	8.7	156	$ 28,000
298	10.05	257	$196,000
1/91-6/91 143	7/91-2/92 7.08	7/91-2/92 226	$489,000
300	3.45	11/11/91-1/31/92 37	
—	10.5	11/11/91-1/31/92 29	
—	8.25	12	$438,000
		TOTAL	$2,289,000

†Incremental revenue calculated by Don Modzewleski, Assistant Vice President, Finance.

Nursing, medicine, social work, administration, patient representatives, operations, and finance were among the departments that participated in the change to a case management delivery system. In some cases, specific medical or surgical departments or specialties were targeted for the development of MAPs. These plans incorporated all professional disciplines in management of the patient's care and ensured outcome-related quality services. In other cases, specific diagnoses or DRGs were targeted for significant reductions in length of stay (Table 22-1).

The Pareto chart, a statistical tool that can be used to determine which diagnoses or procedures to target, was used for the development of managed care plans and financial analysis (Fig. 22-1). If an annual review is being conducted, the number of cases for the top volume DRGs can be tallied. These are then placed on the chart in the form of a bar graph in descending order. On the right side of the chart the percentage of the total cases that each number of cases represents is placed on a cumulative line graph. For example, DRG 707 represented 63 cases, or 31% of the total number of cases. The next highest volume, DRG 277, represented a total of 50 cases, or 24% of the total number of cases. These two percentages are represented cumulatively as 55% of all cases. This means that these two DRGs represented 55% of all cases admitted to the unit. In most instances, one would study the top 80%, in this case DRGs 707, 277, 708, and 89, which represent approximately 80% of all cases. In this way it is clear that a fair representation of all cases has been included.

Non-unit-based case management teams are committed to following all patients of a specific case type who are admitted to the medical center. They are also responsible for monitoring length of stay, resource use, and quality. The teams also

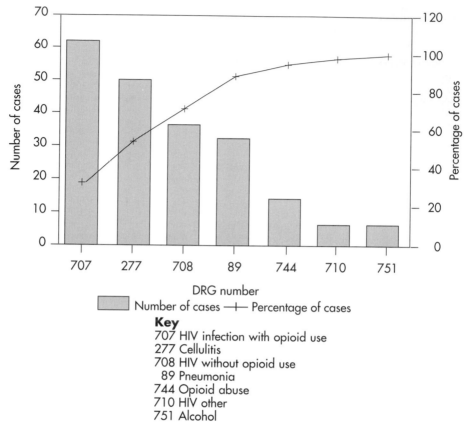

Fig. 22-1   DRG Pareto chart showing patient cases for 1991.

provide in-service training sessions to house staff and nursing personnel to maintain appropriate treatment of these patients.

Two teams, one for diabetes and one for asthma, consisted of several physicians, a nurse case manager, a nurse clinician, and other clinically relevant disciplines. In the case of the diabetes team a nutritionist was included and functioned as a full-time member who saw all patients assigned to the team.

The managed care plan is used to guide care and to provide a framework for keeping the length of stay in check. The length of stay on the plan is determined by studying the region, state, and federal lengths of stay for those DRGs relevant to the diagnosis or procedure. The physician practice patterns are then reviewed, and length of stay for the institution is established for that diagnosis.

Two groups for case management, unit-based case managers and non-unit-based case managers, were developed. The unit-based case managers assumed the same role as the non-unit-based case manager. However, the unit-based manager's primary responsibility was on an individual unit level and involved more than one diagnosis and many different physicians. The unit-based case manager can be equally effective because that person sees the patient several times during the day, intervening whenever necessary. The non-unit-based case managers, on the other hand, may spend a portion of the day traveling from one unit to another. Therefore their time with each patient is more limited.

Both groups, the non-unit-based case managers and the unit-based case managers, were able to demonstrate significant cost reductions within the first few weeks and months of implementation. Once the targeted diagnoses had been identified, the institution's prior length of stay history was obtained. These data allowed the team to determine what the expected length of stay would have been if the conventional model of patient care had been used.

After implementation of case management the length of stay was tracked on a monthly basis for those patients followed by the case management approach. Patients with certain diagnoses or surgical procedures were targeted and followed by the case manager.

Stringent data collection was necessary for accurate cost accounting. Preimplementation length-of-stay data provided the framework for determining whether the length-of-stay goals were achieved.

RELATIVE WEIGHTS AND FINANCIAL ANALYSIS

Some diagnoses fall within a single DRG. For example, pneumonia will almost always be coded within DRG 89. Conversely, many surgical procedures can be classified within a number of DRG categories. For example, laminectomy can be coded within as many as seven DRGs. Each of these DRGs may have a different financial weight.

The weights applied to each DRG are called *relative weights*. The relative weight is a value applied to the DRG based on the average complexity and resource consumption for patients within that DRG. The relative weight for carpal tunnel release will be much lower than the relative weight for major chest procedures, which is one of the most highly weighted DRGs. The relative weight will apply differently for Medicare versus other third party payers.

Institutions performing a larger number of procedures with higher relative weight values will see a higher overall reimbursement, reflected in the case mix index (CMI) for each department and ultimately the institution. The CMI provides an indication of the relative costliness of providing care and is determined by taking an average of all the service intensity weights over all discharges for the institution. The service intensity weights are the average of all the weights of all DRGs seen on a particular service.

For example, transplants carry an extremely high relative weight. Therefore a large number of transplants will inflate the overall CMI, resulting in a better financial appearance. Complexity and intensity form the basis of the CMI system. Although there is no clear definition of complexity, it generally refers to the types of services rendered, while intensity refers to the number of services per patient day or hospital stay (Luke, 1979).

There is some incentive in this system for health care organizations to bring in larger numbers of patients whose DRG will be of a higher relative weight. Often therefore hospitals emphasize these types of services to the detriment of lower paying groups.

Beth Israel Medical Center used the relative weight values as a basis for determining the financial gain or loss of each of the diagnoses or procedures tracked under the case management system. If the diagnosis being evaluated falls within one DRG, the process is much easier. In the case of endocarditis the length of stay for case managed patients decreased from 14.4 days in 1990 to 8.7 days in 1991. This length-of-stay reduction was analyzed against the number of cases at the shorter length of stay and the relative weight for the DRG.

A relative cost weight is obtained by dividing the adjusted national cost per DRG by the adjusted national cost per case for all DRGs. The larger the relative cost weight, the greater the relative costliness of a DRG (Grimaldi & Micheletti, 1983).

An assumption was made that for each day's reduction in length of stay, the bed was "back-filled" with a patient falling into a DRG with the same or greater relative weight. In this way, although the length of stay was decreased, available beds were utilized.

In other cases the surgical procedure being analyzed fell under more than one DRG, as in the case of laminectomies. In this circumstance the relative weight for all possible DRGs must be averaged.

With case management teams that potentially could be managing several DRGs, the same process would be followed. The average relative weight would be averaged for all possible DRGs, again assuming the beds would be back-filled with similar patients.

Although this type of cost-accounting system is not precise, it does give a good indication of the approximate incremental revenue savings for the diagnosis or surgical procedure under analysis.

IMPLICATIONS FOR FURTHER RESEARCH

All the studies reviewed share common implications for clinical and professional practice. One implication is in the area of assessing the quality of the critical path analysis and MAPs. Both the critical path and MAP were used to set clinical resource and cost standards and were responsible for most of the planning, coordination, and integration activities of the nursing case management model. Future research would be helpful for evaluating the critical path's and MAP's reliability and validity. Additional research should also focus on the treatment and practice protocols developed by the critical path and MAP analysis as they relate to patient care and clinical practice outcomes.

One other major implication is in objectively measuring the contributions of the nursing case management model to the quality of patient care, in particular, its effects on patient care resources, and in assessing patient and provider satisfaction. Additional research is needed to look at the effects of nursing case management on professional autonomy and decision-making opportunities for nurses, collaborative practice arrangements between nurses and physicians, nursing case management staffing and assignment allocations, payment and reimbursement mechanisms for nursing case management services, and the types of nursing case management interventions used and the effects of these interventions on patient outcomes. Other general implications for nursing follow:

▼ The changes in practice patterns associated with nursing case management can help to reduce overall expenditures related to hospitalization.

▼ Nursing case management can provide substantial improvements in the cost-effectiveness of patient care.

▼ Nursing case management focuses on collaborative practice arrangements between nurses and physicians to help shorten length of hospital stay and maintain effective use of money and materials, thereby having a significant effect on the hospital's fiscal bottom line and viability.

▼ Nursing case management has the potential to equate the effects of clinical nursing services and outcomes with resource allocation, costs, and reimbursement systems.

▼ Nursing case management has the potential to positively affect the present nursing care shortage by reorganizing delivery systems to maximize professional decision-making opportunities for nurses and allowing for continuity of patient care.

▼ Nursing case management can relate the cost savings of nursing interventions to specific patient populations in the acute care setting.

▼ Nursing case management can enhance the management of nursing services and substantiate the economic accountability and contribution of nurses to consumers of health care services.

Nursing case management provides the baseline for further research and evaluation of the functional competencies and uses of different skill levels in delivering nursing care services to patients and their families. This approach allows for more efficient integration of various levels of support staff by defining role expectations. Cohen's (1990) study successfully used the registered nurse as the case manager and case associate with the nursing assistants as support staff. The nurse case manager coordinated, assessed, evaluated, and participated with the case associates in the delivery of patient care. The nursing assistants carried out tasks associated with the patients' activities of daily living as delegated by the nurse case manager.

REFERENCES

American Hospital Association. (1990). *1990 report of the hospital nursing personnel survey.* Chicago: Author.

Bair, N., Griswold, J., & Head, J. (1989). Clinical RN involvement in bedside-centered case management. *Nursing Economics, 7*(3), 150-154.

Cohen, E. (1990). *The effects of a nursing case management model on patient length of stay and variables related to cost of care delivery within an acute care setting.* Dissertation Abstracts International, 51-07B, 3325 (University Microfilm No. 90-33878), Ann Arbor, Mich.: University Micro Films International.

Cohen, E. (1991). Nursing case management: Does it pay? *Journal of Nursing Administration, 21*(4), 20-25.

Grimaldi, P.L., & Micheletti, J.A. (1983). *Diagnosis related groups.* Chicago: Pluribus Press.

Health Care Advisory Board. (1990). Tactic #1 potential savings of more than $1 million from change in delivery system, use of critical paths for two DRGs. Superlative clinical quality: Special review of pathbreaking ideas, clinical quality (1) (pp. 23). Washington, D.C.: Advisory Board Co.

Luke, R.D. (1979, Spring). Dimensions in hospital case mix measurement. *Inquiry, 16,* 38-49.

McKenzie, C., Torkelson, N., & Holt, M. (1989). Care and cost: Nursing case management improves both. *Nursing Management, 20*(10), 30-34.

Stillwaggon, C. (1989). The impact of nurse managed care on the cost of nurse practice and nurse satisfaction. *Journal of Nursing Administration, 19*(11), 21-27.

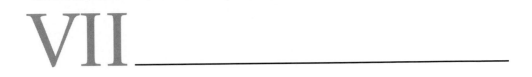

VII

CLINICAL OUTCOMES

23

LINKING THE RESTRUCTURING OF NURSING CARE WITH OUTCOMES

CONCEPTUALIZING THE EFFECTS OF NURSING CASE MANAGEMENT

ARTHUR E. BLANK

▼ *CHAPTER OVERVIEW*

Government, employers, and insurers are trying to restructure the delivery of health care. This restructuring of care has created opportunities for innovation as well as questions about the consequences of altering the delivery of health care. Nursing case management is one such innovation and as such needs to be studied. The Medical Outcomes Study (MOS) approach offers a conceptual guide to assessing the impact of nursing case management, but the MOS is not specific enough to document adequately the consequences of nursing case management. To make the MOS approach more germane, nursing case managers need to accomplish three tasks: (1) identify how case managers change the structure and process of care, (2) identify what clinical, administrative, physiological, and patient outcomes are influenced by these changes, and (3) develop reliable and valid measures. Accomplishing these three tasks will enable hospitals, nurses, and policy makers to assess whether nursing case management has "worked." Some ideas about how to proceed with each of these tasks are presented. ▲

Health care is in flux. National, state, and local governments are redefining the financing and delivery of health services to slow growing public expenditures. Employers are restructuring employee benefits and premiums to control their escalating health benefit costs per employee. And under pressure from employers, insurance companies, and government, health care providers are working to become more cost-effective without sacrificing quality.

These efforts to redefine how health care is provided and paid for have also engendered counter pressures. Employers, government, health care providers, and patients or consumers have started to question whether health care choices are being arbitrarily restricted, whether the quality of care is being sacrificed, and, in everyone's worst nightmare, whether lives are being unnecessarily jeopardized. These apprehensions remind us that change is taking place within another, more abstract context, one of uncertainty. We are not trading one well-defined system of care for another. We are trading for a system of care whose basic parameters are still undefined.

As providers or consumers of care, we are in the midst of a societal, institutional, and personal struggle to balance opportunity and fear, or, more modestly, concern: opportunity, because the structural pressures to reconfigure the delivery of care supports leaders who are willing to innovate; concern, because the consequences of these changes, whether they be at a societal, institutional, or personal level, will not be known for some time.

How can we as health care professionals, as researchers, as policy makers, and as citizens assess the consequences, or outcomes, of these various and varied attempts to reconfigure the delivery of health care? Currently one way is to conduct outcome studies. These studies describe how the structure and process of medical care have been refashioned and identify a set of measures—outcomes—that can be used to determine the consequences of those changes. When done well, these studies tell us how well opportunity and concern have been balanced, and the results become part of a broader social metric. But these studies can be part of the metric only if we identify and measure how components of the structure and process of care are conceptually linked with outcomes of care—health as well as financial—and at a societal as well as an institutional or personal level.

What has all of this to do with nursing case management? It suggests that the MOS approach be used as a conceptual guide for studying the consequences of nursing case management. After all, nursing case management is fundamentally an alteration in the structure and process of care.* As such it is an intervention, an opportunity to reshape the delivery of in-patient care.† But it is also an intervention whose consequences are unknown (Lamb, 1995). The task then is not only to define and identify the organizational changes in the structure and process of care that nursing case management has brought about but also to articulate our concerns so we can link the restructuring of care with its consequences, with its outcomes.

Traditionally, clarifying the conceptual relationships between shifts in the organization of care and the outcome(s) of care is a critical step in designing a research study. But there is a complementary step, one that is often not well attended to in health care: ensuring that our design appropriately measures the relationships and constructs we are interested in. At a technical level the challenge is about the *validity* of our measures: are they conceptually nuanced and robust enough to reflect the relevant dimensions of change introduced by nursing case management.‡ Unfortunately, designing valid measures is no less daunting a task than is designing a rigorous study.

---

*Because *nursing case management* is not a term that means the same thing in every institution where it is practiced, these local variations are important to identify and document if we are to understand how the structure, process, and outcomes of care are linked.

†This chapter presumes nursing case management is being used in a hospital setting.

‡The concern in this chapter is with developing measures for, not the design of, outcome studies. Clearly both the study design and the measures will determine the scientific credibility of the results.

This chapter then has four objectives: (1) to briefly review how valid measures are constructed, (2) to review how the MOS both conceptualized the structure, process, and outcomes of care and developed valid health status measures, (3) to raise questions about whether the definitions and measures used in the MOS research can be directly applied to the study of nursing case management, and (4) to suggest some directions and issues for nursing case management research.

A PARTIAL* MEASUREMENT REFRESHER: DEVELOPING VALID MEASURES

For many years, health care's consequences were assessed by measures of morbidity and mortality. Identifying the time of death, diagnosing whether the individual has an infection, or interpreting a particular laboratory result, for example, was—and is—relatively straightforward. When our measures were this concrete, little attention needed to be devoted to thinking about whether we were capturing what we intended to measure. But as health professionals' interest in the consequences of care became nuanced and abstract, more attention had to be devoted to guaranteeing that we measured what we wanted to (Stewart, Hays, & Ware, 1992; Streiner & Norman, 1989) and ensuring that we knew how to interpret the results (Kane, 1992; Messick, 1995; Streiner & Norman, 1989). For example, measuring blood pressure is straightforward, as for the most part is the interpretation of the result. When we measure depression or patient or job satisfaction, we may be both less certain that we have accurately assessed the construct and less certain about how to interpret the resulting score. Some measures of inpatient satisfaction, for example, focus on hotel services such as the food, cleanliness of the room, and efficiency of the admitting or discharge process. Yet other measures focus on the nurses' responsiveness to pain, the clarity of information provided by physicians or nurses, and the compassion of the staff. Is one measure a more valid measure of satisfaction than the other? How do we measure and feel intellectually confident that we are correctly measuring and interpreting these more abstract consequences of health interventions?

As we approach our consideration of validity, it is essential to remember that there is a critical, interrelated step: to define, or more pointedly limit, what we are referring to when we talk about "outcomes." The concept of outcomes is broad and nonspecific and takes on a precise meaning only in the context of a particular intervention. Although sometimes overlooked, outcomes theoretically should be related to the intervention. This simple setting of boundaries, these definitional decisions, must not be made lightly. In the psychometric or scale development literature, defining the boundaries of the concept is usually treated as the purview of the expert. The expert's knowledge is based on his or her experience in the field as well as on a knowledge of the literature. This expertise will help determine which conceptual domains should be included or excluded. For example, are measures of pain, patient satisfaction, functional status, well-being, cost of care, hospital readmission, and length of stay conceptually relevant when we want to document the effects of nursing case management?

---

*This discussion is partial because it deals only with validity. There is no discussion of reliability, about how to write scale items, or about how to statistically assess the information collected.

If a peer-reviewed literature exists, experts are clearly beneficial. But they may be less helpful if the topic is new or if the literature is out of date. In this context, convening a panel of experts and "users" to discuss the concept's boundaries may help. This need to harness the experience of a diverse group of individuals can be important even in well-established areas of study. For example, the outcome measures discussed in the MOS have been criticized by some as capturing outcomes more sensitive to the work of physicians than of nurses (Kelly, Huber, Johnson, McCloskey, & Maas, 1994), which raises a caution and a simple reminder: definitions set limits. They decide what to include and exclude. These decisions should be explicit and public, not tacit and hidden.

Once we know the domains we want to assess, the issue of whether our scales and surveys measure what we intend them to measure falls under the rubric of validity (Crocker & Algina, 1986; Nunnally, 1978; Portney & Watkins, 1993; Streiner & Norman, 1989; Thorndike, 1982). For abstract constructs, developing valid instruments is time consuming and difficult. Validity is usually discussed in terms of four different types: (1) face, (2) criterion, (3) content, and (4) construct validity.

Face validity, the weakest form of validity, is perhaps the easiest to use and develop. With face validity, items on a survey or questionnaire *appear* to address the question we are interested in. There is, however, no empirical test of this assumption. Content validity tries to ensure that the various *items* that comprise the measure, or which tap the conceptual domain, adequately *sample* the content of the concept or domain being measured. Some of the questions raised earlier about patient satisfaction surface here. Should patient satisfaction include hotel services as well as the thoroughness and clarity of the information provided? Part of the answer would be to review existing instruments, but it would also be useful to convene a panel of experts* to ensure that important items or concerns not be excluded inadvertently. But however the items are put together, content validity, like face validity, is still primarily subjective. The advantages of content validity are that the item pool has been documented thoroughly and that the items reflect the concept being assessed *before* the measure is administered.

More rigorous—that is, more empirically based—tests of validity are possible with both criterion and construct validity. Criterion-related validity indicates that the test developed can be used in place of an already established test—a "gold standard." We may be interested, for example, in constructing a shorter version of a longer, more time consuming scale. To determine whether the shorter test is valid, both tests are administered on the same set of subjects, and if the two sets of scores are highly correlated, the shorter test is valid. Although this is an objective way to proceed, for many abstract constructs such as satisfaction a gold standard is not available. In these cases another approach, construct validation, is called for. Part of construct validity relies on content validity: that is, we have to have an item pool that adequately assesses the complexity of the concept. But the thrust of content validity is to confirm that the

---

*Experts need to be thought of broadly. For example, the Picker Commonwealth Survey of Patient Satisfaction used patient focus groups to identify the dimensions of care that were important to them (Gerteis, Edgman-Levitan, Daley, & Delbanco, 1993).

measure accurately captures the construct by empirically ascertaining whether the new measure correlates with hypothetically related constructs.

Construct validity can be approached from a number of directions, but one common approach is that of convergent and discriminant validity (Cronbach and Meehl, 1955). Simply put, like measures should correlate highly with other measures of the same or similar theoretical constructs—convergent validity—but should not correlate, or show low correlations, with measures of dissimilar constructs—discriminant validity. If researchers are constructing a new measure to assess the impact of an illness on a person's life, the new measure should correlate highly with comparable illness burden measures but only minimally with measures of quite different constructs. The pattern of correlations documents whether the new measure is succeeding. But in the absence of a gold standard it is hard to absolutely know how well we have done. Consequently for some researchers construct validity is an ongoing process, needing always to refine and test the measures (Messick, 1995; Stewart et al., 1992; Streiner and Norman, 1989). Within this framework, construct validity cannot be decided with the results of a single study.

THE MOS APPROACH: AN EXAMPLE OF HOW TO LINK THE STRUCTURE, PROCESS, AND OUTCOMES OF CARE

If we are to use the MOS approach as a guide for conceptualizing how to gauge the consequences of nursing case management, it is beneficial to review that study with two aims in mind: (1) to see how the components of structure, process, and outcomes were defined and (2) to see how a new generic measure of a patient's health status was validated.

The MOS was a "2 year observational study designed to help understand how specific components of the health care system affect the outcomes of care" (Tarlov et al., 1989). The study was conducted at multiple sites across the United States and sampled 502 physicians in group and solo practice, in health maintenance organizations (HMO), and in fee-for-service (FFS) systems of care. Information was collected from physicians using self-administered forms and telephone interviews. Patient data were collected using surveys, clinical examinations, and telephone interviews.

The MOS study was unique, in part because of its explicit emphasis on developing measures that could capture the consequences of medical care from the patients perspective (Stewart & Ware, 1992; Tarlov et al., 1989). In arguing for the need to supplement traditional clinical outcomes such as mortality, laboratory values, and symptoms and signs, the MOS study faced issues comparable to those case management research now faces: MOS researchers had to define outcomes, in this case from the patients' perspective, which should be conceptually responsive to changes in the structure and process of care. Of course, MOS researchers also had to clarify how the components of structure and process would be measured.

For the concept *structure of care*, three broad domains were identified: (1) system characteristics, (2) provider characteristics, and (3) patient characteristics (Tarlov et al., 1989). System characteristics identified five components, including financial incentives, access or convenience, and specialty mix. Provider characteristics included seven components: age, gender, specialty training, economic incentives, job satisfaction, preferences, and beliefs and attitudes; and the eight patient characteristics included age, gender, diagnosis, severity, comorbidity, health habits, beliefs and attitudes, and preferences. The *process of care* had two broad categories: technical and interpersonal style. Technical style included among its eight items medications, referrals, test ordering, expenditures, continuity, and coordination of care; and interpersonal style's four items were communication level, counseling, patient participation, and interpersonal manner. The *outcomes of care* had four components: clinical endpoints, functional status, general well-being, and satisfaction with care. As with the structure and process of care, each of these components was specified in more detail. For example, a patient's functional status was described by measuring a patient's physical, mental, social, and role functioning.

To develop and test the generic patient-centered health outcome measures being sought by the MOS, researchers built upon scales that had been developed as part of RAND's Health Insurance Experiment (HIE) or by other researchers (Stewart & Ware, 1992). Over time the MOS staff examined the existing literature on measures of physical functioning, psychological distress or well-being, health perceptions, social and role functioning, pain, and physical and psychophysiologic symptoms (Stewart & Ware, 1992). By incorporating new items and including a multitude of already developed measures into their study design, MOS researchers could test the validity of their measures.* Face validity was not discussed, and content validity was checked by assessing the literature to determine whether the relevant concepts were captured in the set of measures being used. Criterion validity was used, when available, to see how new measures compared to established old measures. For example, would a new shorter measure of depression correlate with a gold standard measure of depression (e.g., the Diagnostic Interview Schedule in the third edition of the *Diagnostic and Statistical Manual of Mental Disorders* [DSM-III] published by the American Psychiatric Association) or would a shorter measure of physical functioning correlate highly with a longer measure of physical functioning (Hays & Stewart, 1992; Stewart et al., 1992)? Both convergent and discriminant validity were used to examine the construct validity of the measure. In principle, if we are developing new measures of well-being or pain, these measures should correlate highly with scales that measure similar constructs. But we would not expect these measures to correlate with those unrelated to either well-being or pain. More specifically, as the MOS authors indicate, "measures of physical functioning, mobility, and satisfaction with physical abilities were expected to correlate at least moderately with one another because they all assess physical functioning. [and] physical functioning would not be expected to be highly related to a measure of depression or of loneliness" (Stewart et al., 1992, p. 315).

Under construct validity, Stewart et al (1992) also discuss known-groups validity. Identified by Kerlinger (1973), known-groups validity involves comparing groups of individuals who should differ on the concept being measured. So, for example, on a measure of pain, mean scores should be higher for those patients

---

*The MOS covers more than the four types of validity identified in this chapter. Furthermore, it breaks down content, criterion, and construct validity in more detail than is offered here (Stewart & Ware, 1992). Even though there are important refinements that can be made, the general points and theme do not change.

known to be in pain than for those who are not. Of course, the difficulty is knowing that the groups differ on the construct being measured.

This approach to developing an outcomes scale resulted in the MOS Short Form (SF-36). The MOS SF-36 is a generic 36-item measure of the patients' perception of their health status. This measure can be used across populations and across illness to measure the consequences of changes in the structure and process of care. The scale, demonstrated to be reliable and valid, captures eight health care concepts: (1) limitations in physical activities because of health problems, (2) limitations in social activities because of physical or emotional problems, (3) limitations in usual role activities because of physical health problems, (4) bodily pain, (5) general mental health (psychological distress and well-being), (6) limitations in usual role activities because of emotional problems, (7) vitality (energy and fatigue), and (8) general health problems (McHorney, Ware, & Raczek, 1993; McHorney, Ware, Rachael Lu, & Sherbourne, 1994; Ware & Sherbourne, 1992).

NURSING-BASED CHALLENGES TO THE MOS

The MOS's tripartite *conceptualization* of the delivery of health care has become an important framework for assessing the restructuring of health care. But we should not uncritically accept the specific details of the MOS approach without reassuring ourselves that the definitions of the structure, process, and outcomes of care are germane to studying the effects of nursing case management. Does the MOS approach define and capture what is unique to case management?

Nursing-Based Criticisms of the MOS Outcomes

With the successful development and validation of the SF-36, changes in the structure and process of care can now, in principle, be captured from the patients' perspective. For those interested in the patients' perspective, the SF-36 is a valuable addition to a researcher's measurement tools. The question remains, however, as to whether the SF-36 is sufficiently sensitive to reflect the *specific* structural and process changes introduced by nursing case management. If we assume that nursing case management has some similarities to nursing care in general, the articles by Brooten & Naylor (1995), by Kelly, Huber, Johnson, McCloskey, and Maas (1994), and by Naylor, Munro, and Brooten (1991) suggest the answer is no.

Two different concerns are raised in these articles: First, the SF-36 is dominated by outcome measures sensitive to physician practices. Consequently there is a need to construct measures that can capture "nurse sensitive patient outcomes" (Brooten & Kelly, 1995). And second, since the research was begun before all the current changes in the health care environment took place, the MOS—as an approach to effectiveness research—neglects a number of important domains, especially the effects of provider mix, that is, that many different professionals care for the patient (Kelly et al., 1994). This latter point is critical. For we not only must identify what these nurse-sensitive measures are but also must assure ourselves that these measures reflect only what nurses offer and not what other providers of care offer. This chore becomes harder to accomplish, and perhaps is not even achievable, as patient care becomes more interdisciplinary.

Some Suggested Nursing Case Management–Sensitive Outcomes

In their discussion of how to measure the consequences of nursing care, Brooten and Naylor (1995) identify a number of potential indexes: functional and mental status (these two domains are captured on the SF-36), stress level, satisfaction with care, caregiver burden, and the cost of care. Brooten and Naylor expand their suggested list of nurse-sensitive outcomes by incorporating a number of outcome categories identified in Lang and Marek's review of outcomes: physiologic status, psychological status, behavior, knowledge, symptom control, quality of life, home functions, family strain, goal attainment, utilization of service, safety, resolution of nursing problems, patient satisfaction, and caring (cited in Brooten & Naylor, 1995).

These suggested outcome measures continue in the tradition of developing patient-focused outcomes, but there are other outcomes introduced by nurses or nursing case management that also need to be documented. Perhaps most basically, reconfigurations in health care have meant a redefinition of nursing responsibilities. What does this imply for nurses? Will they be more or less integrated in the delivery of care? Will they feel less autonomous or more autonomous in their roles, more or less fragmented with their varied responsibilities? Will nurses leave their jobs more often? Will sick leave increase or decrease? These too are outcomes of changes in nursing case management and should not be slighted when we identify the range of outcomes to be studied.*

Of course, comparable questions could be asked of physicians, especially as their relationships with nurses change. It must be stressed that identifying outcome categories does not end the process; it starts it. The task is to move from the outcome categories to valid outcome measures.

Nursing Case Management and the Structure and Process of Care

Clearly outcomes studies are critical, as they correct many past oversights. But particular outcomes should not be identified, or agreed to, without it first being specified how they are conceptually linked to the structure and process of care. Functional status, mental status, and relief from pain are important outcome measures because we expect them, under certain conditions, to be responsive to medical treatment, to the process of medical care. Similar conceptual linkages are required to measure outcomes that are responsive to the changes introduced by nursing case management. So just as the MOS description of outcomes may not be fully germane for studying the effects of nursing case management, its description of the structure and process of care may also be deficient for our studying case management. But Lamb (1995) has reminded us that there is a good deal of ambiguity regarding what nursing case managers do. Without knowing what case managers do, it is unclear whether the nursing-sensitive outcomes listed above are sensitive to alterations in the structure and process of care introduced by nursing case management. And it is unclear whether these outcomes are, in the words of Brooten and Naylor (1995), "sensitive to nursing alone." How does nursing case management change the structure and process of care?

---

*The MOS approach characterizes provider satisfaction as a structural component, but in a dynamic environment it should also be considered as an outcome.

We can, in a sense, work backward to answer this question. The outcomes suggested by Brooten and Naylor and others imply certain changes, or perhaps clarification, in some MOS definitions of the structure and process of care. For example, consider the process of care. If an outcome of case management is enhanced patient knowledge regarding his or her illness, we have presumed that nurses are educating their patients. Is this different from what is specified in the MOS component of interpersonal style, which "includes many aspects of the way clinicians relate to patients[?]. It encompasses friendliness, courtesy, respect, and sensitivity; the extent to which patients participate in making decisions and share responsibility for their treatment; whether the clinicians counsel patients about their health habits, the need to comply with treatment recommendations, and personal and emotional problems, and the overall level of communication" (Tarlov et al., 1989). Is nursing education distinctive enough to be considered a unique component of the process of care? Do nurses engage in this process differently than other clinicians? Furthermore, do nursing case management programs change how the process of care is organized, a topic that would fall under the MOS idea of technical style? Related questions could be asked about relief from stress, reductions in care-giver burden, or the cost of care? What is it about the process of care that would reduce a patient's stress level, alter a caregiver's burden, or reduce the costs of care?

These questions can also be used to inquire about needed modifications in how the MOS study defined the structure of care. The MOS study, under system characteristics, talks about specialty mix. But Brooten and Naylor's (1995) argument that nurses are working in environments where the skill mix of nursing staff has changed suggests that the idea of specialty mix needs to be expanded. In addition, the interdisciplinary nature of case management suggests that how care is organized may need to be amplified. Questions about team structure and about how well teams function may need to be incorporated into the MOS's definition of the structure and outcomes of case management.

PUTTING IT ALL TOGETHER: SOME FUNDAMENTAL QUESTIONS

Brooten and Naylor's (1995), Kelly et al.'s (1994), and Naylor et al.'s (1991) critiques are forceful, not because they question the conceptual framework of the MOS approach or the validity of the SF-36 but because they pose fundamental questions about definitional and conceptual boundaries regarding the structure, process, and outcomes of care as it relates to, in our case, nursing case management. These critiques suggest the need not only to augment the MOS categories but also to construct measures that capture the unique aspects of nursing case management, the unique role of nurses, and unique nurse-sensitive outcomes that are conceptually distinct from those identified in the MOS approach.

In essence, just as the generic SF-36 should be used in conjunction with specific illness measures so that researchers can capture nuances not measured by the SF-36, the MOS conceptualization of structure, process, and outcomes needs to be modified according to the specific intervention being studied. To use the MOS approach to its full advantage, we need to formally conceptualize the linkages among the structure, process, and outcomes of care that are specific to nursing case management.

The need to articulate how nursing case management reshapes the delivery of patient care and the need to document the impact of those changes is underscored in Lamb's (1995) recent review of the case management literature. Lamb raises a series of questions that should be undertaken as a challenge:

> The task of researchers is complicated by the popularity and visibility of case management. As the number of professions and individuals with a stake in the future of case management expands, it is increasingly difficult to cut through the debate and rhetoric to get to some basic questions, such as: What is case management? Who needs it? Who provides it? For how long? What are its outcomes? What are its costs? Does it save money by keeping people from higher levels of care?

Lamb's questions bring us full circle: if we are to study the consequences of nursing case management, we must know what nurse case managers do. What are the linkages among the structure, process, and outcomes of care?

•   •   •

For the past few years there have been research studies at our institution to try to determine the consequences of various nursing innovations. Part of our charge, as usual, was to determine if the innovation "worked." This charge is difficult in the best of circumstances but is especially difficult in dynamic environments. With the need to develop cost-effective institutions, hospital administrators are introducing multiple innovations, are introducing them system wide, and are concerned with knowing what worked. Administrators were quite willing to listen to researchers' caveats and hesitancies about proceeding, and in some cases we mutually decided that it did not pay to do an analysis, since the results would be uninterpretable. Reaching this decision was part of the job and was not particularly the hard part of the job. The hard part was trying to get staff to detail what they did and what they thought were the specific consequences of their efforts.

Rather than presume we knew what the "right" consequences were or that the literature had the "right" concepts, we would ask staff to describe their jobs and to tell us whether they thought they were having the impact they had expected to have. This was our way of trying to ensure that we were capturing the correct domains and also a way to start thinking about our item pools. For most staff this effort, conducted in lay terms, was not at all straightforward. Of course, some staff were adept at helping us. At times we used the MOS study descriptions as a foil, as a way of probing whether the specifics of what staff were doing was different from how the MOS defined the structure, process, and outcomes of care.

Although we did not systematically interview or sample staff, when answers regarding nursing interventions were provided, they seemed to fall into three categories: (1) helping the patient relax and making him or her less anxious, (2) being more attentive to a patient's and the family's emotional well-being, and (3) educating patients about their illness. Of course, all staff felt they were helping patients with their physical well-being. Clearly the nurses we spoke to may be atypical, but note that two of these items—helping a patient relax and being attentive to a patient's emotional needs—may be different from the list of nurse-sensitive outcomes mentioned earlier in the chapter.

These conversations all worked to frame the questions raised earlier. We struggled with nurses to have them specify what they did, to have them detail the consequences of what they did, and to have them suggest how we could measure these activities and outcomes. It took us some time to resolve these issues, and in many ways they remain unresolved. But it was this specific need to identify how particular nursing innovations could be analyzed within the framework of the MOS approach that generated in a pragmatic way all the more abstract questions raised earlier. We struggled with every measure, concerned with whether it reflected the effect of nurses alone and with whether we were measuring what we thought we were measuring.

It was also clear that telling our story about what "worked" would be enhanced to the extent that we could document that we had the "right" measures and the "correct" outcomes. As we grappled with these issues, other institutions facing similar innovations approached us asking for assistance. So we quickly learned we were not alone.

This chapter, then, puts our struggle in reverse order. It raises general issues about studying the effects of nursing case management as if it preceded our efforts. Rather these concerns followed our efforts. Our efforts drove home the point that the MOS approach provides a general framework for assessing the consequences of care. The real effort is to develop valid measures that capture the interrelations among the structure, process, and outcomes of care that are germane to the particular intervention being put in place. If we can accomplish this, we can truly gauge the unique consequences of nursing case management.

REFERENCES

Brooten, D., & Naylor, M.D. (1995). Nurses' effect on changing patient outcomes. *IMAGE: Journal of Nursing Scholarship, 27*(2), 95-99.

Crocker, L., Algina, J. (1986). *Introduction to classical and modern test theory.* New York: Harcourt, Brace, Jovanovich.

Cronbach, L.J., & Meehl, P.E. (1955). Construct validity in psychological tests. *Psychological Bulletin, 52,* 281-302.

Gerteis, M., Edgman Levitan, S., Daley, J., & Del banco. (1993). *Through the patient's eyes.* San Francisco: Jossey-Bass.

Hays, R.D., & Stewart, A.L. (1992). Construct validity of MOS health measures. In A.L. Stewart & J.E. Ware (Eds.), *Measuring functioning and well-being: The Medical Outcomes Study approach* (pp. 325-342). Durham, N.C.: Duke University Press.

Kane, M.T. (1992). An argument-based approach to validity. *Psychological Bulletin, 112*(3), 527-535.

Kelly, K.C., Huber, D.G., Johnson, M., McCloskey, J.C., & Maas, M. (1994). The Medical Outcomes Study: A nursing perspective. *Journal of Professional Nursing, 10*(4), 209-216.

Kerlinger, F.N. (1973). *Foundations of behavioral research* (2nd ed.). New York: Holt, Rinehart & Winston.

Lamb, G.S. (1995). Case management. In J.J. Fitzpatrick & J.S. Stevenson (Eds.), *Annual Review of Nursing Research, 13* 117-136.

McHorney, C.A., Ware, J.E., Rachael Lu, J.F., & Sherbourne, C.D. (1994). The MOS 36 Item Short-Form Health Survey (SF-36): III. Tests of data quality, scaling assumptions, and reliability across diverse patient groups. *Medical Care, 32*(1), 40-66.

McHorney, C.A., Ware, J.E., & Raczek, A.E. (1993). The MOS 36-Item Short-Form Health Survey (SF-36): II. Psychometric and clinical tests of validity in measuring physical and mental health constructs. *Medical Care, 31*(3), 247-263.

Messick, S. (1995). Validity of psychological assessment. *American Psychologist, 50*(9), 741-749.

Naylor, M.D., Munro, B.H., Brooten, D.A., (1991). Measuring the effectiveness of nursing practice. *Clinical Nurse Specialist, 5*(4), 210-214.

Nunnally, J. (1978). *Psychometric theory.* New York: McGraw-Hill.

Portney, L.G., & Watkins, M.P. (1993). *Foundations of clinical research: Applications to practice.* Norwalk, CT: Appleton & Lange.

Stewart, A.L., Hays, R.D., Ware, J.E. (1992). Methods of validating MOS health measures. In A.L. Stewart & J.E. Ware (Eds.), *Measuring functioning and well-being: The Medical Outcomes Study approach* (pp. 309-324). Durham, N.C.: Duke University Press.

Stewart, A.L., & Ware, J.E. (1992). *Measuring functioning and well-being: The Medical Outcomes Study approach.* Durham, N.C.: Duke University Press.

Streiner, D.L., & Norman, G.R. (1989). *Health measurement scales: A practical guide to their development and use.* New York: Oxford University Press.

Tarlov, A., Ware, J.E., Greenfield, S., Nelson, E.C., Perrin, E., & Zubkoff, M. (1989). The Medical Outcomes Study: An application of methods for monitoring the results of medical care. *Journal of the American Medical Association, 263*(7), 925-930.

Thorndike, R.L. (1982). *Applied psychometrics.* Boston: Houghton Mifflin.

Ware, J.E., & Sherbourne, C.D. (1992). The MOS 36-Item Short-Form Health Survey (SF-36): I. Conceptual framework and item selection. *Medical Care, 30*(6), 473-483.

24

EXPANDING OUR HORIZONS

MANAGING A CONTINUUM OF CARE

JEAN NEWSOME

▼ *CHAPTER OVERVIEW*

Patient education, a case management model of care, and continued outpatient contact and support have a positive effect on outcomes in the care of the diabetic patient. This chapter explores the driving forces behind the assessment of care outcomes at Brookwood Medical Center, Birmingham, Alabama: improving the quality of life for the diabetic patient, assessing and meeting consumer needs, providing holistic care, and expanding the focus on health and wellness. Among the topics considered herein are organizational factors such as evaluating and improving resource utilization, decreasing the cost of care, increasing the value of services provided, positioning the institution for increased competition, and positively influencing the morbidity, mortality, and hospital length of stay of the diabetic population.

▲

As with most chronic illness, diabetes presents multiple challenges to the patient and the health care providers. Those challenges are manifested in all areas of the life of the patient and his or her family as well as within the health care environment. Maintenance of quality of life, preservation of wellness, inhibition of deterioration, and management of financial impacts of the disease act singularly and in combination to create the need for holistic plans of care with which the patient willingly participates and contributes. A number of authors writing on care of the diabetic population have recognized the need for long-term patient follow-ups following educational and therapeutic interventions, yet those projects have yet to be well represented in current literature (Ary, Toobert, Wilson, & Glasgow, 1986; Glasgow, McCaul, & Schafer, 1987; Glasgow, Wilson, & McCaul, 1985; Johnson, 1992; Kurtz, 1990; Rosenstock, 1985). It has been well documented in the literature addressing other chronic illnesses, however, that continued education and outpatient support increase compliance rates and decrease rates of complications from the given illness.

The long-term effects of diabetes on the individual body systems vary from person to person with little consensus regarding factors that provide predictability of those effects. Past research in the area of complication avoidance has failed to demonstrate health-related behaviors or patterns that conclusively correlate with minimizing diabetic complications. Consistently low glycosylated hemoglobin levels, however, have appeared to offer a measure of avoidance of diabetic complications (American Diabetes Association, 1994; Haas, 1993; Jacobson, Adler, Derby, Anderson, & Wolfsdorf, 1991; Orchard et al., 1990; Walsh & Roberts, 1993). The Diabetes Outcomes Project recognized this variable as a critical indicator of the quality of the education and monitoring of the diabetic patient.

An appropriate summation of the goals of this project team was found in Johnson's 1992 study: "Adherence behaviors have not been examined in relationship to health-related daily functioning. More adherent patients may be hospitalized less, miss school or work less, and experience fewer debilitating or distressing symptoms" (p. 1664).

Based on desires to improve patient compliance, decrease rates of diabetic complications, and realize financial improvements for the diabetic population at Brookwood Medical Center in Birmingham, Alabama, a longitudinal project was initiated, targeting improvement in all of the areas identified. That approach to evaluating patient outcomes has been recommended by a number of authors (Ary et al., 1986; Jacobson et al., 1991; Johnson, 1992; Mazzuca et al., 1986; Rosenstock, 1985).

The Diabetes Outcomes Project at Brookwood Medical Center was based on the conceptual model presented in Fig. 24-1.

Determining the Clinical Process Variables

The Diabetes Outcomes Project team identified several variables as the most accessible and measurable within the time frame of their project. The variables were chosen for both their impacts on patient morbidity as well as their impacts on the cost of patient care. The design of the project called for evaluation of the process variables at the time of the patient's initial hospitalization (with diagnosis-related group [DRG] 294), and again at 3 months, 6 months, and 12 months following that hospitalization. The project team recognized that the variables were not all inclusive in the complication, morbidity, and mortality rates of diabetes mellitus. Compliance with physician follow-up visits and patient education were considered inherent in the successful outcome of each area. Certain variables were targeted as reflections of long-term outcomes that could be positively influenced by patient education along with regular professional intervention and support (see box).

IDENTIFYING CLINICAL OUTCOMES

The clinical outcomes to be evaluated at the end of the 12-month tracking period were based on known potential complications of diabetes as well as on assumed consequences of that disease. Following are the clinical outcomes selected by the project team:

▼ Patient morbidity
▼ Patient mortality
▼ Cost of care
▼ Length of stay

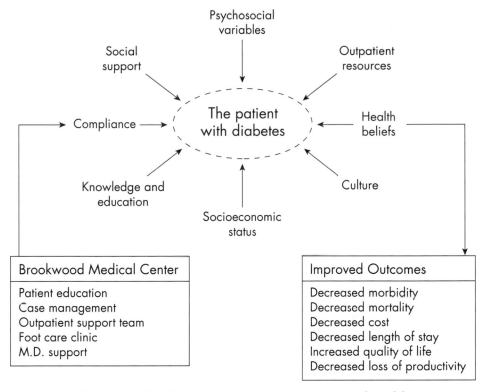

Fig. 24-1 The Diabetes Outcomes Project conceptual model.

CLINICAL PROCESS VARIABLES

▼ Compliance with recommended physician office visits
▼ Self–blood glucose monitoring (SBGM) practices
▼ Blood pressure monitoring
▼ Weight control adherence
▼ Adherence to caloric restrictions
▼ Compliance with recommended ophthalmologic appointments
▼ General well-being scores
▼ Hospital days since initial hospitalization
▼ Emergency room visits since initial hospitalization
▼ Work or school days missed since initial hospitalization
▼ Incidence of lower extremity cellulitis
▼ Incidence of urinary tract infections
▼ Incidence of lower extremity amputation

Caring for the Diabetic Patient

Compliance by the typical diabetic patient is similar to that of patients with other chronic illnesses. Unique to the diabetic population though are the complexity of the treatment programs and their direct impact on all body systems. Although past re-search on diabetic compliance is inconclusive, several themes may be identified. In general, rates of compliance and noncompliance reveal no patterns or predictability among individuals or subgroups within the diabetic population; compliance within one or two areas of diabetes self-care does not reflect or guarantee compliance within others; trends in patient-identified barriers to compliance have been tentatively iden-tified and are currently being tested for validity; and the greater the complexity of diabetes and self-care, the less the rate of consistent adherence to those self-care practices.

Psychosocial Factors

The psychosocial variables associated with positive outcomes in diabetic care have not yet been clearly identified or researched. The fact that diabetic care is long term does not appear to present the same set of psychosocial patterns that often emerge in persons with other chronic illnesses. Social support, education, and overall outlooks and adaptive responses have been only tentatively identified as indicators of positive outcomes in the diabetic population. The questions of psychosocial influences on long-term behaviors and outcomes of diabetic patients remains one that deserves exploration and elaboration.

Patient Education

Educating the diabetic patient is without question an essential element of care, yet current research in that area is lacking evidence of long-term results. Studies reported vary in the amount of importance placed on education as it affects metabolic control, and most studies are prompt to point out that education and metabolic control must not be viewed synonymously. There is, however, agreement within the literature that increased efforts must be made by health care professionals to evaluate the effects of education on overall patient outcomes and over longer periods of time than have been reported previously. At least one study has demonstrated positive outcomes by a diabetes educator on hospital length of stay (LOS) (Feddersen & Lockwood, 1994).

Morbidity and Mortality

Macroangiopathy is responsible for 60% of the deaths in diabetes (Vinicor, cited in Haas, 1993, p. 72). Strokes are at least twice as common in the diabetic person as in the general population and also are accompanied by a higher rate of recurrence and mortality. Coronary artery disease is also more severe in the diabetic patient. Morbidity and mortality rates for both strokes and coronary artery disease are highest in patients with poor glucose control (American Diabetes Association, 1993; Haas, 1993). The Centers for Disease Control (1991) estimates that over 945 diabetics will have lower extremity amputations each year in Alabama alone; Haas (1993) writes that more than 50% of nontraumatic lower limb amputations result from diabetes mellitus. More than 250 cases of blindness will occur each year in Alabama (Centers for Disease Control, 1991), and there will be approximately 12,000 new cases of legal blindness throughout the United States as a result of diabetes (American Diabetes Association, 1993). Nephropathy will progress to end-stage renal disease (ESRD) in up to 40% of patients who have type I diabetes; up to 60% of diabetic patients will develop symptomatic neuropathy (Haas, 1993). Waclawski (1990) conducted a study that demonstrated a striking difference between diabetic and nondiabetic employees in working days lost because of illness.

The Centers for Disease Control (1991) estimated that
▼ Over 2000 Alabamans will die each year from diabetes
▼ Alabama's death rate per 100,000 persons ranks forty-sixth highest among all states and the District of Columbia
▼ Approximately 47,000 annual hospitalizations in Alabama are directly related to diabetes
▼ Diabetes will cost the state of Alabama at least $375 million per year in medical care and lost productivity

Financial Implications

On a national level, the cost of diabetes is staggering. The American Diabetes Association (1993) reports that over $37 billion was spent on diabetes inpatient care, with a total cost of $90 billion for the United States in 1992. Chronic complications of diabetes cost $410 billion for inpatient care. Almost 48,000 persons were permanently disabled because of diabetes in 1992, resulting in lost productivity and premature mortality.

The consequences of diabetes mellitus, and certainly of diabetes mellitus that is not well controlled, are far reaching and dramatic for both patients and health care providers. Early and consistent education, support, and intervention have proved effective in altering negative outcomes from both anecdotal and professional reports.

SAMPLE AND SETTING

Adult patients admitted to Brookwood Medical Center with the diagnosis "diabetes out of control" (DRG 294) were asked to participate in the project during that hospitalization. Only adults 18 years of age or older who were not mentally impaired were included.

The project was designed to begin during hospitalization and to include incidence of the variables under study for 1 year following that hospitalization. All subjects had read and signed a standardized informed consent document before their involvement in this project. Our practice patterns of initiating diabetic education while the patient was hospitalized and of providing consistent outpatient support and education were hypothesized to positively influence many outcomes of the diabetic population we serve.

The final sample consisted of 28 adults, ranging in age from 39 to 80 years. Seven of those adults were newly diagnosed with diabetes at the time of the hospitalization. The length of known diabetes among the remaining 21 participants ranged from 2 to 23 years, with an average of 9.5 years.

INSTRUMENTATION

Three instruments were used in this project to collect and evaluate information pertinent to the patient population. The standardized Diabetes Teaching Outline, the General Well-Being Instrument, and the Diabetes Outcome Data Collection Tool were employed with each patient who participated.

    The Diabetes Teaching Outline, a two-page outline used for diabetic teaching at Brookwood Medical Center, had been used for several years before this project began. The outline consisted of categories of information, with each category itemizing specific areas of instruction to be addressed. The categories were self-monitoring, medications, hypoglycemia, hyperglycemia, exercise, diet, personal care, complications, sick days, and psychosocial factors. Subjects were graded competent, requires assistance, or no knowledge. Competent family was another grading option.

    The General Well-Being Instrument, a two-page standardized multiple-choice questionnaire, was designed to evaluate general attitudes and outlook. Validity of the instrument was determined by its concurrent comparison with several other self-report scales. The General Well-Being survey demonstrated statistical significance in its ability to differentiate emotional status of subjects within an overall sample. The General Well-Being Instrument was either self-administered by the patient or verbally administered by the diabetes educator.

    The Diabetes Outcome Data Collection Tool was developed in 1993 by an interdisciplinary health care team at Brookwood Medical Center in anticipation of this project. Both inpatient and outpatient information that it was deemed essential to monitor by that team was formatted into a one-page data collection form. That form allowed information to be recorded at the time of hospitalization and at 3 months, 6 months, and 1 year after hospitalization.

    Information on the data collection form was recorded at each of the proposed time intervals. Patient information was recorded in the outpatient diabetes center to allow follow-up phone contacts at the proposed intervals following hospitalization. The outpatient diabetes center director and the internal medicine case manager regularly reviewed charts and data collection forms for consistency and accuracy within the process. Regular team meetings of the case management specialty nurses and outpatient diabetes center staff were conducted to discuss patient criteria, to problem solve, and to maintain consistency in process. A number of limitations were recognized by the data collection team involved in this project.

OBJECTIVE OUTCOMES

Following is a brief discussion of the findings of the Diabetes Outcomes Project, along with graphs that depict results for some of the variables. Table 24-1 summarizes the findings for variables that are not accompanied by a graph.

Table 24-1   Summary of project outcomes*

VARIABLE	OUTCOME
Average number of physician office visits per quarter	3.24 before educational intervention 1.76 after educational intervention
Hospital days associated with diabetes	No newly diagnosed patients rehospitalized during project 1 patient with preexisting diabetes rehospitalized
Average number of emergency room visits per quarter	No appreciable change
Missed days of school or work	23 days during 3 months before project began None after project began
Cost of care per case during hospitalization	No appreciable change; remained stable throughout project
Education outcomes: test scores before and after teaching session	Average test score at initial hospitalization: Before teaching session 27% After teaching session 98% Average test score 12 months after hospitalization: Before teaching session 82% After teaching session 97%
Average length of hospital stay (ALOS)	ALOS throughout project remained less than critical path projection of 5 days
Mortality	2 patients died before 3-month follow-up (deaths not directly attributable to diabetes)
Medical benefits	3 patients experienced significant weight loss; 2 of them were able to discontinue insulin therapy; the third patient could discontinue hypertensive medication
Cellulitis	No occurrences in year preceding or during project
Urinary tract infections (UTI)	1 patient had a UTI during year of project 1 patient had a UTI during 3 months after project began and 2 UTI's between 6- and 12-month follow-up
Lower extremity amputations	None in year preceding or during project

*Number of patients in study = 28.

Physician Office Visits. There was a definite decline in physician office visits related to problems with diabetes following the on-going educational intervention. The average number of physician office visits concerning problems with diabetes before the educational intervention was 3.24 per quarter; following the on-going education, the average number of visits reported was 1.76.

Hospital Days Associated with Diabetes. Patients with new-onset diabetes were not rehospitalized during this project. Only one patient with preexisting diabetes was rehospitalized during the project time period.

Emergency Room Visits. There was no appreciable change in the average number of emergency room visits per quarter.

Missed Days of Work or School. Sixteen of the 28 project participants were retired or disabled. Of the 12 participants who were employed or were students, none reported missed work or school days after the project began.

Education Scores. Tests were given before and after each teaching session at the time of hospitalization, and at 3 months, 6 months, and 12 months following that initial hospitalization. The preteaching session test scores of those patients with newly diagnosed diabetes were not averaged into the first set of preteaching session tests. During the initial hospitalization, preteaching session test scores of those persons with preexisting diabetes ranged from 15% to 74% with an average score of 38%.

Cost Per Case. There was no appreciable change in cost of hospital care per case.

Length of Stay. The critical path for DRG 294 at our hospital projects a length of stay of 5 days. The average length of stay (ALOS) during the project time period was fractionally less than that critical path projection.

Mortality. Two participants died before the 3-month follow-up session; neither of those deaths was directly attributable to diabetes.

Medical Benefits. Three patients experienced dramatic medical benefits because of their lifestyle changes. Two of those three lost a significant amount of weight and were able to discontinue insulin therapy. The third participant lost weight and no longer required antihypertensive agents.

Cellulitis. No participants in the project experienced cellulitis during the year preceding the project or during the actual project.

Urinary Tract Infection. One participant reported a urinary tract infection within 1 year of the hospitalization; another participant reported a urinary tract infection within 3 months following the hospitalization; that same subject reported two urinary tract infections between the 6-month and 12-month follow-up assessments.

Lower Extremity Amputation. No participant in this project underwent amputation before or during the project.

PSYCHOLOGICAL OUTLOOK

Psychological outlook was measured by the General Well Being Instrument during the hospitalization and at 3, 6, and 12 months following that stay. That instrument consisted of 14 questions. Eight of those questions referred to negative outlooks or emotions. (Example: Have you been anxious, worried, or upset?) Five of those questions assessed positive outlooks or emotions. (Example: Have you been feeling emotionally stable and sure of yourself?) The questionnaire assessed reports of nervousness, self-control, sadness, stress, personal satisfaction, anxiety, alertness, discomfort, health fears, and fatigue.

The final analysis of the General Well Being Instrument provided surprising results. All participants had essentially no change in their self-perception of the measured variables over the year of data collection. Those who began with high negative responses remained so, as did those with high positive responses. Approximately one half of the population scored high negative consistently, and the other half scored low negative consistently. Only two questions demonstrated a significant decline in negative responses: Have you been bothered by nerves? and Have you felt sad, discouraged, or hopeless?

Those persons scoring high negative consistently were not found to be only the persons who were noncompliant or with low preteaching test scores. Although neither statistically sound nor scientifically controlled, these outcomes present an interesting premise: a person's self-perceived negative well-being does not negatively impact (certain) health care behaviors or knowledge levels.

COMPLIANCE BEHAVIORS

Participants diagnosed with new-onset diabetes (seven participants) at the time of hospitalization were not included in the initial compliance assessment. It is interesting to note that those subjects' compliance behaviors were those consistently adhered to by all the project participants for the year following the diagnosis.

Self–Blood Glucose Monitoring. Before hospitalization, SBGM was markedly poorly maintained, with half of the project participants reporting regular noncompliance. A significant increase in SBGM compliance was reported during the actual project. The greatest decline in compliance was between the 6-month and 12-month follow-up contacts. The cost of glucometer strips was reported as a reason for noncompliance by three subjects as the year progressed (Fig. 24-2).

Caloric Adherence. Poor adherence to prescribed caloric intake was reported by two thirds of the participants before hospitalization. There was a dramatic increase in the reports of compliance 3 months after hospitalization, but that behavior slowly declined as the time period progressed. The greatest decline was noted between the 6- and 12-month follow-up contact (Fig. 24-3).

Weight Control. As would be expected, weight control was also consistently an area of poor compliance before the hospitalization (noncompliance in 70% of subjects). Compliance in that behavior was markedly improved by self-reports, with approximately 70% of the participants compliant during the project (Fig. 24-4).

Ophthalmology Examinations. Recommended eye examinations were poorly complied with before hospitalization according to patient reports. Reported compliance rose by 20% during the project, with a notable drop between the 6- and 12-month follow-up contact (Fig. 24-5).

Blood Pressure Monitoring. An overwhelming majority of patients in this project sample reported consistent compliance with blood pressure monitoring as prescribed by their physician.

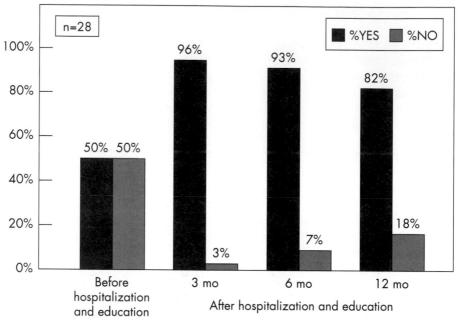

Fig. 24-2   Maintenance of self–blood glucose monitoring over a 1-year period.

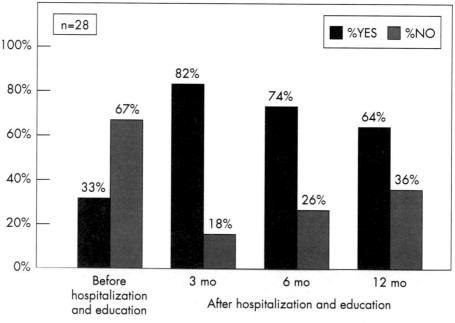

Fig. 24-3   Caloric adherence over a 1-year period.

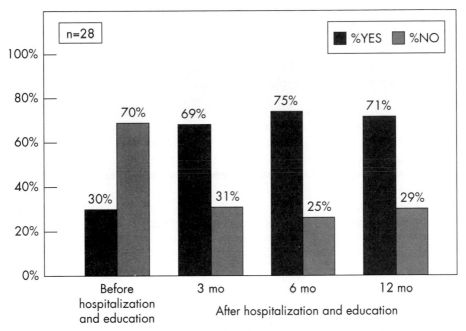

Fig. 24-4   Weight control goals met over a 1-year period.

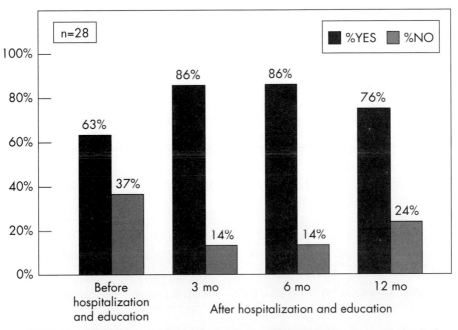

Fig. 24-5   Compliance with ophthalmology examinations over a 1-year period.

Physician Office Visits. Almost universal compliance with physician visits also was reported for this study sample. Two of the three noncompliant subjects stated that finances were the reason for not visiting their physician as recommended.

SUMMARY OF THE PROJECT'S RESULTS

The project was designed to evaluate the impact of educational efforts and regular follow-up contacts by a team of diabetes educators at Brookwood Medical Center. It was theorized that greater educational efforts would decrease the overall incidence of complications, rehospitalization rates, and cost per case and length of stay for hospitalizations. Increases in knowledge scores, compliance behaviors, productivity, and psychosocial well-being perceptions were anticipated.

The final outcomes demonstrated no complications, with the exception of urinary tract infections, which plagued two of the participants. No patient in the project was rehospitalized during the year of the study.

Knowledge scores and self-reported compliance behaviors did indeed improve dramatically and were well maintained. It is notable that the greatest decreases in those two areas occurred between the 6- and 12-month follow-up contacts consistently, leading to the assumption that a 6-month delay in caregiver contact is detrimental to patient outcomes. The number of missed days of work or school decreased, and psychological well-being perceptions did not change.

The project was an aggressive attempt to improve the quality of care, quality of life, and efficiency in resource utilization for the patient with diabetes. The outcomes of that project, while not scientifically sound, deserve consideration in the planning of optimum care for the diabetic patient.

Acknowledgment

The Diabetes Outcomes Project at Brookwood Medical Center was a progressive and successful attempt to positively affect quality of the overall care for a patient with diabetes. That project was successful only because of the committment and excellence of the members of the Diabetes Outcomes Project:

▼ Patsy Kanter, RN, Certified Diabetes Educator
▼ Judy Baker, RN, Diabetes Educator
▼ Nancy Martin, RN, Diabetes Educator
▼ Debbie Miller, RN, Case Manager
▼ Joye Taylor, M.S., Registered Dietitian, Certified Diabetes Educator
▼ Anita Floyd, Registered Dietitian

REFERENCES

American Diabetes Association. (1994). *Diabetes 1993 vital statistics.* (ISBN #0-945448-23-6).

Ary, T., Toobert, D., Wilson, W., & Glasgow, R. (1986). Patient perspectives on factors contributing to nonadherence to diabetes regimens. *Diabetes Care, 9*(2), 168-172.

Brown, S. (1988). Effects of educational interventions in diabetes care: A meta-analysis of findings. *Nursing Research, 37*(4), 223-230.

Cassileth, B., Lusk, E., Strouse, T., Miller, D., Brown, L., Cross, P. & Tenaglia, A. (1984). Psychosocial status in chronic illness: A comparative analysis of six diagnostic groups. *The New England Journal of Medicine, 311*(8), 506-511.

Centers for Disease Control (1991, May). Diabetes in the United States: A strategy for prevention. U.S. Department of Health & Human Services.

Cerkoney, K., & Hart, L. (1980). The relationship between the health belief model and compliance of persons with diabetes mellitus. *Diabetes Care, 3,* 594-598.

Chandalia, H., & Bagrodia, J. (1979). Effects of nutritional counseling on the blood glucose and nutritional knowledge of diabetic subjects. *Diabetes Care, 2*(4), 353-356.

Davis, M. (1966). Variations in patients' compliance with doctors' orders: Analysis of congruence between survey response and results of empirical investigations. *Journal of Medical Education, 41*(11), 1037-1048.

Diabetes Education Record. Birmingham, Alabama: Brookwood Medical Center, Outpatient Diabetes Center.

Diabetes Outcome Data Collection Tool. (1993). Birmingham, Alabama: Brookwood Medical Center, Outpatient Diabetes Center.

Feddersen, E, & Lockwood, D. (1994). An inpatient diabetes educator's impact on length of hospital stay. *the Diabetes Educator, 20*(2), 125-128.

Garrard, J., Mullen, L., Joynes, J., McNeil, L, & Etzwiler, D. (1990). Clinical evaluation of the impact of a patient education program. *The Diabetes Educator, 16*(5), 394-400.

General Well-Being Schedule. (1977). (DHEW Publication No. HRA 78-1347) U.S. Department of Health, Education and Welfare. National Center for Health Statistics, Hyattsville, Maryland.

Glasgow, R., McCaul, K., & Schafer, L. (1986). Barriers to regimen adherence among persons with insulin-dependent diabetes. *Journal of Behavioral Medicine, 9*(1), 65-77.

Glasgow, R., McCaul, K., & Schafer, L. (1987). Self-care behaviors and glycemic control in Type I diabetes. *Journal of Chronic Disease, 40*(5), 399-412.

Glasgow, R., Wilson, W., & McCaul, K. (1985). Regimen adherence: A problematic construct in diabetes research. *Diabetes Care, 8*(3), 300-301.

Haas, L. (1993, March). Chronic complications of diabetes mellitus. *The Nursing Clinics of North America, 28*(1), 71-85.

Holmes, D. (1986). The person and diabetes in a psychosocial context. *Diabetes Care, 9*(2), 194-206.

Jacobson, A., Adler, A., Derby, L., Anderson, B., & Wolfsdorf, J. (1991). Clinic attendance and glycemic control: A study of contrasting groups of patients with IDDM. *Diabetes Care, 14*(7), 599-601.

Johnson, S. (1992). Methodological issues in diabetes research. *Diabetes Care, 15*(11), 1658-1667.

Korhonen, T., Huttunen, J., Aro, A., Hentinen, M., Ihalainen, O., Majander, H., Siitonen, O., Uusitupa, M., & Pyorala, K. (1983). A controlled trial on the effects of patient education in the treatment of insulin-dependent diabetes. *Diabetes Care, 6*(3), 256-260.

Kurtz, S. (1990). Adherence to diabetes regimens: Empirical status and clinical applications. *The Diabetes Educator, 16*(1), 50-56.

Legge, J., Massey, V., Vena, C., & Reilly, B. (1980). Evaluating patient education: A case study of a diabetes program. *Health and Education Quarterly, 7*(2), 148-158.

Mazzuca, S., Moorman, N., Wheeler, M., Norton, J., Fineberg, N., Vinicor, F., Cohen, S., & Clark, C. (1986). The diabetes education study: A controlled trial of the effects of diabetes patient education. *Diabetes Care, 9*(1), 1-10.

Orchard, T., Dorman, J., Maser, R., Becker, D., Ellis, D., LaPorte, R., Kuller, L., Wolfson, S., & Drash, A. (1990). Factors associated with avoidance of severe complications after 25 years of IDDM. (1990). *Diabetes Care, 13*(7), 741-747.

Rosenstock, I. (1985). Understanding and enhancing patient compliance with diabetic regimens. *Diabetes Care, 8*(6), 610-616.

Rubin, R., Peyrot, M., & Saudek, C. (1989). Effects of diabetes education on self-care, metabolic control, and emotional well-being. *Diabetes Care, 12*(1), 673-679.

Rubin, R., Peyrot, M., & Saudek, C. (1991). Differential effect of diabetes education on self-regulation and life-style behaviors. *Diabetes Care, 14*(4), 335-338.

Stevens, J., Burgess, M., Kaiser, D., & Sheppa, M. (1985). Outpatient management of diabetes mellitus with patient education to increase dietary carbohydrate and fiber. *Diabetes Care, 8*(4), 359-366.

Waclawski, E. (1990). Sickness absence among insulin-treated diabetic employees. *Diabetic Medicine, 7,* 41-44.

Walsh, J., & Roberts, R. (1993, November). Uncomplicating diabetes. *Diabetes Interview,* 14, 8.

Watkins, J., Williams, F., Martin, D., Hogan, M., & Anderson, E. (1967). A study of diabetic patients at home. *American Journal of Public Health, 57*(3), 452-457.

Wilson, W., Ary, D., Biglan, A., Glasgow, R., Toobert, M., & Campbell, D. (1986). Psychosocial predictors of self-care behaviors (compliance) and glycemic control in non-insulin-dependent diabetes mellitus. *Diabetes Care, 9*(6), 614-622.

25

DEVELOPING OUTCOME MANAGEMENT STRATEGIES

AN INTENSIVE DRG-FOCUSED STUDY

BILL BRODIE

▼ *CHAPTER OVERVIEW*

In July 1994 the Department of Psychiatry at Brookwood Medical Center, Birmingham, Alabama, initiated an intense diagnosis-related group (DRG)–focused outcome study that would involve patients who met the American Psychiatric Association's *Diagnostic and Statistical Manual of Mental Disorders* 3rd ed. rev. (DSM IIIR) criteria for DRG 426, depressive neurosis. The goal was a 6-month study of 70 patients to identify and prioritize opportunities for measurable improvement in the delivery of patient services. This study was the first attempt ever undertaken at this medical center to identify areas on which to focus to improve quality in the areas of medication compliance and discharge planning.

The DRG 426 outcome team, which included psychiatric case managers, identified several measurable variables that would best represent barriers to achieving the desired outcomes: decreased readmission rates, increased functional capacity, increased medication compliance, decreased cost of care, decreased length of stay, and increased understanding of symptom management. Tracking of these variables and review of the final data revealed two key areas that if addressed would help achieve major improvements in care delivery: (1) the patient's ability to pay for medications and (2) educational deficits related to symptom management during and after hospitalization. In the future the outcome team will undertake a more detailed study of the outcomes identified and will further evaluate some new interventions that the team introduced.

▲

Patients who are diagnosed with DRG-426 depressive neurosis typically consume a large amount of inpatient resources, as well as a large proportion of limited public mental health care resources. This concern led a DRG-focused team at Brookwood Medical Center to perform an intense clinical and financial review of patients frequently hospitalized and rehospitalized within the department of psychiatry. A retrospective chart review revealed that patients diagnosed with depressive neurosis have high readmission rates, high rates of self-harm, poor compliance with outpatient medication regimens, poor attendance at inpatient therapeutic activities, an unstable home environment, a lack of understanding of the disease process, longer lengths of stay, and higher cost.

The following resources were used to further substantiate these initial chart findings:

▼ A cost analysis report for DRG 426 provided by the medical centers' cost accounting department

▼ Resource consumption trending reports for DRG 426 provided by the data processing and adjunctive therapy departments

THE STUDY

In June of 1994 this DRG 426–focused team from the Department of Psychiatry at Brookwood Medical Center in Birmingham, Alabama, began to develop what would be a 6-month study of 70 patients diagnosed with depressive neurosis. The goal of this team was to identify and prioritize opportunities for measurable improvement in the delivery of patient care services within the department of psychiatric services. The DRG 426 outcome team consisted of health professionals with various clinical back-grounds, including psychiatrist, psychologist, psychiatric case managers, pharmacist, occupational therapist, and psychiatric registered nurses. The qualifications for team members included leadership ability, clinical expertise, knowledge of case management principles, continuous quality improvement experience, and point of care contact with patients.

Input was elicited from the cost accounting department, the psychiatric quality assurance committee, and the psychiatric strategic business unit committee to assist in the profiling of potential participants. These committees confirmed DRG 426 depressive neurosis as a population of psychiatric patients who were not only high volume but also high cost and problem prone. In addition, the quality assurance committee and a medical focus group had identified these patients as having high rates of recidivism and poor outpatient follow-up compliance. Further input from the cost accounting department demonstrated that DRG 426 accounts for 28% of all inpatient psychiatric admissions and lengths of stay of 9.02 days.

On the basis of the quality assurance committee's and the medical focus group's recommendations, patients diagnosed with DRG 426 depressive neurosis would be the identified population for the intense DRG outcome study.

CLINICAL OUTCOMES

The outcome team identified eight measurable outcomes to be evaluated during the time frame of their study:

1. Decreased readmission rates
2. Decreased acts of self-harm
3. Increased compliance with inpatient therapeutic treatment activities
4. Improved functional capacity

5. Increased medication compliance
6. Increased understanding of symptom management at discharge
7. Decreased cost of care
8. Decreased length of stay

METHODS USED

The outcome study began July 1, 1994, and initial data collection lasted through August 31, 1995. During this time 70 patients who met the DSM IIIR criteria for DRG 426 depressive neurosis were asked to participate in a 6-month outcome study. Only patients 18 years of age and older who exhibited no associated axis 1 diagnosis or no associated medical complications were included in the outcome study. The outcome study began during hospitalization and would conclude 6 months after that initial hospitalization.

Each participant read and signed a consent form for participation in the DRG 426 depressive neurosis outcome study. All records reviewed and collected by the outcome team were kept in secured areas of the hospital. Only persons directly involved with the outcome study were permitted access to patient materials. Patients also agreed to be interviewed and to take the Beck Depression Inventory (BDI) on admission, discharge, and at 3- and 6-month intervals after discharge. Additionally, each participant was informed that this intense study would require that they divulge information relating to their family or social structure, social and economic levels, medication compliance or noncompliance, treatment plan compliance, and discharge teaching comprehension. Postdischarge compliance and any identified acts of self-harm would be assessed by the outcome team during scheduled follow-up telephone interviews. This information was necessary because the findings would assist the outcome team in determining whether these variables played any role in positively or negatively influencing the outcomes of the psychiatric patients studied.

Two data collection instruments were used during this outcome study to collect and evaluate information relevant to the study population. The BDI and the Depressive Neurosis Data Collection Measurement Tool were used with each patient who was enrolled in the outcome study.

The BDI measures the affective variables of anxiety and depression. The inventory can be completed by the subject in as short a time as 5 minutes. The BDI inventory, therefore, is an excellent quick and easy aid in detecting the individual suffering from depression in cases where an evaluation might otherwise not be made (Beck & Beamesderfer, 1974).

The Depressive Neurosis Data Collection Measurement Tool (Fig. 25-1) was developed by the outcome study team. The final tool was implemented after revisions were made during a 10-patient pilot period. The final two-page tool addressed 15 key areas. Each key area captured information relevant to the expected patient outcomes. The tool itself would be used to record both inpatient and outpatient information over the 6-month study period. Confidentiality was of upmost importance to this study population and outcome team.

DRG/IC-9:

Patient Name: _____   Insurance Company: _____
Medical Record #: _____   Unit: _____
Patient Date of Birth: _____   Admitting Physician: _____
Planned Admit: _____   Emergency Admit: _____   Attending Physician: _____

I. Criteria For Admission
A. Symptoms met DSM III R Criteria   Yes ____   No ____

II. Previous Admission   *Please Check*
A. Within last month   _____
B. Within last 3 months   _____
C. Within last 6 months   _____
D. More than 6 months ago   _____
E. More than 1 year ago   _____

III. Family Social Structure
A. Care provider   _____
B. Relationship to patient   _____
C. Current living arrangements   _____
   alone _____   domiciliary _____
   with family _____   nursing home _____
   foster homes _____   boarding home _____
D. Service assistance
   dept. human resources _____   case worker _____
   home health care _____   other _____

IV. Social Economic Level
Vocation _____
Social Security _____   Social Sec. disability _____
Retirement/Pension _____   Other _____
Est. monthly income _____

Please check
<$12,000/year _____ $15,000-$25,000/year _____ $25,000-$35,000/year _____
$35,000-$50,000/year _____   >$50,000/year _____

DATA COLLECTION

Case Manager: _____
Specialty Nurse: _____
Open Adult: _____
Geriatrics: _____

V. Level of Cognition
Mini Mental Score _____

VI. Medication Compliance/Noncompliance
(Prehospitalization)
A. Taken as prescribed   Yes ____   No ____
B. Multiple medications prescribed (list) ____

_____
_____

C. List most bothersome side effects ____

_____
_____

VII. On admission was
A. Previous medical record available   Yes ____   No ____
B. Social history obtained   Yes ____   No ____
C. Previous therapies reviewed   Yes ____   No ____
   • Previous activities (list)
   _____

   • Assigned activities (list)
   _____

VIII. Functional Capacity
Beck Depression Inventory Scale   *Please indicate score*
   • Admit day   _____
   • Day of Discharge   _____
   • 3 months after discharge   _____
   • 6 months after discharge   _____

IX. Inpatient Therapeutic Treatment Plan Compliance

A. Standard process (prevention) % activities attended

100%_____ 75%-100%_____ 50%-75%_____ <50%_____

B. Inpatient therapeutic treatment plan compliance

Reasons for nonattendance

refused_____

disruptive_____

unavailable_____

C. Interrupted process (after intervention) % activities attended

100%_____ 75%-100%_____ 50%-75%_____ <50%_____

Interventions/strategies to increase attendance:

1.1 intervention_____   MD order_____

Other_____

X. Discharge Understanding Teaching/Screening

(able to verbalize)

A. Has a management of symptoms plan   Yes_____ No_____

B. Understands disease process   Yes_____ No_____

C. Has clear discharge goals   Yes_____ No_____

List:_____

D. Interventions and strategies planned to meet education deficit

List:_____

E. Were discharge criteria met?   Yes_____ No_____

XI. After Discharge -- Did Patient Comply with

A. Prescribed office visits   Yes_____ No_____

B. Support group attendance   Yes_____ No_____

If no, indicate why:_____

XII. Prescribed Medication

A. Inpatient. List:_____

B. At discharge. List:_____

XIII. Acts of Self-harm

Use scale

1 0-3 months **3** >6 months

2 3-6 months **4** During hospital stay

A. Overdose_____

B. Self-inflicted wound_____

C. Ideation_____

D. Suicide/death_____

XIV. Inpatient Tracking

A. Estimated length of stay_____

B. Actual length of stay_____

C. Total cost per case_____

D. Variable cost per case_____

E. Variance from critical path_____

Please indicate all diagnostic testing/consultations

_____

XV. Other Treatment Used

A. Electroconvulsive therapy   Yes_____ No_____

#_____

B. Individual psychotherapy   Yes_____ No_____

Fig. 25-1   Depressive Neurosis Data Collection Measurement Tool developed by the DRG 426 outcome team.

SUMMARY OF DATA ANALYSIS

▼ 18.6% of study patients previously had been hospitalized with the same diagnosis twice within a 6-month window.

▼ 27.3% of study patients had annual combined household incomes of $25,000 or less.

▼ 5.6% of study patients had annual combined household incomes of $12,000 or less.

▼ 9.4% of study patients were unable to convey an understanding of their disease process on discharge.

▼ 15.8% of study patients were unable to identify a management-of-symptoms plan on discharge.

▼ 22.4% of study patients were unable to identify clear discharge goals.

▼ 17% of study patients admitted to a self-harm act within the 6 months following hospitalization.

▼ 22.5% of study patients had not complied with their inpatient treatment plan.

▼ 37.9% of study patients self-reported noncompliance with medication administration.

BECK DEPRESSION SCORES

COMBINED STUDY PATIENT SCORES (N=70)

▼ Admission score = 36
▼ Discharge score = 23
▼ 3-month postdischarge score = 28
▼ 6-month postdischarge score = 22

DEPRESSION SEVERITY LEVELS

▼   0-9 Minimal
▼ 10-14 Borderline
▼ 15-20 Mild to moderate
▼ 21-30 Moderate
▼ 31-40 Severe
▼ 41-63 Very severe

STUDY RESULTS

In November of 1995 the 6-month data collection period ended for all 70 participants. Final data analysis is presented in the boxes that appear above.

The outcome team reviewed the final data analysis and divided the data into three categories:

1. Patient economics

2. Educational deficits
3. Medication compliance
       These three categories allowed the outcome team to capture the clinical picture and patient management needs of this defined patient population. Each category was then further analyzed, and the data indicated the following:
1. *Patient economics:* 32.2% of the study patients have combined household incomes of less than $25,000.
2. *Educational deficits:* 47.6% of the study patients have no clear discharge plans
3. *Medication compliance:* 37.9% of the study patients reported noncompliance with medication administration.

OUTCOMES EVALUATION

In November of 1995 the outcome team presented the final data analysis and outcome questions to the psychiatric quality assurance team and the department of psychiatry chairperson. All persons present at the meeting agreed that the data findings and literature review would support the associations between medication compliance and patient education as predictors of patient outcomes. The outcome team also hypothesized that improving medication compliance and patient education among this population of patients would reduce readmission rates and increase treatment plan compliance.

       To substantiate this hypothesis the outcome team was challenged to develop tools that could address these two identified areas of patient outcome improvement. The two tools that the team developed were a Psychotropic Medication Cost Card (Fig. 25-2) and a Patient Education/Orientation Manual.

       The Psychotropic Medication Cost Card indicates costs for 30-day outpatient prescriptions. Cost codes are provided for high and low dosing. The card includes generic availability for the listed medications and common adverse side effects. The card also identifies outpatient mental health care centers' formulary codes to ensure medication availability as the patient moves from the inpatient setting to the outpatient setting. The card does not include every medication available for each category, but it includes most medications prescribed within the department of psychiatric services.

       During the course of inpatient management, study patients revealed that noncompliance with outpatient medication has a variety of causes, including inability to tolerate adverse side effects of certain medications and insufficient funds to buy some prescriptions. The Psychotropic Medication Cost Card could serve as a reference card for the psychiatrist prescribing medications. The admitting psychiatrist can discover the patient's financial status on his or her admission by reviewing the financial statement provided by our financial planning liaison. The psychiatrist could take this information into consideration when prescribing the patient's medication as well as the availability of the medication at the patient's outpatient mental health care center and his or her side-effect tolerance.

ANTIDEPRESSANTS

Price	Drug
$$-$$$	**Wellbutrin** (bupropion HCl)
$$$-$$$$$	**Prozac** (fluoxetine)
$$$-$$$$$	**Paxil (paroxetine)***
$$$-$$$$$	**Zoloft (sertraline)***
$$$-$$$$$	**Luvox** (fluvoxamine)
$$-$$$	**Serzone** (nefazodone HCl)
$-$$$$	**Elavil (amitriptyline HCl)***
$	Anafranil (clomipramine)*
	Sinequan, Adapin (doxepin HCl)*
$$-$$$	**Tofranil (imipramine)***
$$-$$$	Surmontil (trimipramine)
$$-$$	**Asendin (amoxapine)**
$$-$$$$	**Norpramin (desipramine)***
$	**Aventyl HCl, Pamelor (nortriptyline)***
$$$-$$$$$	Vivactil (protriptyline)
$$$-$$$	Effexor (venlafaxine)
$$-$$$	**Ludiomil (maprotiline HCl)**
$$$-$$$$$	**Desyrel (trazodone)**
$$$	Nardil (phenelzine)
$$-$$$	Parnate (tranylcypromine)

ANTICONVULSANTS

Price	Drug
$	**Tegretol (carbamazepine)**
$	**Depakene (valproic acid)**

ANTIANXIETY AGENTS

Price	Drug
$	**Equanil (meprobamate)**
$	**Xanax (alprazolam)***
$	**Librium (chlordiazepoxide)***
$	**Tranxene (clorazepate)***
$	**Valium (diazepam)***
$$-$$$	Paxipam (halazepam)
$	**Ativan (lorazepam)***
$$-$$$$$	**Serax (oxazepam)***
$$$$	**Klonopin (clonazepam)**
	BuSpar (Buspirone HCl)
$	**Atarax (hydroxyzine HCl)**
$	**Vistaril (hydroxyzine pamoate)***
$$-$$$$	**Sinequan, Adapin (doxepin HCl)**
$$-$$$$$	Trancopal (chlormezanone)

SEDATIVES/HYPNOTICS

Price	Drug
$$	Ambien (zolpidem tartrate)
$$-$$$	**Noctec (chloral hydrate)**
$	Placidyl (ethchlorvynol)
$	**Dalmane (flurazepam HCl)**
$	**Restoril (temazepam)***
$	**Halcion (triazolam)***
$$	Doral (quazepam)
$	**Phenobarbital**
$	**Nembutal sodium (pentobarbital sodium)**

ANTIPSYCHOTICS

Price	Drug
$	**Haldol (haloperidol)***
$$-$$$$$	Moban (molindone HCl)
$-$$$$	**Loxitane (loxapine)**
$$$$	Clozaril (clozapine)
$$$$	Risperdal (risperidone)
$-$$$	Orap (pimozide)
$-$$$$	**Thorazine (chlorpromazine HCl)***
$-$$$$	**Sparine (promazine HCl)**
$	**Mellaril (thioridazine HCl)***
$-$$$$	Serentil (mesoridazine)
$-$$$	**Trilafon (perphenazine)**
$-$$	**Prolixin (fluphenazine HCl)**
$-$$	**Stelazine (trifluoperazine HCl)**
$	**Navane (thiothixene)***
$	**Eskalith (lithium carbonate)***
$-$$	Lithobid (lithium carbonate)

PSYCHOTHERAPEUTIC AGENTS

Price	Drug
$	**Etrafon, Triavil (perphenazine and amitriptyline HCl)**
	Hydergine (ergoloid mesylates)
$-$$	**Ritalin (methylphenidate HCl)**
$$-$$$	Cognex (tacrine HCl)
$$$	Deprol (meprobamate and benactyzine HCl)
$$$-$$$$$	**Limbitrol DS 10-25 (chlordiazepoxide and amitriptyline)**

*A good, effective medication recommended for treatment of specific disorders.
Bold Print: Generic drug availability

COST CODE   The Cost Code provides approximate cost information for a 30-day prescription. Pharmacy prices will vary.

$ <$ 25.00 $$ <$ 50.00
$$$ <$ 100.00 $$$$ >$ 100.00
$$$$$ The drug is inexpensive at low doses but becomes expensive with higher doses.

MEDICATION INFORMATION

1. Selective serotonin reuptake inhibitors (SSRIs) are emerging as the preferred first-line option for panic disorder. Of these agents, when a patient requires 50 mg/d, sertraline 100 mg tab (½ tab/d) will be less expensive. Otherwise, Paxil may be least expensive.

2. Imipramine and clomipramine are useful in panic disorders. Imipramine is inexpensive, and clomipramine becomes costly at higher doses.

3. The recommended steady-state serum lithium levels are 0.8-1.0 mmol/L during acute mania, and 0.5-0.8 mmol/L for prophylaxis. Lithium is excreted renally. Risk factors, e.g., reduced sodium intake, dehydration; signs of lithium toxicity, e.g., slurred speech, unsteady gait, coarse tremor.

4. Antipsychotics control manic symptoms; side effects (e.g., extrapyramidal, anticholinergic, antiadrenergic, neuroleptic malignant syndrome) may not be well tolerated.

5. Recommend triazolam (Halcion) for short-term insomnia. Zolpidem (Ambien) costs 4 to 5 times more than triazolam and should be reserved until patient has failed treatment with a benzodiazepine for 10 to 14 nights in a 14-day period.

6. Clomipramine (Anafranil), fluvoxamine (Luvox), paroxetine (Paxil), and fluoxetine (Prozac) are FDA approved for treatment of obsessive-compulsive disorder. Presently, clomipramine (Anafranil) is the least expensive, then paroxetine (Paxil).

7. **Common side effects:** Benzodiazepines, sedation; tricyclic antidepressants, anticholinergic effects, orthostatic hypotension, sedation, sexual dysfunction, weight gain; SSRIs, nausea, headache, nervousness, insomnia, sexual dysfunction; MAO inhibitors, food and drug interactions; lithium, nausea, fatigue, tremor, thirst, edema, weight gain; chlorpromazine, sedation, postural hypotension, weight gain, anticholinergic and occasional extrapyramidal effects; antipsychotic drugs, extrapyramidal effects.

8. Antidepressants require several weeks to achieve maximum therapeutic benefit.

9. Clozaril may be effective in schizophrenic patients resistant to other antipsychotics. Check with manufacturer for assistance with expense for this drug.

Fig. 25-2   Psychotropic Medication Cost Card developed by the DRG 426 outcome team.

Development of the Patient Education/Orientation Manual was based on the identified need to improve inpatient treatment plan compliance and to address deficits identified in discharge planning. The Patient Education/Orientation Manual would serve as a patient guide throughout the patient's hospitalization and after discharge.

The patient would be requested to record his or her experiences within the therapeutic milieu daily. The staff, along with the patient, would use this tool as a teaching and learning guide.

The Patient Education/Orientation Manual is divided into several clinical sections. Each section focuses on the patient's individual treatment plan. Therapeutic activities and program group descriptions are defined. Both short- and long-term patient goals are also identified. Each section clearly defines the patient's treatment plan, diagnosis, and medication management and treatment objectives. Upon discharge the manual is reviewed with the patient, with emphasis placed on discharge goals, inpatient therapeutic educational deficits, outpatient management, support mechanisms, and follow-up medical appointments. The Patient Education/ Orientation Manual helps the care provider ensure that after discharge the patient has a management of symptom plan, a follow-up appointment, a clear understanding of the necessity to take the medication as prescribed, and the means to purchase the medication.

Implementing the first step of the DRG 426 study and reviewing the final data analysis made it clear that a major contribution to the delivery of care can be made by addressing the economic ability of patients to pay for medications at the beginning of hospitalization and by identifying educational deficits related to symptom management during and after hospitalization. Nurse case management played an important role in achieving the project's desired outcome of identifying areas on which to focus to improve medication compliance and quality in discharge planning.

FUTURE STUDY

The next step for the outcome team is to undertake a more detailed study of the clinical outcome benefits of the Psychotropic Medication Cost Card and the Patient Education/Orientation Manual. The information gained will enable the outcome team to develop optimal outcome management strategies to predict which patients are most at risk for noncompliance with medication administration and poor outpatient symptom management leading to readmissions. It is anticipated that the DRG 426 depressive neurosis study will continue collecting further data for the next 6 months. Further study is necessary to investigate the refinements made in the delivery care to these patient types.

The DRG 426 Depressive Neurosis Study was the first attempt at improving quality in the areas of medication compliance and discharge planning ever undertaken at the Department of Psychiatry, Brookwood Medical Center. This outcome study was the first progressive initiative to combat the traditional questions and answers with user responses that would produce true patient outcomes. Through this experience the outcome team learned the value of a focused study and how that allows one to uncover areas of intervention never before realized. Finally, realizing the continuum of care involved in a chronic illness, we took steps to positively affect that entire continuum.

Acknowledgments

There are so many uncharted waters within nursing case management. Taking the voyage into psychiatric case management was not without risk. For this reason I would like to recognize those brave individuals who not only took the voyage but are charting its future course. These individuals, together with the patients who volunteered for this study, are developing a navigation map for mental wellness. The hope of the Depressive Neurosis Outcome Study Team's collaborative effort is to create a map that will decrease the symptoms endured and prejudices experienced by those who suffer from mental illness.

▼ To Glenda Brogden and Derek Spellman, two people who "mastered the risk" and provided the vision and support necessary to implement nursing case management successfully within psychiatry.

▼ To the DRG 426 Depressive Neurosis Outcome Study Team: Dr. Ed Logue, Albertha Lyas, Jean Newsome, Linda Lind, Gloria Sandlin, Sara Romano, Sue Trant, Sharon Beal Fowler, Gary Tate, Joan Witt, Karen Litwiniec, and Ellen Hitchcock, who provided the expertise, guidance, and professional assistance that allowed us to meet the goals and initiatives identified for this study.

▼ A personal thank you to Elaine L. Cohen for being my long-distance friend and for recognizing the efforts and contributions that nursing case management is bringing into the twenty-first century.

REFERENCE
Beck, A.T., and Beamesderfer, A. (1974). Assessment of depression: The depression inventory. *Psychological Measurements in Psychopharmacology, 7,* 151-169.

VIII

ISSUES FOR CONSIDERATION

26

Organized Labor and Case Management

▼ **CHAPTER OVERVIEW**

Nursing administrators generally believe that nursing case management models cannot be implemented in unionized facilities. This chapter demonstrates that these two concepts are not mutually exclusive. Nurse administrators in unionized environments can use the strategies discussed in this book to implement case management models in their hospitals. It is also worthwhile to consider organized labor's own interest in containing the costs associated with providing health care for union members. The concepts of nursing case management are of interest to organized labor because the model provides those *in* the union with high-quality, cost-effective care.
▲

CASE MANAGEMENT IN UNIONIZED FACILITIES

For those departments of nursing represented by collective bargaining unions or state associations, special consideration is needed when case management is implemented. Initial planning for the model will require determining whether the case manager position will be a union or management position. This decision probably will depend on the job description and philosophy of the position.

If the case manager position is one that will be filled by a staff nurse, it would then be rational to leave it within the union. However, if clinical nurse specialists are used as case managers or if the case manager position is not considered to be an option on the career ladder, it may then be more appropriate to designate it as a nonunion position.

If the staff nurses of the institution are represented by collective bargaining, leaving the position in the union as a staff level position may result in the forfeiture of some of the position's autonomy. For example, the staff level nurse will be limited by rules and regulations concerning work hours, vacation and holiday time, conference time, and time off the unit. The nature of the case manager job requires the nurse to spend additional periods of time off the unit meeting with other professional disciplines, doing research for the managed care plans, or attending in-service programs. This freedom of movement will be restricted by collective bargaining agreements to which every staff nurse must conform.

On the other hand, removing the position from the bargaining unit may send a negative message that indicates to staff and others that excellence can only be achieved by using someone outside the bargaining unit. Conversely, a management position within a unionized facility will mean more autonomy and independence for the case manager.

If it is decided that the position will remain as a career ladder option within the collective bargaining unit, the union must be included as early as possible in decisions regarding salary, job description, and title.

It is likely that there will be minimal resistance from the union if the position is left within the union. The position will provide opportunities to reward outstanding performance with an internal promotion for staff nurses, resulting in an increase in salary and advanced role. By keeping the case manager position as part of the organized union, there will be no erosion in bargaining power for the unit member. If the organization implementing case management desires a quick implementation period, making the position part of the union might be the path of least resistance. Philosophically the message will be made clear. Excellence can occur within the union as well as without, and one does not need to be in a management position to achieve a level of autonomy or accountability.

Negotiations with the union include issues of salary. Other issues to be negotiated should certainly include daytime working hours, rotation, holidays, and weekends. Case managers should be on duty Monday through Friday, when they can have the greatest effect on patient care. It is during these time periods that they are best able to meet with other disciplines, as well as facilitate tests, treatments, or procedures. The transition will be smoother if these issues are negotiated with the union before implementation.

CASE MANAGEMENT: ORGANIZED LABOR'S RESPONSE TO ESCALATING HEALTH CARE COSTS

In discussing the role of organized labor in nursing case management, it may be helpful to consider organized labor's interest in providing high-quality, reasonably priced health care to its own union members.

As health care becomes more expensive, organizations are looking toward case management to assist in managing and controlling spiraling health care costs. Case management and other corporate health care alternatives are being integrated into employees' medical and liability benefit plans, worker's compensation and disability, long-term care and retiree services, and dependent care initiatives (Frieden, 1991b; Katz, 1991). Case management has also been successful in providing and maintaining quality, cost-effective mental health care services, prenatal care, and employee health promotion programs.

Along these lines, labor organizations have also begun to initiate cooperative alliances with management in an effort to contain health care costs (Bell, 1991). Maintaining health care and insurance benefits has become a priority of union leaders according to a survey conducted by Metropolitan Life (Data Watch, 1991).

A 1991 survey by the Health Research Institute showed a willingness by both labor and management groups to develop health care programs that support early prevention and primary care services (Data Watch, 1991).

Other joint arrangements between labor and management have led to the development of initiatives that offer stress and mental health counseling, substance abuse programs, preemployment screening, child and dependent care support, disability, case management, access to health care service networks, such as on-site medical care, outpatient care, home health care, community-based programs, and health awareness education (Bell, 1991; Beresford, 1991; Chelius, Galvin, & Owens, 1992; Jordahl, 1992; Lucas, 1991).

Efforts to maintain employee health-benefit levels while reducing expenses have led some corporations to contract with preferred provider organizations (PPOs) (see Chapter 8). These arrangements have helped ensure accessibility and affordability to needed health care services (Ciccotelli, 1991; Varecha, Barry, & Martingale, 1991).

Organized labor has also begun to launch national health reform campaigns. These efforts are aimed at implementing a national social health insurance plan, controlling medical service reimbursement, providing universal health care coverage, coordinating and managing administrative activities, and providing access to long-term, community-based health care services (Frieden, 1991a).

Innovative approaches to delivering and maintaining health care services will become more prevalent as the economic environment continues to grow more complex and difficult to manage. Hospitals currently involved in restructuring interests have joined with labor groups to focus efforts on providing quality, cost-effective patient care. This goal has been achieved in some settings with the deployment of nursing case management, both in union and management positions.

REFERENCES

Bell, N. (1991). Workers and managers of the world unite! *Business and Health, 9*(8), 26-34.

Beresford, L. (1991). Union wants a soberer image. *Business and Health, 9*(8), 51-54.

Chelius, J., Galvin, D., & Owens, P. (1992). Disability: It's more expensive than you think. *Health, 11*(4), 78-84.

Ciccotelli, C. (1991). Union engineers a better health care system. *Business and Health, 9*(8), 56-57.

Data Watch. (1991). Unions and health care. *Business and Health, 9*(8), 8-9.

Frieden, J. (1991a). Unions rev up health reform engines. *Business and Health, 9*(8), 42-50.

Frieden, J. (1991b). What's ahead for managed care? *Business and Health, 9*(13), 43-49.

Jordahl, G. (1992). Labor/management partnerships foster better employee relationships. *Business and Health, 9*(4), 73-76.

Katz, F. (1991). Making a case for case management. *Business and Health, 9*(4), 75-77.

Lucas, B. (1991). Armour foods thin slices workers' compensation costs. *Business and Health, 9* 9(8), 58-60.

Varecha, R., Barry J., & Martingale, J. (1991). Laboring to manage care. *Business and Health, 9*(8), 35-41.

27

CLINICAL CAREER LADDERS

▼ **CHAPTER OVERVIEW**

Nursing career ladders can be linked intrinsically to a case management model. The case manager position can be integrated as the third or fourth rung of a clinical career ladder. In this way, greater experience and education are rewarded in a bedside position that recognizes and rewards experience. Traditional clinical career ladders often do not accommodate educational and experiential qualifications of the advanced practitioner. The autonomous case manager role is attractive to nurses with experience who wish to remain in bedside nursing but who are looking for a position of increased responsibility and independent practice.

When considering clinical career ladders, institutions need to assess the cost of maintaining a ladder and evaluate the positive effects such a ladder has on recruitment and retention. ▲

GOALS AND OBJECTIVES OF A CLINICAL CAREER LADDER

The nursing case management model can provide the framework for the integration of a true clinical ladder. Traditionally, clinical ladders have not provided a system for promotion at the bedside that included true changes in job title and responsibility.

Most of promotions at the bedside have provided the staff nurse with an elevated title, such as staff nurse level II or senior staff nurse. This change in title may also have included a financial reward and an altered job description. However, analysis of such positions reveals that the actual day-to-day responsibilities remained the same.

Each organization implementing a career ladder will have different goals and objectives for an addition of this kind. Generally the integration of a career ladder will cost the organization money. The long-term savings that come because of decreased turnover or lowered vacancy rates are difficult to measure. Even more difficult is showing a cause-and-effect relationship between the career ladder and the decreased turnover and vacancy rates (Vestal, 1984).

Nevertheless, there are some generic goals and objectives that most organizations will hope to achieve by implementing a career ladder. Whether the achievement of these goals offsets the cost of the increased salaries that accompany the ladder will be a determination each organization must make for itself (Del Bueno, 1982).

An effective clinical career ladder has some inherent benefits:

▼ Provides the opportunity for professional advancement in a direct patient care position
▼ Promotes individual professional growth and development
▼ Attracts nurses to the organization and helps retain them
▼ Rewards individual expertise
▼ Provides a framework for the development of performance evaluation tools
▼ Increases job satisfaction
▼ Positively affects patient care

Most clinical career ladders reflect what the name suggests. The ladders are designed to promote clinical advancement, usually at the bedside. Therefore the emphasis is on the direct care provider, generally the staff nurse. Other ladders may be designed for career or professional advancement, such as administration or education, or they may be a combination of clinical, administration, and education.

Each step or level must be defined by specific behaviors and levels of performance that are identifiable and measurable. They should also be realistic and achievable (AORN, 1983).

Advancement in the clinical ladder is initiated by the nurse through a request. It is the nurse's responsibility to produce documents supporting a claim for advancement to the next level. Evaluation will then take place through a review of the documents. The documents should include the nurse's periodic evaluations and any other evidence of professional education, certification, and the like.

The documents are weighed against the performance expectations of the level to which the nurse is striving. Theorectically any nurse who has met the criteria should be eligible for advancement. In a true career ladder situation there should be no quota of positions per level, and any qualified nurse should be eligible for the advancement.

All nurses within the career ladder should be evaluated periodically. These evaluations result in advancement, retention in the current position, or demotion (AORN, 1983).

Incentives for promotion include advanced title, salary benefits, and heightened status. Each promotional level should move the nurse toward a higher level of empowerment and self-actualization.

Just as there are benefits to the implementation of a ladder, there also are some problems (McKay, 1986). As already mentioned, the cost/benefit ratio may not be suitable for the organization. There is always the potential for a ladder to have a negative effect because it implies a hierarchical organizational structure.

For the ladder to produce a truly supportive environment and improve the quality of care, staffing patterns for each day and for each shift should incorporate representatives from each level. This may not always be feasible or realistic, particularly on the evening or night shift when staffing levels are low.

Monetary awards are often greater for those advancing within an administrative career ladder than for those advancing within a clinical ladder.

Other difficulties arise if the nursing department is represented by a union. The goals of the department and the goals of the clinical ladder must meld with those of the union. Each aspect of the ladder needs to be negotiated for integration into the bargaining union contract. Nursing departments represented in this way should include union representatives in the negotiations from the very beginning. In most cases the institution of a clinical career ladder will be best implemented at the beginning of a new contract.

The number of levels of any ladder will depend on the philosophy, goals, and budget of the organization. Following are qualifications a nurse from a particular level should have.

Level I
▼ Entry level capabilities
▼ A license or temporary permit to practice professional nursing
▼ An understanding of the hospital policies and procedures
▼ A basic familiarity with patient care
▼ General skills needed to function at a beginning level of nursing practice

Level II
▼ A more holistic understanding of patient care delivery
▼ A career orientation with goals and direction
▼ An ability to prioritize needs of patients and families and to delegate responsibilities to other members of the nursing staff as appropriate
▼ An ability to act as a resource for other nursing staff members
▼ An understanding of the relationship between career goals and personal growth

Level III
▼ Ability to act as a resource for the health care team
▼ Self-directed in most aspects of learning
▼ Involvement in professional committees or organizations
▼ An understanding of the health care team as a whole that comes together to meet mutual patient goals
▼ A change agent for the institution within the department of nursing
▼ An active seeker of additional professional responsibility
▼ Commitment to nursing as a career
▼ Ability to plan patient care based on current and future patient care needs
▼ Ability to plan for appropriate discharge
▼ Financial awareness incorporated into daily practice, including resource use, length of stay, and discharge planning needs

The level I registered nurse is expected to apply basic nursing theory to practice. Nursing care is delivered to the nurse's assigned group of patients based on actual needs, physician orders, and nursing diagnoses. The registered nurse at level I is able to complete all required treatments for a particular shift in accordance with the policies and procedures of the organization. This nurse may begin to learn the skills necessary to assess patient and family learning needs and to begin meeting those needs (Barr & Desnoyer, 1988).

The level II practitioner begins to shift from actual patient problems to identifying potential problems and applying interventions that will prevent those problems from occurring. At this level the nurse's organizational skills begin to develop. Focus becomes more global as the nurse develops an awareness not only of the nurse's own patients but also of those throughout the unit. Patient problems are seen on a health care continuum that extends beyond hospitalization (Barr & Desnoyer, 1988).

The level III practitioner sees the health care team as a whole and seeks to begin to bring the team together to meet patient needs and to provide the best possible care. At this level the nurse begins to take a more active leadership role on the unit, serving as preceptor and informal leader. The registered nurse at this level is involved in seeking advanced education in some specialty or certification category. The nurse applies this knowledge and skill in practice and becomes an expert in the chosen area. This knowledge is used by the expert nurse to create an environment for positive change both on the unit and in the department (Barr & Desnoyer, 1988).

Differentiated practice is a personnel deployment model designed to better use the skills and education of the experienced nurse. An educational requirement within a clinical performance framework is incorporated into the differentiated practice model. By using a differentiated practice modality, the design of the clinical ladder can clearly delineate the evolving knowledge base and expanded level of functioning of the experienced nurse. Some institutions may want to include criteria for educational level and mandate that those at the third or fourth level have a master's degree. Using this model within a clinical career ladder bases employees' roles on both educational preparation and clinical performance.

In other models the fourth or fifth level is that of the clinical nurse specialist. If this role is seen as a bedside clinical position and not as a management or educator position, it belongs in a clinical career ladder. Once again, this depends on the perception of the role within the department (Metcalf, 1984).

THE CASE MANAGER POSITION WITHIN THE CLINICAL LADDER

The case manager position provides the opportunity for the development of a true career ladder, one that integrates a title change and financial incentive with significant changes in job description and job responsibilities.

The staff nurse position incorporates all the direct nursing tasks associated with providing nursing care. Included among these are the physical assessment, vital signs, medication administration, blood drawing, wound care, skin care, ambulation, and patient feedings.

The generic nurse case manager role removes the staff nurse from direct nursing functions. Her role becomes one concerned with the indirect nursing tasks provided to patients. Among these are patient and family teaching, care planning, coordination and facilitation of patient care and services, and discharge planning.

Shifting the focus to these functions also involves a substantial increase in the number of patients that can be taken care of on a daily basis. A case manager's focus is much broader than just the tasks at hand. The case manager must constantly focus on the plan of care for the days ahead by coordinating and facilitating services whether for discharge planning or patient teaching.

For the first time, this group of nurses has been given responsibility for controlling costs and length of stay. In this position, nursing holds the purse strings of health care.

Furthermore this is the first time a registered nurse who wishes to remain at the bedside can do so while accepting promotion and change in job status. This position can be attractive to nurses who are not interested in positions within administration or education but who are looking for a change that still involves bedside nursing. In other cases the position might be attractive to a nurse who has been in the field for 1 or 2 years but who does not yet have the skills or education needed to advance to administrative or educational roles.

The case manager position is usually found at the third or fourth level of a clinical career ladder. The position empowers the staff nurse to create an environment for change in the organization, and it has the potential to generate a tremendous amount of job satisfaction. Research shows that longevity and job satisfaction are related (Malik, 1992). The career ladder, therefore, provides an incentive for the more experienced nurse to remain in a clinical position. Increased job satisfaction may have a trickle-down effect on the other staff nurses on the unit.

The autonomous case manager role may be the best argument thus far for creating clinical career ladders. Malik (1992) reports that clinical career ladders may not provide a position that affords the experienced staff nurse the opportunity to use her advanced skills and knowledge. The case manager role, which requires a higher level of functioning and skills, may serve to fill this gap.

REFERENCES

AORN. (1983). Guidelines for developing clinical ladders. *AORN Journal, 37*(6), 1209-1224.

Barr, N.J., & Desnoyer, J.M. (1988). Career development for the professional nurse: A working model. *The Journal of Continuing Education in Nursing, 19*(2), 68-72.

Del Bueno, D. (1982, September). A clinical ladder? Maybe! *Journal of Nursing Administration,* 19-22.

Malik, D.M. (1992). Job satisfaction related to use of career ladder. *Journal of Nursing Administration, 22*(3), 7.

McKay, J.I. (1986). Career ladders in nursing: An overview. *Journal of Emergency Nursing, 12*(5), 272-278.

Metcalf, J. (1984, Fall). The clinical nurse specialist in a clinical career ladder. *Nursing Administration Quarterly,* 8-19.

Vestal, K.W. (1984, Fall). Financial considerations for career ladder programs. *Nursing Administration Quarterly,* 1-8.

28

CASE MANAGEMENT AND INFORMATION TECHNOLOGY

ROY L. SIMPSON

▼ *CHAPTER OVERVIEW*

Information technology will be pivotal to the future success of case management because of its potential to help professional nurse case managers perform their jobs more effectively and efficiently. This is especially true for those who are involved in beyond-the-walls case management, which still depends heavily on paper-based processes. Because of its pervasiveness, information technology's greatest opportunity for case managed care lies in the development of a national information network that links nursing information systems with patients in their own homes via computers. Such a network would allow nursing professionals to satisfy the patient's need for confidentiality and 24-hour access to information support while meeting nursing's need to reach ever-growing patient populations.

   Among innovative efforts already underway that successfully offer case managed care via computer networks to patients with diseases such as AIDS and Alzheimer's is ComputerLink, a special computer network designed to help nurses support home-based care. The computer's capacity to offer daily follow-up contact, to serve as a medium for asking and answering questions, to provide voice reminders or alarms to signal anything from medications to checkups, and to contain costs are characteristics that will contribute to the success of networks that both case management professional and patient alike can access. The acceptance of a universal nursing minimum data set to codify nursing knowledge will also be crucial to this process. ▲

Despite advances in information technology, case management in the mid-1990s continues to be a largely manual, labor-intensive process. Yet information technology, like no other tool available to professional nurse case managers, promises to make case management more viable, effective, and powerful. To be sure, technologically sophisticated hospitals utilizing within-the-walls case management protocols likely are already benefiting greatly from existing clinical information systems and patient tracking systems. In these institutions, automation primarily is used for documentation assistance and for managing patient follow-up schedules.

309

When it comes to beyond-the-walls case management, however, few institutions have the information technology tools needed to liberate professional nurse case managers from intensive paper-based processes. Yet it is precisely in this area—in case management beyond the walls of the institution—that information technology holds the greatest promise.

The real opportunity for case managed care lies in the direction in which technology is currently and rapidly moving—toward the advent of *pervasive* technology or pervasive health care information networks or infrastructures.

A pervasive technology is one that is more noticeable by its absence than its presence, in the same way that automobiles, televisions, and telephones are today. In other words, a hotel room—or even a hospital room—today without a phone or television would be an unpleasant surprise. Yet it is likely that within 10 years, a hotel room or a hospital room without a *computer as well* will also be an oddity. The wild excitement over the Internet and the World Wide Web is only a hint at how powerfully the information superhighway is beginning to permeate the consciousness of American society.

This is particularly true of younger generations who are as comfortable with computers as toddlers of previous generations were with telephones. With this in mind it is important to remember that only people born before a technology becomes pervasive think of it as "technology"; all others think of it as part of the environment. Thus today's schoolchildren do not think of television and telephones as technology; they simply cannot imagine life without them. They are part of the landscape of modern existence. Tomorrow's children—and tomorrow's nurses—will feel the same way about computers.

In this march toward pervasiveness, technology historically passes through four predictable stages:

1. Development as experimental curiosities as individuals try to solve a particular problem in laboratories or—in the case of computers—in their garages or basements
2. Usage by a small number of specialists to solve a specific problem
3. Mass development as it becomes manufacturable and commonplace (although still used primarily by a small fraction of the population who have specialized training)
4. Total pervasiveness and accessibility by the average citizen, as exemplified by telephones, televisions, and radios.

Although health care technology will never move beyond the third stage (after all, it will always require individuals with specialized training to operate), the *network* in which information is shared will indeed become pervasive. One need only look at the explosion of current interest in the Internet and the World Wide Web to get a glimpse at the way in which information networks will pervade American society. Indeed the technology to deliver multimedia services over telephone wires via the television has existed since the early 1990s. Cable television companies and telephone operating companies are fighting it out to determine who will "own" the ability to deliver information technology services to the home. In other words, this convergence of technology means that the television—the current focus of entertainment in most

American homes—will also be the focus for computer interaction (i.e., the television will also *be* the computer—it will be possible to go from watching a TV show to attaching a keyboard to the set and to instantly begin "surfing" information networks or communicating with caregivers via bulletin boards).

The development of a pervasive national information network has tremendous ramifications for the nurse case manager. A national network will link nursing information systems and, as a result, nurse case managers to patients in their own homes via computers (or multimedia centers—the TV as computer or vice versa). It is even imaginable that within 10 years all homes will come equipped with a TV, just as they come equipped with ovens. Prognosticators also predict that there will be a computer company or information company, similar to the phone company, that individuals will call to get their computer turned on and linked into the network (just as one calls the power company to get the power turned on). Taken to its logical conclusion, this prediction sees an information utility company just like the phone or electric utility. This information utility will likely be run like any other utility, with some sort of public service commission in charge and with hefty governmental laws that regulate distribution of services.

NETWORK LINKAGE AND HOME CARE

With network linkage linking patients with each other and with nurses through a computer network the nursing professional can satisfy the patient's need for confidentiality and 24-hour access to informational support. Network linkage also supports nursing's need to reach out to an ever expanding patient population. Today nurses are already experimenting with case-managed care via computer networks for such diseases as AIDS and Alzheimer's with immensely positive results.

Consider the work of Patricia Brennan, PhD, RN, FAAN, associate professor of nursing and systems engineering at the Frances Payne Bolton School of Nursing at Case Western Reserve University, who used computer networks to link AIDS and Alzheimer's disease patients' family caregivers to nurses and with each respective subgroup. Participants in the study were provided with terminals and modems and given access to ComputerLink—a special computer network designed to help nurses support home-based care. Users were free to access the network any time of the day or night at no cost. Each participant was provided with 1.5 hours of free training and ongoing assistance in using the system.

The ComputerLink network offered three primary modules:
1. A communications module, which included a bulletin board area for "conversing" with others in the same predicament and a question-and-answer section for anonymous postings to nurses
2. A decision support model, which helped participants make self-care choices using a structured decision analysis method
3. An information module, a database filled with encyclopedic data about the disease.

A project nurse was assigned as chief moderator, responsible for reading all public "conversations" and notations (and therefore for assessing information gaps in the participating populations), maintaining the currency of the electronic encyclo-pedia, troubleshooting for all participants, and acting as clinical expert in all capabilities.

The results were positive. The typical user got on the system 125 times, or an average of four to five times a week. According to Brennan, "testimonial evidence of perceived support abounded in both groups of participants. Postings on the public forum contained messages of encouragement, ideas for self-care and for managing with the formal health system, and counsel to peers" (Simpson, 1994).

There were also many nursing benefits. Case managers were able to dissemi-nate information to patients more easily and quickly. Nurses could also control misinformation by ensuring that outdated information was not accessible to users. Privacy over the network ensured that all users could learn from an interaction, not just one patient at one time.

Brennan's research project proved that "continuity of care in home care can be achieved through both traditional and non-traditional means,—sending nurses out to the homes or through novel use of existing technology such as computer terminals" (Simpson, 1994).

NETWORK LINKAGE AND CASE MANAGEMENT

Having a network that can be accessed by case management professionals and patients alike will be key to the success of case management in the future. If computers do indeed become as ubiquitous as phones and televisions in people's homes, case management beyond the walls becomes a viable reality. Without ever leaving the hospital, nurses could have daily contact with patients for follow-ups, questions about medications, patient follow-through, and so on.

With voice or sound computer-generated reminders or alarms, nurses could remind patients or family members about everything from taking insulin shots, to changing their dressings, to coming in for a check-up. Via the same network, patients could report to the caregiver unusual symptoms or concerns about their care. Although such communications could never replace the personal contact and personal care that is so important to the professional practice of nursing, they would certainly alleviate the strain on nurses who must manage the details involved in community-based health care delivery.

In addition, using networked computers would support the institution's desire to contain costs. If day-to-day communications and educational issues are addressed via computer, resources could be allocated more cost effectively, ensuring that nursing professionals spend their face-to-face time with more critical situations.

Once a nationwide network of health care information is in place, it can be surmised that "back office" linkage will be an important part of the network. And it will likely be expected that the case manager will manage the various critical pathways and treatment protocols outlined by different payers. In this way the case manager truly becomes an advocate for the patient and an intermediary for the institution—ensuring not only that the patient receives the best care but also that the institution follows prescribed protocols to obtain reimbursement.

Insurance companies and third-party payers are already playing a big part in the development of the health care information network so that benefit and financial information can be managed quickly and efficiently on the patient's behalf. Payers and institutions alike will likely be the focus for collecting all the data related to patient care, performing variance analyses and indicating benchmark outcomes in an ongoing attempt to determine the best protocols while containing costs. The debate as to who will set critical pathways and treatment protocols continues to rage (i.e., the payers or the providers?). To have a strong voice in this process, nursing must be able to identify and codify nursing services and outline its contributions to the patient's outcomes.

The result of establishing benchmarks and of being held to standards of care will be profound. For example, if 3 patients out of 10 with a cholecystectomy develop a nonsocomial infection after surgery and the benchmark is 1 out of 10, the competence of the nursing care will be closely scrutinized. Nurse managers and case managers must be prepared for this eventuality.

Clearly a pervasive network of this kind will empower nurses, particularly case managers, at the same time that it makes them more accountable for their actions. The case manager of the future need be an expert not only in clinical care but also in critical analysis of enormous amounts of data upon which decisions will be based.

PREPARING FOR THE FUTURE

A common health care network would not, and could not, replace nursing contact. However, it would serve as a powerful support tool in the evolution of case management. It may be 10 years or more before a pervasive network is in place whereby nursing would have both the informational infrastructure and the ability to contact and communicate with patients electronically. The advent or acceptance of a universally accepted nursing minimum data set is critical to this process. Nursing must be able to codify its knowledge in order to be able to properly use computer networks and share nursing information and outcomes with other medical and nonmedical caregivers.

Nursing has always been able to adapt to technological advances. Fifty years ago there was no such thing as an intensive care unit (ICU). Today, nurses are critical to the success of ICUs. In the same way we must prepare for a future that will be dramatically different—a future of vast computer connections that can link patients with caregivers, caregivers with each other, and more. The promise of case management will be achieved by using informational technology to share information and communicate with patients and caregivers beyond the walls of the institution. It is up to nurses *today* to prepare themselves for such a future.

REFERENCE

Simpson, R.L. (1994, Winter). Computer networks show great promise in supporting AIDS patients. *Nursing Administration Quarterly,* 18(2), 92-95.

29

ETHICAL ISSUES IN CASE MANAGEMENT

SISTER CAROL TAYLOR, CSFN

▼ *CHAPTER OVERVIEW*

This chapter explores the ethical issues related to case management. The essential elements of ethical competence are described, and strategies for developing and evaluating ethical competence are offered. The nurse case manager's potential for influencing the well-being of patients is highlighted with a discussion of advocacy. The principle- and care-based theoretical and practical approaches to clinical ethics are presented with a discussion of the nurse case manager's role in clinical ethics. The chapter concludes with a discussion of moral integrity and with an examination of the six recurrent issues confronting nurse case managers.

▲

Nurse case managers literally hold human well-being in their hands. Repetitious execution of the multiple administrative and clinical tasks that make up the workday of each nurse case manager often blinds us to the truth of this statement. Renewed attention to what we do and reflection on *why* we do what we do will quickly remind us that the "cases" we "manage" are actually people with unique life histories and needs. Moreover, we will readily see the links between who we are and how we conduct ourselves professionally and the well-being of those society entrusts to our professional care. This concluding chapter examines why ethical competence is essential for nurse case managers, explores the role of the nurse case manager in clinical ethics, and examines specific challenges to the professional and personal integrity of nurse case managers.

ETHICAL COMPETENCE AND THE NURSE CASE MANAGER
Ethical Competence as a Core Competence

Is ethical competence a core or an elective competence? Is it like knowing the general principles of asepsis or like knowing how to run a neonatal intensive care unit?

Content adapted from Taylor, C. (1997). *The morality internal to the practice of nursing.* Unpublished doctoral dissertation, Georgetown University, Washington, D.C.

Although some nurses continue to think about ethical competence as a specialized expertise that nurses can choose to develop, the American Nurses Association (ANA) in 1991 published standards of professional performance that hold all nurses accountable for ethical practice. The accompanying boxes present the ANA Code of Ethics and Standards of Professional Performance. Today nurses are legally liable if their practice is ethically deficient.

Elements of Ethical Competence

Part of the difficulty in holding ourselves and one another accountable for ethical competence lies in the failure to define exactly what it is that constitutes ethical competence. When hiring a new nurse case manager, we generally have a clear idea of the intellectual, clinical, and administrative competencies essential to the successful execution of the role. Rarely, however, are the requisite ethical competencies clear in our mind, and we thus fail to evaluate candidates in this arena. Listed below are some basic characteristics of the ethically competent nurse case manager. Following the list are reasons why these characteristics are important and ways they can be evaluated in a prospective employee interview. Ethically competent nurse case managers are able to

▼ Be trusted to act in ways that advance the best interests of the patients entrusted to their care
▼ Hold themselves and their colleagues accountable for their practice
▼ Act as effective patient advocates
▼ Mediate ethical conflict among the patient, significant others, the health care team, and other interested parties
▼ Recognize the ethical dimensions of practice and identify and respond to ethical problems
▼ Critique new health care technologies and changes in the way we define, administer, deliver, and finance health care in light of their potential to influence human well-being

Commitment to Patient Well-being. This element of ethical competence would seem to be self-evident, since all those in helping professions in general and in health care professions in particular have as their reason for being commitment to human well-being. Unfortunately the health care system is changing in ways that make it increasingly difficult to assume this orientation. The nurse case manager's first challenge and core responsibility is to keep the entire system of care and the caregiving team focused on meeting the needs of the patients it purports to serve. One nurse case manager voiced frustration when she was unable to find a bed on the unit a patient with AIDs requested when he was being readmitted for new complications. She was quickly told that worrying about which unit had a bed was not "her job." She quickly responded to her colleague that if this was important to the patient, then it was important to her because she didn't know who else was going to worry about it.

> *Example.* Nurses working in an oncology unit are discovering that patients enrolled in certain managed care companies have had their access to mental health services severely restricted. Their options are to accept the restricted services as a given or to begin to gather the data that will demonstrate that these restrictions are dramatically

THE AMERICAN NURSES ASSOCIATION'S CODE OF ETHICS

1. The nurse provides services with respect for human dignity and the uniqueness of the client, unrestricted by considerations of social or economic status, personal attributes, or the nature of health problems.
2. The nurse safeguards the client's right to privacy by judiciously protecting information of a confidential nature.
3. The nurse acts to safeguard the client and the public when health care and safety are affected by the incompetent, unethical, or illegal practice of any person.
4. The nurse assumes responsibility and accountability for individual nursing judgments and actions.
5. The nurse maintains competence in nursing.
6. The nurse exercises informed judgment and uses individual competence and qualifications as criteria in seeking consultation, accepting responsibilities, and delegating nursing activities to others.
7. The nurse participates in activities that contribute to the ongoing development of the profession's body of knowledge.
8. The nurse participates in the profession's efforts to implement and improve standards of nursing.
9. The nurse participates in the profession's efforts to establish and maintain conditions of employment conducive to high quality nursing care.
10. The nurse participates in the profession's effort to protect the public from misinformation and misrepresentation and to maintain the integrity of nursing.
11. The nurse collaborates with members of the health professions and other citizens in promoting community and national efforts to meet the health needs of the public.

From American Nurses Association. (1985). *Code for nurses with interpretive statements*. Kansas City, MO: The Association. (EDMNA, Appendix C, p. 266).

THE AMERICAN NURSES ASSOCIATION'S STANDARDS OF PROFESSIONAL PERFORMANCE

STANDARD V. ETHICS: THE NURSE'S DECISIONS AND ACTIONS ON BEHALF OF CLIENTS ARE DETERMINED IN AN ETHICAL MANNER
Measurement criteria
1. The nurse's practice is guided by the *Code for Nurses*
2. The nurse maintains client confidentiality
3. **The nurse acts as a client advocate**
4. The nurse delivers care in a nonjudgmental and nondiscriminatory manner that is sensitive to client diversity
5. The nurse delivers care in a manner that preserves/protects client autonomy, dignity, and rights
6. The nurse seeks available resources to help formulate ethical decisions

From American Nurses Association. (1991). *Standards of clinical nursing practice*. Washington, D.C.: The Association.

influencing the health and well-being of the patients being served. If commitment to the health and well-being of patients is their primary commitment, they will not allow this change in the system to go unchallenged.

Responsibility and Accountability. As systems for delivering health care continue to fragment, it is not unusual for patient health problems to go undiagnosed or when diagnosed, to be ignored or inadequately addressed. The diffusion of power and authority in complex caregiving teams makes it easy to assume that "someone else" is responsibly monitoring the problem. By virtue of the coordinating role they play in the caregiving team, nurse case managers are well positioned to monitor the effectiveness of the plan of care and to call to accountability those whose efforts remain uncommitted: If I hold myself accountable for the well-being of those committed to my care, I need more than a task orientation to each day's work. It isn't enough for me to be "busy" doing professional activities. These activities must be contributing to the well-being of those I serve. My workday is complete when I am confident that everything necessary is being done for those entrusted to my care. This critical distinction is often overlooked in practice today.

> *Example.* Nurses on your unit are pleased that the newly implemented critical pathway for women undergoing a modified radical mastectomy seems to be streamlining care and ensuring a better quality of care for all. Each staff nurse has been encouraged to keep women "on the path" postoperatively so that discharge outcomes can be met within specified time intervals. One nurse voices a concern that one patient seems to need more time and that she is afraid that nurses are impatient with her lack of outcome achievement. The nurse case manager who assumes responsibility for patient well-being is able to counsel staff nurses about the importance of respecting individual patient needs and about their need to assume responsibility for advocating that patients receive the time they need to meet critical outcomes. At issue is our ability to remember that we are first accountable to the patient and then to a new system of care.

> *Example.* Although everyone in your hospital knows something about advance directives and some are even enthusiastic about their potential for eliminating or reducing conflict over end-of-life decision making, the hospital has not identified who is responsible for actually helping patients to specify their preferences in a meaningful way. Each patient receives literature on advance directives in the admitting office but after that is at the mercy of any health care professional who elects to pursue this conversation. More often than not no one pursues this concern. You can elect to raise this issue and attempt to change the system to ensure that this need is being addressed or accept the status quo.

Ability to Act as Effective Advocate. Most of us have heard stories from friends or acquaintances about someone's terrifying hospitalization. "I don't know how people in hospitals survive without a family member in constant attendance to make sure the patient gets the ordered care and to prevent mix-ups!" Although numerous variables influence the amount and type of advocacy required by different patients, it is generally true that someone needs to act as advocate for the patient on multiple levels and in particular for the patient whose self-advocacy is impaired. Again the nurse case manager is in the ideal position to "work the system" both within and outside the hospital to ensure that the patient's needs are met. In the current climate of financial "bottom-line" decision making the need for strong patient advocacy is even more pronounced.

> *Example.* A managed care company decides to reimburse hospitals for only the first 12 to 24 hours after delivery, and nurses begin to find women who need a longer hospital stay after delivering to realize valued maternal-infant outcomes. The nurse case manager must choose whether to advocate for these women. A nurse case manager can decide to accept that some outcomes simply cannot be realized in this short time frame or can work to change the system to ensure that these needs are met either in the hospital or at home. An effective advocate will work with individual patients on a case by case basis as well as try to marshal forces to change the system.

Ability to Mediate Ethical Conflict. Ethical conflict is inherent in health care practice today. Among the forces contributing to this conflict are

> ▼ The multiple therapeutic options available for most health problems and the lack of consensus about their medical effectiveness, benefit, and burdens
> ▼ The raging debate about who should get how much of our scarce health care resources and the increasing tendency to dismiss certain patients as "poor investment risks" or as simply "unworthy" of indicated medical care
> ▼ The condition of moral pluralism; the fact that we seem to grow more heterogeneous daily in our religious and cultural beliefs and values

Ethically competent nurse case managers need to be skilled in identifying patients, families, and caregiving teams that are at risk for ethical conflict and in addressing the factors contributing to this conflict. When nurse case managers can effectively mediate problematic situations or invite ethics consult teams to perform this service, the conflict does not escalate, and the alienation that sometimes results between patient and families and caregiving individuals, team, or institution can be avoided. A chief objective is to identify the sources of common problems and to change the system to prevent their recurrence.

> *Example.* The wife of one of the patients on your unit comes to you and tells you that a gastrointestinal consultant has just informed her that they need to take her husband back to surgery because he has developed a mesenteric infarct. She tearfully tells you that she knows her husband would refuse this surgery if he were able to speak but that no one seems to be listening to her. He did not do well following surgery to remove a recurrent meningioma. She said that he only reluctantly consented to repeat surgery after much pleading from his adult children. You can side with the medical team who seems to be of the mind that this is a reversible problem that needs to be addressed or you can try to find out more about the wife's reluctance to consent and get the caregiving team to sit down with the wife and family to decide what actually is in the patient's best interests. The nurse case manager must choose whether to ignore the conflict (or hope that someone else assumes responsibility for its resolution) or to intervene to mediate the conflict.

Ability to Recognize Ethical Dimensions of Practice. The ethical dimensions of practice range from sensitivity to threats to human dignity in the caregiving environment to concerns about limited access to basic health care services.

The nurse case manager who recognizes the ethical dimensions of practice and who knows how and when to intervene can provide effective leadership in this domain.

> *Example.* Nurses in a medical intensive care unit are voicing frustration with the unevenness with which ethical dimensions of care are addressed in the unit, depending on which attending is leading the resident team that month. Two of the four attendings who make rounds with the residents are supportive of and encourage discussion of ethical questions, whereas the other two seem to believe that these discussions distract attention from the "critical," that is, medical, aspects of the case. At issue is how comfortable the nurses and medical residents are in addressing the topic of do-not-resuscitate (DNR) orders and in initiating advance planning for critical end-of-life decisions. While one case manager allows the attending to determine what can be discussed in morning rounds, another invites all four attendings to a meeting in which nurses present a plan to make ethical concerns a priority item in the discussion of each patient during rounds. The time gained with patients for whom there are no current ethical questions will allow for a timely discussion of issues when they do present.

Ability to Critique Potential to Influence Human Well-being. A final critical element of ethical competence for the nurse case manager is the ability to critique new health care technologies and changes in the way we define, administer, deliver, and finance health care in light of their potential to influence human well-being. The nurse skilled in this ability remains sufficiently distant from and critical of all aspects of caregiving to evaluate them in terms of their human consequences. Examples of successful intervention in this regard occur in both beginning and end-of-life care. In the not so distant past physicians always interjected the latest medical technology into the processes of childbearing and dying. Although this type of care continues to meet the needs of some high-risk patients, we fortunately now have the options of natural childbirth and hospice care for patients who elect to go a different route. These alternative types of care were made available after reflective health care professionals challenged the need for the latest medical treatment for all beginning and end of life care.

> *Example.* A critical care nurse comments there is almost no need to spend time in the patient's room anymore because sophisticated monitoring equipment allows everyone at the nurses' station to know more than they ever wanted to know about each patient at any moment in time. A nurse case manager listening to this comment begins to wonder how beneficial this equipment is, in its totality, to the patient. How much of it is merely a convenience to the nurses and doctors? What benefits are gained for the patient and at what cost in terms of burden and discomfort? He decides to study this concern and involves other interested nurses. As a result of the data they collect and especially because of what they learn from patient interviews, one type of monitor is "retired" and another is used only for patients with special monitoring needs. When they share their findings with the company who manufactures many of the products they use they discover that the company is interested in the topic of humanizing technology and seeks their collaboration in a research project.

Evaluating Ethical Competence

To evaluate ethical competence in prospective nurse case managers it is helpful to present case scenarios common to the practice setting and elicit their response. Responses should demonstrate their ease and competence in recognizing and addressing ethical concerns. The following box offers sample scenarios for evaluating ethical competence and highlights the specific competencies they test. These scenarios could also be used in an informal or formal staff meeting to spark conversation about ethical competence and to encourage reasoning about how case managers identify and meet ethical obligations to individual patients and to society. After several hypothetical scenarios are explored, staff can be invited to present situations they have experienced so that the team can talk together about different ways of responding. When these discussions are regularly scheduled, they communicate the expectation that ethical competence is critical to the performance of the nurse case manager's roles and that it needs to be consciously developed and updated in the same way that clinical and administrative competencies are approached.

Theoretical and Practical Approaches to Clinical Ethics

Ethics broadly defined concerns itself with right and wrong moral conduct, with how we ought to live (and die) and why. Clinical ethics, a relatively new branch of ethics, addresses ethical issues and problems that arise in the context of caring for actual patients in varied clinical settings, in the hospital, residential facility, clinic, and home. The ethically competent nurse case manager will be familiar with at least two common approaches to clinical ethics: the principle-based approach and the care-based approach. Brief descriptions of these follow, and references are cited for those wishing to learn more about these methods.

Principle-based Approach. One of the leading theories of bioethics and clinical ethics has been termed the four-principle approach. Popularized by Beauchamp and Childress (1994) this approach identifies four ethical principles derived from common moral beliefs and uses them to identify, discuss, and analyze the moral features of particular situations. The four principles include autonomy (self-determination), beneficence (benefiting or helping), nonmaleficence (avoiding harm), and justice (treating fairly). Other theorists list as key principles veracity (truth telling), confidentiality (respecting privileged information), fidelity (keeping promises), and avoiding killing. All of these are held to obligate health care professionals in a prima facie manner; that is, all things being equal, I am obligated to respect patients, benefit them, cause them no harm, treat all fairly, be truthful, and so on. A moral dilemma results when I am unable to simultaneously execute two prima facie obligations. A woman with AIDs begs you not to inform her sexual partner and the father of her child that she has AIDs because she is afraid that he will leave her. While you have an obligation to respect her privacy and to keep privileged information confidential, you also have an obligation to prevent harm to identifiable third parties. Seemingly you cannot do both. Unfortunately there is no agreed upon hierarchy of principles that specifies which principles may supersede others. Clouser and Gert (1994) offer a strong critique of this method, which they term *principlism*. Many nurses have been critical of this methodology because popularized versions seem to promote

EVALUATING ETHICAL COMPETENCE

Sample Case Scenarios for Interviewing Prospective Employees

INTERVIEWER: "Among the competencies we find to be essential for our nurse case managers is ethical competence. I'd like to get a sense of your competence and confidence in responding to some hypothetical situations. I'll describe a situation and invite you to tell me how you would respond if you were the responsible case manager."

SCENARIO 1

The wife of a patient with end-stage cancer seeks you out and tells you that she is afraid that her husband is "losing hope" and "giving up." She tells you that she has just learned that one of the patients on the unit was evaluated for inclusion in a clinical trial that offers some promise of arresting the disease if the patient receives the experimental drug. She wants you to get her husband in this trial and to do whatever you can to ensure that he receives the experimental drug. You are not familiar with the criteria for inclusion in this trial and think that it would probably be futile for her husband given his condition. You have to be at an administrative meeting in 20 minutes. What do you say to her?

Evaluate response for
▼ Commitment to patient well-being
▼ Sense of responsibility and accountability
▼ Ability to be an effective patient advocate

SCENARIO 2

Once of the staff nurses on your unit complains that the medical staff is treating patients differently and that it is making a lot of the nurses "mad." The unit has both wealthy, well-insured patients and a large number of minority, Medicaid, and Medicare patients. She reports that a number of the attendings seem to bend-over backward to ensure that the preferences of the wealthy patients are known and met while doing the bare minimum for other patients. You suspect that she is probably right but also know that this system is well entrenched.

Evaluate response for
▼ Commitment to patient well-being
▼ Sense of responsibility and accountability
▼ Ability to be an effective patient advocate
▼ Ability to recognize ethical dimensions of practice

SCENARIO 3

A woman who has just delivered her first baby and who appears utterly fatigued after a lengthy labor and overwhelmed by the new demands of parenting confides to you that she needs to stay in the hospital for a couple of days until she feels comfortable caring for her newborn. You are concerned about her level of stress but also know that her health maintenance organization will only fund the first 24 hours of care after delivery and that this couple has limited financial resources.

Continued.

EVALUATING ETHICAL COMPETENCE—cont'd

Evaluate response for
▼ Commitment to patient well-being
▼ Sense of responsibility and accountability
▼ Ability to be an effective patient advocate
▼ Ability to critique system's potential to influence human well-being

SCENARIO 4

Marita, a 16-year-old high school junior with congenital heart defects and a long history of hospitalizations, surgical and pharmacologic interventions, and chronic illness, now needs a heart transplant or she will die. She adamantly refuses the transplant and says she prefers death to the ordeal of the transplant. Her mother cannot accept this decision and refuses to even discuss this with her daughter. The staff is split as to whether to side with the patient or her mother and differ in their assessments of the probability of the transplant's ultimately benefiting her. You sense the team's growing frustration and know that if the transplant option is pursued, the sooner it is done the better the prognosis.

Evaluate response for
▼ Commitment to patient well-being
▼ Ability to be an effective patient advocate
▼ Ability to mediate ethical conflict

SCENARIO 5

While making rounds you encounter an 82-year-old patient who was admitted from the local prison with complications secondary to his emphysema. You recognize him from previous admissions and in talking with him listen to his descriptions of how horrible the conditions are in the prison for the aging convicts like himself. Listening to his story you recall other elderly prisoners who have been on your unit during the last 3 or 4 years who have presented with some signs of neglect. He tells you that he will do anything to get admitted to the hospital and that most of the other elderly prisoners would too. "Not even a dog should have to live the way we do." You sense that he is probably being honest and that he does not seem to be manipulative or playing on your sympathies.

Evaluate response for
▼ Commitment to patient well-being
▼ Sense of responsibility and accountability

SCENARIO 6

An 11-year-old Native American boy in the pediatric oncology unit tells you to make sure that "Ellen never takes care of me again." When you question him, he tells you how "mean" she is and that she never treats him nicely like the other nurses do. You respect Ellen's clinical competence and know that this patient has a reputation for being a problem.

Evaluate response for
▼ Commitment to patient well-being
▼ Sense of responsibility and accountability
▼ Ability to be an effective patient advocate

a type of quandary ethics of the to-pull-the-plug-or-not variety, which has not been sensitive to the everyday ethical concerns of practicing nurses.

Care-based Approach. Dissatisfaction with the principle-based approach to nursing ethics combined with attentiveness to Gilligan's (1982) ground-breaking work in moral development led some nurse theorists to begin to articulate an ethic of care (Benner & Wrubel, 1989; Fry, 1989; Watson, 1985). Central to this perspective is the nature of the nurse-patient relationship and attention to the particulars of individual patients viewed within the context of their lives. Operating within this methodology nurses pay attention to the human needs and interests that underlie ethical conflict with the intent of restoring and strengthening bonds between professionals, patients, and families. Characteristics of the care perspective include the following:

▼ Centrality of the caring relationship
▼ Promotion of the dignity of and respect for patients as people
▼ Acceptance of particular patients and health care professional variables (beliefs, values, relationships) as morally relevant factors in ethical decision making
▼ Norms of responsiveness and responsibility
▼ Redefinition of fundamental moral skills (Taylor, 1993)

Ethically Relevant Considerations. Whichever ethical approach the nurse case manager uses, the following list of ethically relevant considerations is helpful in the analysis of ethically problematic cases and in the discussion of these cases with others. Fletcher, Miller, and Spencer (1995) suggest that the following eight considerations offer a bridge between ethical principles, an ethics of caring, and the clinical situation.

1. Balancing benefits and harms in the care of patients
2. Disclosure, informed consent, and shared decision making
3. The norms of family life
4. The relationships between clinicians and patients
5. The professional integrity of clinicians
6. Cost-effectiveness and allocation
7. Issues of cultural and religious variation
8. Considerations of power (pp. 11-13)

Ethical Resources for the Nurse Case Manager

Since clinical ethicists in general and nurse ethicists more specifically are still something of a rarity and infrequently are employed by health care agencies and institutions, nurse case managers who are interested in developing ethical competence may need to look outside their institutions for resources. Many professional nursing organizations such as the American (and states') Nurses Association and the Association of Critical Care Nurses have task forces and committees that deal exclusively with ethical matters. These organizations and others frequently host conferences and seminars that address ethical issues and can refer nurses to the educational resources most likely to address their needs. The following box highlights some of the better known ethics resources. Some geographic areas are served by regional networks of ethics centers or by university-based ethics centers.

ETHICAL RESOURCES

American Nurses Association Center for Ethics and Human Rights
600 Maryland Avenue, SW
Suite 100 West
Washington, DC 20024-2571
(202)651-7055

Publishes the *Ethics and Human Rights Communiqué,* which provides an ongoing
  vehicle of communication for nurses facing ethical and human rights dilemmas
  in practice. *Communiqué* informs readers about important upcoming events and
  resources of interest such as bibliographies, surveys, grants, ANA conferences,
  ethical continuing education offerings, and new ANA publications.

National Reference Center for Bioethics Literature
Kennedy Institute of Ethics
Georgetown University
Washington, DC 20057
800-MED-ETHX

A specialized collection of library resources concerned with contemporary biomedical issues in the fields of ethics, philosophy, medicine, nursing, science,
  law, religion, and the social sciences. Call for bioethics information, BIOETH-
  ICSLINE searches (computerized data base), search strategies, reference help,
  and publication orders.

The Hastings Center
255 Elm Road
Briarcliff Manor, NY 10510
914-762-8500

A nonprofit, nonpartisan organization that carries out educational and research
  programs on ethical issues in medicine, the life sciences, and the professions.
  Publishes *The Hastings Center Report.*

Advocacy and the Nurse Case Manager

Nurse ethicist Sally Gadow defines advocacy as the moral commitment to enhance
patients' autonomy. "Among all of the professionals surrounding a patient, nurses
often are the most capable of fostering patient self-determination. The practice of
advocacy in nursing thus involves development of the nurse-patient relationship as
the medium for expression of patients' values" (1989, p. 535). To function effectively
as a patient advocate, nurse case managers have to understand the basic dynamics in
health care decision making.

Basically there are three models of health care decision making that are "alive
and well" in most clinical settings (Table 29-1). In paternalism or maternalism the
clinician is "boss" and makes decisions to benefit patients, who are viewed as generally
lacking sufficient knowledge to make right decisions. When this model works well,
patients are spared the anguish of making tough decisions, and competent and
compassionate clinicians make good decisions in the patient's best interests. When

Table 29-1   Models of health care decision making

MODEL	DESCRIPTION	PRINCIPLE	JUSTIFICATION	DANGERS
Paternalism	Physician is the boss.	Beneficence	Patients often do not understand enough about medicine to make the "right" decision.	Patients may receive care they do not want and must live with the consequences.
Patient sovereignty	Patient is the boss.	Autonomy (self-determination)	No one knows better than the patient what is in his or her overall "best interests"; right to be self-determining ought always to take precedence.	No one protects patients from a "poor" or "ill-advised" choice; "easy-out" for health care practitioners.
Shared decision making	Patient and health care team work together.	Authentic autonomy	Patient may need support in being authentically autonomous.	Can easily slide into paternalism.

this model does not work well, patients receive unwanted care and live with the consequences long after the clinician exits the scene. The patient sovereignty model evolved to correct the problem of patients' receiving unwanted care. Championing the patient as "boss" and the principle of autonomy, this model claims that no one knows what is best for the patient better than the patient him or herself. In this model, patients get the care they desire or demand, and the chief drawback is that there is often no one to protect patients from their poor or ill-advised choices.

In the early 1980s the President's Commission for the Study of Ethical Problems in Medicine and Biomedical and Behavioral Research rejected both these models and recommended a model of shared decision making. This model is also based on autonomy but respects the fact that both the patient and clinicians bring something of importance to the process of decision making and calls for both to participate in the decision. The objective in this model is not simply that patients choose but that patients make the choice that is right for them, that is, a choice consistent with their values, moral identity, and decisional history. In this model clinicians are obligated to provide the support patients need to make good decisions. It is in this respect that the decision-making model differs from the patient sovereignty model, which is a model of noninterference.

Even this brief introduction of models will make clear why the advocacy role of the nurse is problematic. Although most ethicists agree with the President's

Commission and recommend a model of shared decision making, clinicians may be found who subscribe to each of the three models. Not surprisingly these clinicians differ in their estimate of whether patients and families need advocates and in their acceptance of the differing responsibilities of advocates.

CLINICAL ETHICS AND THE NURSE CASE MANAGER
Promoting Autonomy

Among our most prized human abilities is the freedom to make choices in light of what we value or deem good. Individuals are autonomous to the extent that they are self-determining. Much of the bioethics debate in the United States has focused on how we can safeguard the right of patients to be autonomous. Nurse case managers by virtue of their position and authority in the health care system can play a critical role in safeguarding patient autonomy.

Individuals with an intact decision-making capacity have the right to consent to and to refuse all medically indicated therapy. Since judgments about decision-making capacity ideally are made by those who know patients best, nurse case managers ought to participate in efforts to determine and document capacity. Criteria for decision-making capacity include

1. The ability to comprehend information relevant to the decision at hand
2. The ability to deliberate in accord with a relatively consistent set of values and goals
3. The ability to communicate preferences.

Nurse case managers who are effective advocates will help patients with decision-making capacity to anticipate the types of health care decisions they may need to make in the future and to explore their treatment options. It is important that patient preferences be documented and that nurses be familiar with state law about advance directives. Nurse case managers can play a leading role in making sure that the agency or institution they are affiliated with has a policy that identifies the parties responsible for obtaining and documenting patient preferences.

It is important that case managers working with patients with complex needs support authentically autonomous decision making, that is, ensure that decisions reflect the identity, decisional history, and moral norms of the patient. This frequently will mean walking patients through the various treatment options to see what each will mean for this patient in terms of real-life benefits and burdens. When institutional, caregiver, or family interests interfere with the autonomy of the patient, nurse advocates will support the patient and ensure that his or her interests are protected.

Lack of decision-making capacity does not of itself negate the right to be self-determining. Known preferences of the incapacitated individual are to be respected. Advance directives—a living will or durable power of attorney for health care—legally protect an individual's preferences concerning health care. Case managers advocate for incapacitated patients by supporting their surrogate decision makers. The role of the surrogate decision maker is to be a voice for a patient who can no longer speak for him or herself. Surrogates should be instructed to use their knowledge of the patient and the patient's values to make the choice the patient him or herself would make if he or she were able to do so.

Valid moral surrogates have intact decision-making capacity, understand the information pertinent to the decision at hand, know the patient's preferences to the extent that this is possible, have no undue conflict of interest, and are not experiencing severe emotional problems. Relatives who are legally valid surrogates but who are financially or emotionally dependent on a patient may make treatment decisions based on their own needs rather than on the interests of the patient. Nurse advocates can teach such surrogates that their charge is to be a voice for a now incapacitated patient and that they should decide as the patient would decide. If surrogates persist in making decisions that run counter to the patient's previously expressed wishes, health care professionals may need to explore legal means to challenge the surrogate's decision-making authority.

Promoting Patient Well-being

The first task of the nurse advocate is to work with the patient, family, and health care team to clarify and communicate the appropriate goal of therapy: cure and restoration, stabilization of functioning, or preparation for a comfortable, dignified death. Although this would seem to be a given, often confusion makes it difficult to ensure that all interventions are consistent with the goal. Obviously treatment goals may need revision when a patient makes unexpected progress or fails to progress. In one tertiary medical center a decision was made to terminate aggressive treatment for a man with an advanced, stage IV, glioblastoma. He was transferred out of the neurology step-down unit to a general floor. Unfortunately the transfer was made on a weekend evening when communication was poor, so when the patient spiked high temperatures, an aggressive workup was done and therapy for sepsis was initiated. If the intent of the therapy was comfort and the therapy was consistent with preparing him for a dignified death, the intervention was appropriate. If, on the other hand, it was merely a knee-jerk response to a life-threatening complication and was aimed at restoration and cure, it was inappropriate for this patient. The families of incapacitated, frail, debilitated patients may need great support in determining what is in the best interests of the patient and in deciding when to treat a condition aggressively and when to let nature take its course. Unfortunately there is no clear line to be drawn between promoting life and needlessly prolonging dying.

Pellegrino (1989) recommends analysis of therapy along two lines: effectiveness and benefit/burden ratio. A treatment is effective to the degree that it reverses or ameliorates the natural progression of the disease. Surgical repair has a high probability of being effective treatment for a mesenteric infarct. This is an objective medical determination—to the degree that medicine as a science can be objective. Whether the benefits of that surgery would advance the overall best interests of the patient described on page 318 who had had a recurrent meningioma and outweigh the burdens of the surgery is, however, a subjective determination that can be made only by the patient or by those who know the patient best. Nurses may need to remind physicians that more is at stake in treatment decisions than whether the proposed therapy is "medically indicated." Nurses' knowledge is also critical in the determination of the probability that a particular intervention will contribute to or compromise a goal such as comfort.

Nurses advocating for the patient's interests will also ensure that the patient's priority needs are addressed (biologic, psychosocial, and spiritual needs). As health care reform increasingly fragments services, the likelihood that patients will be cared for by health care professionals, including nurses, who know them well is decreasing. Nurse managers must critique nursing systems of care in which no one nurse is responsible for the overall plan of care and the identification and resolution of concerns of high priority to patients and families. All too frequently the only patient problems receiving attention today are physical problems. It is nursing's charge to ensure that holistic, individualized, prioritized care is a reality, especially for today's elders.

Preventing and Resolving Ethical Conflict

Nurse case managers who wish to prevent ethical conflict will work in care settings where it is established that preventing and resolving ethical conflict falls within the authority of each health care professional engaged in the care of a patient. This conviction will facilitate early recognition of problematic situations and timely communication among all those involved in decision making. When communication among the patient, family, and caregiving team fails to resolve the problem, an ethics consult or meeting of the institutional ethics committee may be indicated. Sensitivity to and the ability to communicate about the factors contributing to ethical conflict are essential to successful mediation of these conflicts. When mediation is not attempted, conflicts tend to escalate, and it is not unusual for patients and families to develop hostile adversarial relationships that all too frequently end in litigation or at the very least in alienation and a distrust of health care professionals that colors future interactions with caregivers. Nurse case managers should be aware of the ethics resources available in their institutions and professional community and use them when needed (review the box on page 324). Mastery of a process of ethical decision making to simplify conflict resolution is also important as shown in the box on page 329. The box on page 330 summarizes critical elements of the advocacy role of the nurse case manager.

MORAL INTEGRITY AND THE NURSE CASE MANAGER

Mark Siegler (1984), a physician ethicist, describes three stages in the evolution of medicine and notes how medicine's focus has changed from one stage to the next. In the first stage, the age of paternalism, physicians focused on the good of the patient **as defined by the physician.** In the second stage, the age of autonomy, the focus remained the good of the patient but **as defined by the patient him or herself.** In the third stage of medicine, which Siegler termed *the age of bureaucratic parsimony,* the good of the patient is weighed against the good of society. Today we can add a fourth stage of medicine to Siegler's list, which might be termed *the age of for-profit medicine* in which health care professionals (or other decision makers) weigh the good of the patient against the good of stockholders. These are profound paradigmatic changes that have the potential to dramatically influence the practice of professional nursing. Nurse case managers who wish to preserve their moral integrity in today's changing health care milieu face multiple challenges. Six of these challenges are explored on pages 331 to 333.

A PROCESS OF ETHICAL DECISION MAKING

ASSESSMENT

Gather and document pertinent medical and nonmedical facts:

▼ **Who:** persons who have the authority for decision making and the responsibility for its consequences and the effect on them personally of the decision needing to be made

▼ **What:** patient's medical condition, prognosis, and therapeutic options and probable consequences of treatment and nontreatment; patient's beliefs, values, interests; related family, caregiver, and institution beliefs, values, and interests; pertinent legal and administrative considerations

▼ **When:** time parameters

▼ **Where:** setting

▼ **Why:** variables creating or fueling conflict

DIAGNOSIS

Identify the ethical issue(s) as clearly as possible. Distinguish ethical problems from communication or general patient care management problems.

PLANNING

1. Identify the objective of doing the ethics workup.
2. List and explore courses of action likely to achieve this goal. Think through the short- and long-term consequences of each.
3. Think of the ethical justification for each course of action and defend it against competing options:
   a. Compatibility with aims of nursing and demands of nurse-patient relationship
   b. Approaches to ethical inquiry: ethical principles, care perspective, virtue theory, communitarianism
   c. Grounding and source of ethics: philosophical (based in reason), theological (based in religion), sociocultural (based in custom)
4. Clearly identify what you believe to be the moral obligations of the nurse.
5. Select the course of action you are best able to defend against counter arguments.
6. Seek assistance if unable to work through the above steps independently.

IMPLEMENTATION

Implement the selected course of action and assess consequences.

EVALUATION

Critique your decision incorporating feedback from involved participants if possible. Decide how you would respond to a similar case in the future. Determine whether you need to do something now to optimize future responses. Interventions may be personal (e.g., learn more about advance directives) or institutional (e.g., clarify the hospital's DNR policy and reeducate caregivers about the policy).

From Taylor, C. (1997). Ethical perspectives. In M.M. Burke & M.B. Walsh (Eds.), *Gerontologic nursing: Care of the elderly* (2nd ed.). St. Louis, MO: Mosby.

ADVOCACY COMPETENCIES

SUPPORTING AUTONOMY

1. Determining and documenting the patient's decision-making capacity; ensuring that agency or institution policies specify how this is to be done and identify responsible parties
2. Protecting the right of patients with decision-making capacity to be self-determining
   a. Facilitate communication and documentation of the patient's preferences
   b. Anticipate the types of treatment decisions that likely will need to be made
   c. Assist in the preparation of advance directives
3. Promoting authentic autonomy; authentic decisions reflect the individual's identity, decisional history, and moral norms
4. Identifying the morally as well as legally valid surrogate decision maker for patients who lack decision-making capacity
5. Supporting the surrogate decision maker, clarifying the surrogate decision maker's role
6. Identifying limits to patient or surrogate autonomy and limits to caregiver autonomy
7. Developing agency or institution policies that identify the caregivers responsible for and the procedures to be used to identify and support the appropriate decision makers

PROMOTING PATIENT WELL-BEING

1. Clarifying the goal of therapy: cure and restoration, stabilization of functioning, preparation for a comfortable, dignified death
2. Determining the medical effectiveness of therapy
3. Weighing the benefits and burdens of therapy
4. Ensuring that all interventions are consistent with the overall goal of therapy
5. Ensuring that the patient's priority needs are addressed (biologic, psychosocial, and spiritual needs)
6. Ensuring continuity of care as patient is transferred among services and within and without the institution
7. Weighing the moral relevance of third-party interests (family, caregiver, institution, society)
8. Identifying and addressing forces within society and the health care system that compromise patient well-being

PREVENTING AND RESOLVING ETHICAL CONFLICT

1. Establishing that preventing and resolving ethical conflict falls within the authority of all health care professionals engaged in the care of a patient
2. Developing awareness of and sensitivity to the conscious and unconscious sources of conflict
3. Facilitating timely communication among those involved in decision making: one-on-one meetings and periodic meetings of the patient, family, and interdisciplinary team to clarify goals and plan of care
4. Documenting pertinent information on the patient record
5. Referring unresolved ethical issues to the ethics consult team or the institutional ethics committee
6. Identifying and addressing system variables that contribute to recurrent ethical problems

From Taylor, C. (1997). Ethical perspectives. In M.M. Burke & M.B. Walsh (Eds.), *Gerontologic nursing: Care of the elderly* (2nd ed.). St. Louis, MO: Mosby.

Challenge 1: Fidelity to the Unique Needs of Individual Patients

When asked to list descriptors of quality care many nurses use words like *holistic, individualized, prioritized,* and *continuous.* It is interesting to reflect on the reality that underlies these descriptors and to ask if we are still able to practice nursing in a way that makes this type of care anything more than interesting rhetoric. Are the type of nurse-patient relationships that make holistic, individualized, and prioritized care possible a reality today or are they mere relics of a bygone past when nurses had the time to really get to know their patients? For example, nurses in a medical center were discussing the care received by a patient who had recently died from end-stage breast cancer. Apparently she was concerned about seeing her two children, ages 17 and 20, who had stopped coming to visit because they were overwhelmed by the degree of her illness, especially since their father had died of a brain tumor 2 years earlier. What the staff realized after she died was that no one had picked up on her requests to see her children and had not arranged a visit, so the patient died without ever seeing her children again. Horrified that this had been allowed to happen, the nurses realized that not one of them had seen this request as his or her responsibility in their attempts to provide highly technical rescue medicine that was responsive to each medical complication and crisis. One nurse caught herself saying, "I am familiar with 'the case' but didn't really know this woman."

Clinical practice guidelines based on aggregate data, critical pathways, and algorithms all seem to draw attention away from individual patients to population aggregates. Each of these standardizing methodologies has the potential to improve patient outcomes by keeping achievable target outcomes consciously before patients and the caregiving team. Whether these methodologies are used to improve care for individual patients or to force individuals to jump through predetermined hoops that may or may not contribute to their well-being may in large part be determined by the stance adopted by nurse case managers. Never before have patients been so in need of nurse advocates who know the system well enough to ensure that it is responsive to the unique needs of individual patients and their families. In the past our lack of skill in "working the system" limited our power to effectively serve as advocates for patients. Today the nurse case manager has the authority to pull together and to coordinate the services each individual patient needs and to modify systems that are unresponsive to patient need. How this authority will be used remains to be seen.

Challenge 2: Competing Loyalties

The nurse case manager's ability to modify the system to meet individual patient needs depends on his or her loyalties. When asked, to whom are you accountable, nurse case managers may reply, to the patient, to the hospital, to my boss, to myself, to the caregiving team. If I see myself as primarily accountable to an employing institution who pays my salary and who is driven by a financial bottom line, I may be reluctant to advocate for a patient who needs additional time to achieve target outcomes before discharge. It is helpful to consciously reflect on one's loyalties and to identify potential conflicts. Once again, the rhetoric of nursing reminds us that our primary concern is the patient. Unfortunately, today it is not uncommon for nursing practice to reflect concern for anything but this reality.

Challenge 3: Resolving Role Conflict

Among other things, the nurse case manager is a service coordinator, an advocate, a counselor, and a gatekeeper. Obviously, where one works, the needs of the patients served, and the mix of professionals on the caregiving team will all influence the roles played by the nurse case manager and the amount of time spent in each role. It can be helpful to use a pie chart to record the portion of time you spend in each role, on average, on any given day and to compare your chart with those of others in comparable positions. Reflection and discussion should yield greater insight into whether your personal mix of roles is adequately serving your patients and your employing institution. An important question to ask is, What determines which of your roles takes precedence when role conflict exists?

▼ The needs of your employer: "Utilization review says she has to be out of here by noon tomorrow at the latest."

▼ The needs of your patient: "We just have to get her pain under better control before she goes home, and this might take another day or two; they just changed her medicine this evening."

▼ Your unique talents: "I don't know how utilization review does it. . . . I could never talk with an already overburdened family about the need to take their mom or dad home before they think they are ready."

Our moral integrity makes it imperative for us never to allow our priorities to be dictated solely by our employing agency or institution. As the health care system changes, we need to reflect more carefully on what may be termed the "nonnegotiables" of our practice. What are those elements of professional nursing care that we cannot surrender without ceasing to be nurses?

Challenge 4: Owning Responsibilities to Underserved Populations

Nurses have both individual and corporate responsibilities to underserved populations. Nurse case managers are uniquely situated to gather the type of data that can be used to demonstrate to policy makers that the needs of select groups of patients are not being adequately addressed. Recurrent admissions of patients whose problems could have been more successfully addressed had the patients been seen earlier should be a signal that health needs are not being adequately met. Whether the patients be homeless men and women; a large population of abused children, spouses, or the elderly; incarcerated individuals; those with psychiatric or mental health problems; or simply those with inadequate insurance, nurse case managers can, if they choose, lead caregiving teams in gathering the type of data that will convince policy makers of the need for system reform.

Challenge 5: Identifying Personal Biases

In the interests of providing care that is just and oriented to giving each person his or her due, it is essential that nurse case managers attempt to identify personal sources of bias or discrimination. Reflection will usually reveal the presence of some factors that positively or negatively predispose us to patients. An air of helplessness in a patient may elicit one nurse's mothering instinct and disgust in another. Similarly, age, gender, body size, occupation, skin color, nationality, culture, religion, financial status, and lifestyle factors can all influence the way we perceive and relate to patients. One nurse case manager who had worked in an AIDS unit for several years confided that she slowly realized after reflecting on her work that she treated patients differently on the basis of how they had acquired AIDS. "I'm much more patient and giving of myself to those who acquired it through sexual transmission rather than by sharing needles." This brief vignette illustrates the importance of identifying our personal biases. We need to be as conscious as we can of what inclines (or disinclines) us to "go to bat" for a patient whose needs are not being met.

Challenge 6: Balancing Care for Others with Appropriate Self-Care

A final word of caution. The tremendous potential nurse case managers have for influencing the delivery of health care in the United States may result in some nurses' literally sacrificing themselves on the altar of quality care for those entrusted to their practice. While responsibility and accountability are essential elements of ethical competence, in excess they can fan the flames of burn-out and quickly reduce a competent, caring professional to a lifeless mannequin. When deficient, nurses poorly serve their patients and colleagues, who quickly learn not to trust nurses who consistently places their needs and well-being over and above the needs of those they work for and with. The ethically competent nurse knows how to balance competing responsibilities to self, family, and work and is able to skillfully meet both professional and personal obligations. This dimension of moral integrity merits ongoing reflection and may be aided by discussion with colleagues. Because no two nurse case managers will view their responsibilities to patients, the caregiving team, and themselves in exactly the same way, discussions about what constitutes acceptable boundaries of responsibility and accountability can be helpful.

• • •

These are exciting times. More individuals than ever before are claiming as an achievable goal quality, affordable care for all. Unfortunately, some of the means being used to achieve this goal are already suspect. Nurse case managers are on the front lines of the revolution in health care. Never before have the everyday choices of practicing nurses had greater potential to set standards of excellence that will serve us all. Ethical competence is not an option for nurse case managers. The health and well-being of all those we serve literally depend on their ethical competence.

REFERENCES

American Hospital Association. (1991). *Put it in writing: A guide to promoting advance directives.* Chicago: Author.

American Nurses Association. (1991). *Standards of Clinical Nursing Practice.* Washington, DC: Author.

American Nurses Association. (1985). *Code for nurses with interpretive statements.* Washington, DC: Author.

Beauchamp, T.L., & Childress, J.F. (1994). *Prin-*

ciples of biomedical ethics, (4th ed.). New York: Oxford University Press.

Benner, P., & Wrubel, J. (1989). *The primacy of caring.* Menlo Park, CA: Addison-Wesley Publishing Co.

Clouser, K.D., & Gert, B. (1994). Morality vs. principlism. In R. Gillon, (Ed.), *Principles of health care ethics.* New York: John Wiley & Sons.

Concern for Dying. (1991). *Advance directive protocols and the patient self-determination act: A resource manual for the development of institutional protocols.* New York: The Association.

Fletcher, J.C., Miller, F.G., & Spencer, E.M. (1995). Clinical ethics: History, content and resources. In J.C. Fletcher, C.A. Hite, P.A. Lombardo, & M.F. Marshall (Eds.), *Introduction to clinical ethics* (pp. 3-17). Frederick, MD: University Publishing Group.

Fry, S. (1989). The role of caring in a theory of nursing ethics. *Hypatia, 4,* 88-103.

Gadow, S. (1989). Clinical subjectivity: Advocacy with silent patients. *Nursing Clinics of North America, 24*(2), 535-541.

Gadow, S. (1980). Existential advocacy: Philosophical foundations of nursing. In S.F. Spicker & S. Gadow (Eds.), *Nursing: Images and ideals: Opening dialogue with the humanities* (pp. 79-101). New York: Springer.

Gilligan, C. (1982). *In a different voice: Psychological theory and women's development.* Cambridge, MA: Harvard University Press.

The Hastings Center. (1987). *Guidelines on the termination of life-sustaining treatment and the care of the dying.* Bloomington and Indianapolis: Indiana University Press.

Jameton, A. (1993). Dilemmas of moral distress: Moral responsibility and nursing practice. *AWHONN's Clinical Issues in Perinatal and Women's Health Nursing, 4*(4), 542-551.

Patient Self-Determination Act of 1990, In OBRA 1990 (P.L.101-508, H.R.5835).

Pellegrino, E.D. (1989). Withholding and withdrawing treatments: Ethics at the bedside. *Clinical Neurosurgery, 35,* 164-184.

President's Commission for the Study of Ethical Problems in Medicine and Biomedical and Behavioral Research. (1982). *Making health care decisions* (Vols. 1-3). Washington, DC: U.S. Government Printing Office.

President's Commission for the Study of Ethical Problems in Medicine and Biomedical and Behavioral Research. (1983). *Deciding to forego life-sustaining treatment: Ethical, medical, and legal issues in treatment decisions.* Washington, DC: U.S. Government Printing Office.

Siegler, M. (1984). Should age be a criterion in health care? *Hastings Center Report, 14*(5), 24-27.

Taylor, C. (1993). Nursing ethics: The role of caring. *AWHONN'S Clinical Issues in Perinatal and Women's Health Nursing, 4*(4), 552-560.

Taylor, C. (1995). Rethinking nursing's basic competencies. *Journal of Nursing Care Quality, 9*(4), 1-13.

Watson, J. (1985). *Nursing: The philosophy and science of caring.* Boulder, CO: Colorado Associated University Press.

INDEX